The Estrogen Question

Know Before You Say "No" to HRT

Sandra Rice, MD

The material in this book is provided for informational use only. It is not intended to replace the advice or recommendations of a woman's health care team but to be a resource to facilitate a productive discussion regarding the benefits and risks of hormone replacement therapy.

Respected medical studies have been summarized to the best of my ability in an effort to make complicated medical information understandable to non-professionals. References to current guidelines reflect the recommendations of various organizations as of 2019 and these guidelines may be updated and revised in the future.

The patient examples in this book are based on actual patient interactions, but the names have been changed to assure medical privacy.

The author and publisher specifically disclaim any liability, loss, or risk that may be incurred as a consequence, directly or indirectly, from the use and application of any of the contents of this book.

All rights are reserved and no parts of this book may be reproduced or transmitted in any form without written permission of the author.

Copyright © 2019 Sandra Rice
All rights reserved.
ISBN: 978-0-578-57413-4

DEDICATION

This book is dedicated to my loyal patients who trusted me and respected my opinions and guidance during their perimenopausal and postmenopausal years. It has been my interactions with them that have given me the clinical wisdom to affirm what I believe – that women benefit immensely from estrogen replacement therapy. Their support and enthusiastic encouragement have been invaluable in motivating me to undertake writing this book.

ACKNOWLEDGMENTS

First and foremost, I want to thank and acknowledge my wonderful husband, Martin Nizlek. It takes a special person to be the spouse of a full-time primary care physician. His unwavering support of my 30-plus year career, with its attendant long working hours and interrupted nights and weekends, in my estimation, merits nothing short of sainthood. Without his help, patience, and encouragement, I would not have been able to accomplish this lifelong goal to write a medical book. In addition to his indulging my passion for this project, he has contributed countless hours of help with editing, formatting, and publishing this book.

I also want to acknowledge my big sister, Janine Shinkoskey Brodine and her husband Marc Brodine, both accomplished writers, for their help in reviewing and editing this book. Janine has helped with structuring the content and reining in my over-technical medical explanations and assumptions. Marc's keen eye for grammatical faux pas has been invaluable.

Finally, I want to include a tribute to the memories of my grandfather, Lyle Cubbage, who instilled a love of words and books at an early age, and my father, Jack Newton Shinkoskey, a career English teacher who, since we were children, insisted his four daughters always speak and write correctly – with phrases ingrained in our heads even today such as *"cakes and pies are done; little girls are finished."*

ABOUT THE AUTHOR

Dr. Sandra Rice is a board certified internal medicine specialist and has been practicing medicine for over 35 years. She has decades-long experience managing menopausal women and is passionate about the benefits of estrogen therapy.

Dr. Rice is reaching out to women through this book to provide them the information they need to make an informed decision about hormone replacement therapy (HRT). Additional information can be found at her website: *www.YourEstrogenQuestions.com*

Table of Contents

INTRODUCTION

"You know, I really don't wish I'd been born a male, but I wish that I didn't have to make a decision whether or not I should take hormones." This is what one of my patients told me. She was 50 years old and hopeful of living another 30 years. She was having horrible hot flashes, not sleeping well and frequently feeling depressed and irritable. None of the remedies she had bought from the health food store made her feel better. She was aware that hormones would help, but she had heard so many bad things about estrogen that she was frightened to consider it.

This is a dilemma thousands of women face every day. Should they take hormone replacement therapy (HRT)? Unlike our male counterparts, the production of our two main female hormones, estrogen and progesterone, abruptly shuts down at midlife as we go through menopause. This causes distressing symptoms as well as a host of medical problems that many women may not even be aware of. The goal of this book is to describe what the loss of our hormones does in our bodies and to help you answer these important questions:

- Should I take hormones when I go through menopause?
- If so, which ones should I take?
- And, how long should I take them?

Who should read this book?

- Women going through menopause who are trying to decide whether or not to take estrogen (especially those getting conflicting advice from family, friends, and physicians).

- Women already taking estrogen and trying to decide if they should continue it.

- Husbands or family members of women taking estrogen who have concerns about whether it is safe.

- Medical students and other professionals looking for an easily readable review of the history and studies on HRT treatment.

- Medical care providers looking for a book about estrogen therapy that they can recommend to their patients.

Why is HRT controversial?

It seems like it shouldn't be a hard decision about whether or not women should take hormone replacement. When we lose any of our other important hormones, such as thyroid hormone, we have no qualms about simply filling a prescription and taking a pill daily. Why is the decision to replace our estrogen and progesterone any different? It has been interesting to me to explore the answer to this question, and it turns out to be very complicated. In a nutshell, it is because the pendulum has swung back and forth regarding whether HRT causes more benefits than risks or more risks than benefits. Countless studies have been done since the 1950's attempting to resolve this question. Many of the earlier studies concluded that women were far better off taking estrogen, primarily due to its remarkable bone-preserving properties which prevented fractures – a major cause of death and disability in older women. This, and that it was a miracle cure for hot flashes and other menopausal symptoms, made estrogen one of the most frequently prescribed drugs of all time. However, with long-term use, it was observed that estrogen appeared to increase the risk of uterine and breast cancer – consequences which landed it the reputation of being a carcinogen, raising doubts about its safety. This concern, however, appeared to be offset by other studies that demonstrated that women taking estrogen had far fewer heart attacks and other cardiovascular complications.

To resolve the uncertainty about whether or not women should be encouraged to use HRT, in 1991 the National Institute of Health launched a landmark study called the Women's Health Initiative (WHI). This was a massive endeavor, enrolling thousands of women, costing millions of dollars and run by a Who's Who list of menopause experts across the U.S. I will be discussing this study and its impacts throughout this book, but the bottom line is that shortly after the results of this study were published in 2002, the way menopause was managed transformed overnight. The study concluded that hormone replacement caused more risks than benefits and should not be recommended as a preventative treatment for heart disease – a complete reversal of what decades of earlier research had told us. The results of the WHI were alarming and totally unexpected. Front-page headlines across the nation blasted admonitions accusing doctors of misleading their patients about the wisdom of taking estrogen. Concerns about the safety of HRT were rekindled in the minds of women across the globe, as well as in the minds of their health care providers.

The aftermath of the WHI

The impact of the WHI study was colossal. Millions of women threw out their hormones. New, guardedly cautious guidelines for estrogen treatment emerged – advising physicians to prescribe only the *lowest dose for the shortest period of time* and only for very symptomatic women. Prescriptions for estrogen drugs plummeted and during the years following the WHI, the percentage of women taking HRT has been a fraction of that in the past. Furthermore, funding for new research on hormone replacement has been significantly curtailed.

Physicians like me, who had always embraced hormone replacement, were in a quandary. Many of us truly believed that estrogen therapy carried many more long-term benefits than risks, but the guidelines generated by the WHI essentially discouraged women from using them other than if absolutely necessary. Sure, no one was going to prohibit us from writing prescriptions for estrogen, but whenever we did, we received pushback from many directions. Insurance companies questioned the rationale for prescribing them and frequently refused payment; pharmacists reluctantly dispensed them. The FDA added black box warnings to the patient inserts – so when women picked up their hormones at the pharmacy, they were warned that the pills they were about to take could increase not only breast and uterine cancer, but possibly cause heart attacks and dementia. All of this led many physicians to simply put on blinders and apply the guidelines to all their patients.

However, many physicians continue to be concerned that withholding estrogen treatment from women is causing more harm than benefit. Why was it that the WHI found there were more risks than benefits when the bulk of earlier studies had come up with the opposite conclusion? Not surprisingly, there has been an intensive effort to explain this conflict, and the WHI conclusions are being challenged. This subject will be discussed in great detail throughout this book and I will illustrate how the WHI study is an example of the "best available science" being inappropriately applied.

However, policymakers rely on large-scale studies to dictate guidelines, and no such undertaking is likely to appear in the near future to address the shortcomings of the WHI. Many roadblocks stand in the way – a lack of funding, ethical considerations, and seemingly apathetic attitudes about this issue from members of the medical community. Even if such an endeavor was undertaken, it would take years to design and implement and even more years before the results would impact the guidelines. In the meantime, women and their providers can either adhere to the WHI-generated guidelines with their uncertain validity, or they can educate themselves about the known benefits and risks of estrogen therapy and make informed decisions about what they feel is the right course of action.

What type of book is this and what does it address?

There are many different books on the market that deal with menopause and hormones, and they come from different perspectives. There are the *"estrogen is bad for you"* books. Some of these promote non-hormone "natural" and holistic ways of managing the symptoms of menopause. Other books are even more extreme and portray estrogen as a toxic substance – so much so that after reading them women can become so "estro-phobic" they are afraid to even drink tap water!

Other books attempt to convince women that they should shun any pharmaceutically-derived estrogen and embrace only bioidentical hormones. While there is some merit to this approach, the authors of books on bioidentical hormones don't always conform to conventional medical practice and can swing pretty far out into the alternative medicine arena – pushing women into clinics that promote propriety hormone preparations and anti-aging supplements.

Then there are the types of books that your family doctor or gynecologist would recommend that you read – books based on peer-reviewed research that reflect the opinions of respected menopause experts. This is the type of book that I have written. *The Estrogen Question* contains up-to-date information based on accepted medical studies that I have attempted to present in a way that women can understand.

In the book, I explain what happens to women going through menopause, review the various types of hormone preparations used for treatment, and describe what has shaped and changed our attitudes about hormone use over the years. I describe how hormones affect the brain, the bones, the breasts, the heart, and just about every other area that has been studied. Each section contains some background medical information to help you understand the body system being addressed and how hormones affect each area. For instance, what exactly is osteoporosis and how does estrogen make the bones stronger? Or, what causes a heart attack and how can taking estrogen prevent one?

Rather than just telling you what hormones do, I want you to understand how they work to help you decide if it makes sense to take them after your body no longer produces them. Estrogen is not just responsible for our female bodily changes and menstrual periods. It plays a vital role in maintaining healthy bones, brain cells, and blood vessels. The loss of estrogen has widespread consequences. It causes the skin, vaginal tissues, and bones to thin; it alters how our body handles blood sugar and cholesterol, and affects where fat gets deposited. These are things women need to know before they say "No" to HRT.

How does this book help you decide what to do?

Within each chapter are descriptions of the studies that have assessed how hormone treatment affects women's health. My goal is to not just recite the conclusions of this research but to give you an idea of the characteristics of the women studied, the types of hormones used, and the magnitude of the risks and benefits that resulted. Too often the actual degree of risk that a treatment carries is not fully clarified. When making a decision, especially when weighing risks and benefits, a one-in-one-hundred chance of a negative outcome is far different than a one-in-ten-thousand chance. You should also know the details of the participants in the study. Every woman has unique health issues and circumstances. What may apply to one group of women may not apply to women who are more like you. You need to know this type of information and not just accept a study's conclusion that HRT carries "significant" risk.

Years of discussing these issues with thousands of patients has made me realize that there is always one more question that women wished they had an answer to. While the amount of information in this book may seem overwhelming, my goal is to answer as many questions as possible about hormone replacement that my readers may have. At the end of most chapters, you will find a section called the *Decision Making Helper.* This lists the most important key factors in the chapter to help guide you in your assessment of how the benefits and risks of HRT apply to you.

Why you should read this book now

If women are to reap the many benefits of taking hormone replacement, they need to start taking them close to the time they enter menopause. Waiting for a period of years beyond menopause may not be advisable because we are learning that our bodies don't react to hormones in the same way after prolonged estrogen deprivation. In fact, that is what may actually cause more risk than benefit when it comes to taking HRT. This is why I feel there is a sense of urgency to disseminate this information. If a woman delays treatment, she may not be a candidate for taking hormones down the line – and miss an opportunity to significantly improve her health situation, and even prolong her life!

Why did I write this book?

I practiced medicine for two decades before the WHI study and almost two decades after and have treated thousands of menopausal women. It has been difficult for me to ignore the huge amount of research and studies that have shown the beneficial effects of estrogen because of one pivotal point in HRT history, the WHI. I am concerned that by discouraging HRT we are doing a major disservice to our patients and depriving them of future health benefits.

I've struggled with how to best manage my patients under this cloud of uncertainty – which to this day I can't escape. My approach has been to present as much information as I can squeeze into an office visit and let each patient decide what is best for her. But frequently the final decision comes down to, "So, Dr. Rice, what would you do if you were me?" I respond by saying that I started HRT at the time of my menopause and continue to take it. It has been encounters like these with my patients that have spurred my desire to write a comprehensive, yet patient-friendly, book on menopausal hormone treatment – to help women make the right decision.

Why am I qualified to write this book?

I am a board certified internal medicine specialist, have practiced medicine for over 37 years, and have been very interested in menopause throughout my career. I have closely followed this field as new data and new studies have emerged. Years of treating and following my menopausal patients has given me much experience – observing firsthand how women respond to hormones, how to best prescribe them, and how to monitor them during treatment. I am a member of the two major societies devoted to menopause management and research, the North American Menopause Society and the International Menopause Society.

If I was looking for a good book on hormones, I would want a book written by someone who has nothing to gain other than the unselfish desire to share important health information. I can assure you that this is my mission. I am not employed by any pharmaceutical company and have no financial ties to any of them. I am not selling some proprietary hormone cream or other product for financial gain.

I am not employed by a large academic institution. While this may lessen my credibility as an expert in this field, it also gives me some unique advantages. I believe I can speak more freely about the benefits of estrogen. The academic experts who have written the guidelines are constrained to some degree from voicing their personal opinions. They are expected to base their recommendations on only the "highest quality" of evidence based on the "gold standard" of studies, as agreed upon by a consortium of colleagues. The problem that I see with respect to guidelines on HRT is that the only "gold standard" study that we have is the WHI, and as you will learn reading this book, the way its findings have been applied has its shortcomings. One of my goals is to educate you why the recommendations based on the WHI's conclusions may not apply to you.

In discussing this book proposal with an agent, I was told that I would have more credibility in my qualifications to write this book if I was a gynecologist. I was floored! I politely explained to her that gynecologists spend much of their time performing surgeries, delivering babies, and caring for younger women during their fertile years. As internists, most of what we do is care for mid-life and older women, who have "graduated" from their gynecologists' practices and have multiple chronic medical problems – the very problems that are greatly affected by menopause. Internists are trained not only in gynecology, but cardiology, endocrinology, rheumatology, neurology, and geriatrics – all areas where hormone treatment has major impacts. As an internist, I am in a unique position to address all these areas and assess how hormones can help women achieve the best quality of life possible for as long as possible.

The choice to take HRT is a personal one – each woman needs to consider her health, family background, goals, and personal preferences in deciding what is best for her. My hope is that the information in this book will help you make a well-informed decision; one that will allow you to maximize your quality of life and your enjoyment of the many years you will live beyond menopause.

Chapter 1
Anatomy and Physiology – My Favorite Subjects

I have always been fascinated by the human body. When I was in grade school, while other girls were playing with dolls, I was carefully painting and putting together plastic anatomical models. You may remember them. There was the *Visible Man* and the *Visible Woman*. I was particularly intrigued by her because she came with an "optional feature" – a small box labeled the *organs of generation*. This contained a fully developed miniature fetus tucked inside an oversized uterus, complete with an interchangeable baby bump tummy plate. I was tickled that I owned both non-pregnant *Ms. Visible Woman* and very pregnant *Mrs. Visible Woman!*

My mother went to extremes to find new additions for my collection which I displayed on shelves in my bedroom. By the time I left for college, I had over 25 pieces including various nonhuman models such as a cow, a fish, and even a grasshopper. Also on display was a larger than life plastic eyeball, a rendering of a skin biopsy, and a football-sized human cell featuring a DNA filled nucleus, its energy-producing mitochondria, and other essential structures. Needless to say, my three sisters thought I was weird. So it is no surprise that I set my sights on a career in medicine at an early age.

I loved medical school, especially the first two years which were devoted primarily to anatomy, which is the study of the structure of the human organs, and physiology, which is the study of how they function. Each course addressed a different body system ranging from the brain and nervous system to the bones and musculoskeletal system. The two systems that I will address in this chapter are the ones that involve our sex hormones – the *endocrine system* (organs involved in making hormones) and the *genitourinary system* (organs involved in reproduction and urinary function).

The endocrine system

The endocrine system is a collection of glands – notably the ovaries, testicles, thyroid, pituitary gland, and adrenal glands, among others – that produce hormones. Hormones are chemical messengers made by one of our endocrine glands. They are released into the bloodstream to seek specific cells and organs to stimulate specific actions. Collectively hormones regulate almost every process in our body.

The principal female sex hormones are estrogen and progesterone. The primary source of production of these hormones is the ovaries, thus classifying the ovaries as endocrine glands. Our sex hormones are primarily responsible for our sexual development and reproduction, but they also play vital roles in many areas of our bodies as you will learn in the coming chapters. Hormones work by connecting to specific sites on our cells called *receptors*. An important point to be aware of is that a hormone can't exert any effect unless it finds and interacts with its receptor. This unique hormone-receptor interaction unlocks the cellular machinery to produce myriad types of biological actions. This fascinating process and the critical role it plays in hormone therapy are discussed in detail in Chapter 7.

The other endocrine gland pertinent to this discussion is the pituitary gland, which is a grape-sized appendage that sits at the bottom of the brain. The pituitary releases hormones into the circulatory system where they specifically seek out our various endocrine glands such as the thyroid and adrenal glands as well as the ovaries. The pituitary hormones that target the ovaries are *FSH (follicle-stimulating hormone)* and *LH (luteinizing hormone)*. Their roles in reproduction and menopause are described later in this chapter.

The reproductive organs, menstruation, and pregnancy

The uterus is a pear-sized, mostly made-of-muscle organ that sits right above the vagina. The primary function of the uterus is to provide a nurturing environment for the fertilized egg and become the womb for the developing fetus. Each month, stimulation from estrogen transforms the lining of the uterus into a cushion of blood-enriched tissue to support a potential pregnancy. If fertilization doesn't occur, the lining sloughs off in the form of the menstrual flow.

On either side of the uterus are the two apricot-sized ovaries. The ovaries have two main functions – producing hormones and storing and releasing our eggs. Whenever I cut open a cantaloupe and see the inside packed with seeds, I think about my ovaries! However, a woman's eggs are tiny, measuring 0.1 millimeters at the time they are fully developed, which is the thickness of a human hair. Each egg lies in a tiny fluid-filled nest lined by a coating of cells, known as a follicle. The follicular cells are the main source of estrogen production.

Our eggs remain in a dormant state until menstruation occurs and the reproductive cycle begins. Each month six or seven follicles start to slowly enlarge and move toward the outer edge of the ovary. By mid-month, only one of the follicles becomes the dominant one that will go on to release an egg. The others shrink and fade away. By mid-cycle, the dominant follicle is poised on the edge of the ovary and has grown into a fingernail-sized cyst. Then at ovulation, the cyst pops open releasing the egg, which is caught by the arms of the fallopian tube and is transported down to the uterus. After the egg is released, the follicle stays behind and is transformed into the *corpus luteum*. This entity then becomes the source of progesterone production that occurs after ovulation. If an egg is not fertilized, it is flushed out with the lining material inside the uterus as part of the monthly menstrual flow. After the menstrual period ends, a new set of follicles is selected and the cycle repeats itself.

If a sperm finds its way into the uterus it travels into the fallopian tube and if it happens to be mid-cycle when an egg is making its journey, fertilization occurs. The DNA from both parents unites and cell division begins. Soon a bundle of cells called an embryo is formed. This then drifts back down into the uterus and settles into the uterine lining where a placenta is formed along with the developing fetus. The placenta is the lifeline between the growing fetus and its mother. It provides oxygen and nutrients and removes waste material. It also becomes the major source of estrogen and progesterone production during pregnancy and produces increasing amounts of human growth hormone (which is the factor measured in the standard pregnancy tests).

If the fetus has two X chromosomes tiny ovaries appear. Within a number of weeks, they become stocked with some five to seven million eggs. Strangely, most of these waste away and less than a million are present at birth. By the time we reach puberty we only have about 300,000 eggs remaining. This mysterious egg depleting process continues throughout life – such that by the time a woman approaches menopause she has less than 50 eggs left, and then after menopause she has none. I find it interesting to reflect on the fact that, since we only ovulate 12 times a year, and this goes on for about 40 years, only about 500 out of those millions of eggs ever have the potential to become a new person! The physiologic mechanism that is behind the disappearing act of our eggs is unclear but appears to be some sort of a preprogrammed self-destructive process. Without eggs there are no follicles and no corpus luteum – thus the major source of hormone production is gone – which is the hallmark of menopause.

Some comments on ovulation

Some women can feel when they ovulate, the moment the follicular cyst pops and releases the egg mid-cycle. It is perceived as a sharp or dull pain deep on the right or left side of the lower abdomen. Occasionally this can be mistaken for a case of appendicitis and I admit that I was fooled a couple of times until the diagnosis was confirmed by an ultrasound. Sometimes the follicular cysts don't pop and just grow. These eventually can slowly leak and resolve, or get so big they rupture. This can cause extreme pain and sometimes require emergency surgery.

In the syndrome known as *polycystic ovarian syndrome*, the follicles don't ever seem to reach maturity, and thus many follicles develop and fill up the ovary – causing an ovary full of cysts. This is an interesting syndrome because the abundant follicular cells produce excessive amounts of male hormones. This causes acne and facial hair, which are characteristic features of this disorder.

Women having difficulty conceiving frequently need to resort to fertility treatments. Basically, this involves administering drugs that stimulate follicles to develop. This often causes multiple follicles to mature at once – thus increasing the chance of multiple births – twins, triplets and more!

Our sex hormones and how they fluctuate

We can measure the level of sex hormones in the blood. The results for progesterone and estrogen are usually reported out in *"ng/ml"* (*nanograms per milliliter*) or *"pg/ml"* (*picograms per milliliter)*. These are very tiny units – the total amount of circulating hormones in our body probably could fit on the top of a pinhead!

The levels of our sex hormones fluctuate over our life spans, with major changes occurring during puberty, pregnancy, and menopause. We have very low amounts of estrogen and progesterone during childhood, but after puberty, our bodies produce significantly higher levels. Once monthly ovulation starts, the levels of estrogen and progesterone bounce up and down. They are low during and right after the menstrual flow and then peak at ovulation with levels of estrogen reaching up to 350 pg/ml and progesterone up to 20 ng/ml. Then they drop down to levels of about five to ten percent of their peak values at the time of the next menstrual period.

During the reproductive years, the dramatic fluctuations of the hormones that occur throughout the month can create daily changes in a woman's body. High hormone levels stimulate breast tissue, cause fluid retention, and increase our appetites. These physiologic changes are triggered because our hormones are gearing the body up for pregnancy. However, if fertilization doesn't occur, women simply have to put up with the breast tenderness, bloating, and weight gain as part of the monthly ritual. These changes, plus a tendency to be moody and irritable, contribute to the notorious premenstrual syndrome, PMS.

Once a woman reaches menopause, the production of estrogen and progesterone declines to a fraction of earlier levels. The small amounts remaining come primarily from the adrenal glands. The loss of hormones leads to many body changes. The uterus and ovaries shrink in size, the lining of the vagina thins, and the glands and ducts in the breast regress and are replaced by fat. In addition, many other changes occur. These changes, and how they impact our health, will be discussed in the coming chapters.

A few words about testosterone

Besides estrogen and progesterone, male hormones are also present in women's bodies throughout their lives, although only about one-tenth of the levels found in men. Testosterone production ramps up in girls as they reach adolescence and that is why young women have to deal with oily skin and acne along with the other challenges of puberty. Our male hormone levels peak around age 35 and then gradually decline over the next 20 years. So unlike estrogen and progesterone, which drop precipitously around age 50, testosterone doesn't change that much once a woman reaches menopause.

The other genitourinary organs

To complete our anatomy lesson of the GU system let's look at the other genitourinary organs – the bladder, the urethra, the vagina, plus the outer female parts referred to as the external genitalia – which are the vulva, clitoris, and labia. Since the lining of these tissues is stimulated by estrogen, women will note changes in these areas at various stages of life.

With the onset of puberty, the vulvar skin thickens and the vagina becomes more corrugated in texture, the clitoris enlarges, and the bladder and urethra mature.   These organs remain in this "youthful" condition as long as the ovaries continue to function.   On the other side of life, the disappearance of estrogen after menopause leads to thinning and loss of elasticity in these tissues.   This causes vaginal dryness, discomfort with intercourse, bladder leakage, and an increase in the risk of bladder and vaginal infections. More on the effects of menopause on these organs will be covered in Chapter 16.

The role of the brain and pituitary gland

Although not considered a part of the genitourinary system, the brain plays a pivotal role during the reproductive and postmenopausal years. A special section of the brain, the hypothalamus, sends chemical messengers to the pituitary. At puberty, these special brain hormones instruct the pituitary to cyclically release high levels of FSH and LH. FSH stimulates the ovarian follicles to mature and stimulates estrogen production. At the time of ovulation, the estrogen level peaks. This high level then turns off further FSH production through a feedback mechanism. Similarly, the high level of progesterone that was produced after ovulation by the corpus luteum shuts down LH release. If pregnancy doesn't occur, the estrogen and progesterone levels fall. Cells in the hypothalamus detect this and command the pituitary to secrete FSH to begin the cycle again.

When a woman reaches menopause, her ovaries, depleted of follicles, no longer generate hormones. Sensing low estrogen, the pituitary churns out more FSH to flog the ovaries into action. But, because they are unable to respond, the FSH level continues to rise. An elevated FSH level is one of the hallmarks of menopause and can be helpful in confirming if a woman has indeed passed this milestone.

This concludes our anatomy and physiology lesson. Throughout the coming chapters, I will be referring to the organs in our endocrine and reproductive systems frequently and will be discussing in greater detail how our hormones affect just about every other system in our body.

Chapter 2
What Is Menopause?

Understanding the terminology

There are a lot of terms used to describe a woman's hormonal life cycle and these can be very confusing, especially the ones referring to the time before and after menopause. So let's review them.

As a girl makes the transition into womanhood, she goes through *puberty*. Most of us know a lot about this phase. In addition to the host of bodily changes that are encountered, the first menstrual cycle appears, which is called the *menarche*. After a year or more of irregularity, monthly menstrual cycles commence and from ages 14 to 50 (or so) we say a woman is in her *reproductive years*.

The period of a woman's life shortly before the occurrence of menopause is called the *perimenopause*, and this can last several years. During this time the ovaries don't consistently release an egg and the sex hormones tend to rise and fall unevenly and unpredictably. This leads to a number of physical symptoms such as irregular menstrual cycles and emotional symptoms such as mood swings. Another term that describes this period of declining fertility is the *climacteric*.

The term *menopause* refers to the point in time when a woman's ovaries have ceased to function. The production of estrogen and progesterone dramatically drops, and she is no longer fertile. Menopause heralds the cessation of monthly menstrual cycles assuming the woman still has her uterus. (Technically I've always thought it should be called *"menostop"* instead of *menopause*. Others like the word *"womenopause"* – but we won't go there!). Because a woman can't know which menstrual cycle will be her last, it has been decided to designate that menopause officially occurs once 12 months elapse without a menstrual period. A woman is considered to be *postmenopausal* once she has gone through menopause.

Natural menopause is the term we use for menopause that occurs all by itself and not due to some external factor. *Surgical menopause* is the term used if the ovaries are removed for some medical condition. Menopause can also be brought on by anything that causes permanent damage to the ovaries such as a severe infection, an autoimmune disease, or cancer treatment involving radiation or chemotherapy.

When does menopause happen?

As you enter your late 40s, you may ask: "How do I know which will be my last monthly cycle?" The truth of the matter is – you really can't. We can measure your hormone levels to get a general idea about where you are, but these levels fluctuate so much during any given month that they are not good predictors. I tell patients: "If it has been six months since your last period there is roughly a 50% chance you may have another one, but if it has been 12 months, there is a 99.9% chance that you are done, so welcome to menopause!"

For the many women who have had a hysterectomy, knowing whether they have reached menopause is even trickier. As will be discussed below, a woman's age, the onset of menopausal symptoms, and results of blood tests that assess ovarian function generally are used to make a determination.

Invariably, the next question patients ask is when they should stop using birth control. It goes without saying that most women prefer not to become pregnant at this point in their lives. The concern is not irrational, because almost everyone has heard about someone who had an unexpected late-in-life "surprise." Some women think they are no longer fertile after age 50, but this is not true. In fact, a woman can become pregnant right up until the time of menopause. So to be absolutely safe, it is wise to use birth control until a woman has gone a year without a menstrual period.

The median age of natural menopause is 51.4 years. This means that half of all women have stopped menstruating by that age and half will still be flowing. Interestingly, whereas life expectancy has increased tremendously since ancient times, it appears that women have always reached menopause around this age.[1] For 90% of women, natural menopause will occur sometime between the ages of 45 and 55. Of the rest, 5% stop menstruating between ages 40 and 44, and the other 5% will make it past 55 before their menstrual cycles end. (We don't have reliable data on who may hold the record for being the oldest woman to reach menopause, but likely she would be age 59). If women go through menopause younger than age 40 we refer to this as *primary ovarian insufficiency* or *premature ovarian failure*. Certain genetic abnormalities and autoimmune conditions can cause this, but 75% to 90% of the time the reason is unknown.[2]

Many factors can influence when a woman has natural menopause. Lifestyle issues contribute to the timing. It has recently been noted that women who work night shifts tend to go through menopause earlier than women on normal daytime schedules. Smokers generally go through menopause earlier by one to two years, and women who live at high altitudes tend to have an earlier menopause. Although women who are undernourished and women with low body fat tend to go through menopause earlier, being overweight or obese has not been shown to consistently correlate with a later menopause.

At the time of natural menopause, approximately one in three women will already have had surgical removal of their uterus (i.e., a hysterectomy). Even though the ovaries are left in place, these procedures tend to cause an earlier menopause than expected – by as much as five years.[3,4] This likely is related to some impairment of the blood supply to the ovaries caused by the surgery, although other factors may be involved. Recently, it also has been shown that just removing one ovary can bring on menopause about one to two years earlier than normal.[5]

If early menopause runs in your family, odds are you will also experience it earlier than average.[6] As we are learning more about the genetic code, we are pinpointing some of the genes that may be responsible for this.[7] While we often tell women that there is a relationship between when her menses started and when she undergoes menopause, this is controversial. Some studies have shown a relationship, but many have not.[8]

Even though most of the patients in my practice consisted of mid-life women, it wasn't until late in my career that I made an extra effort to note and record at what age my patients had their final menstrual periods. It is surprising how many women can't recall the exact date. The significance of being aware of this is actually very important and will become more apparent as you read this book. Although it has long been known that women who go through menopause early have a higher risk of osteoporosis, more and more evidence shows that they also have higher risks of other health problems such as heart diseases and diabetes. An even lesser-known fact is that having an early menopause is associated with a shorter life span![9]

Menopause chemistry and physiology

Regardless of when menopause occurs, the hallmark is a loss of ovarian function. The ovaries' production of hormones diminishes, and ovulation stops. The brain tries to stimulate the unresponsive ovaries by secreting more and more FSH (follicle-stimulating hormone) into the bloodstream. During the reproductive years the FSH level is generally below 20 IU/L (international units per liter), whereas in postmenopause, the level can be as high as 140 IU/L. So the laboratory features of menopause are low levels of estrogen and high levels of FSH. Measuring these levels can be particularly useful in assessing for menopause in a woman who has had a hysterectomy, who doesn't have monthly menses as a means of identifying where she is with respect to menopause.

There is considerable variation in the degree of estrogen and FSH levels among postmenopausal women. We know that certain factors such as the amount of body fat affect estrogen levels, but the cause for the variation in FSH levels is unclear. It is interesting that symptoms don't necessarily correlate with these levels and the exact mechanism behind the various menopausal symptoms is an area of ongoing research.

For years we have primarily focused on FSH's role in ovulation. However recent research is revealing that it may have effects in other areas. It is possible that the high levels of FSH affect bone and cholesterol metabolism, and may contribute to some of the symptoms and changes in the body that occur after menopause. We are a long way from fully understanding the significance of this, but in the future a woman's FSH level may dictate how we fine-tune the management of menopausal women.

Another relatively new test that correlates with our ovarian reserve is the *anti-Mullerian hormone* (AMH) level. This test basically indicates how many viable eggs remain in the ovaries and is being used in some situations to help predict when a woman may go through menopause. About five years prior to menopause the AMH level drops, and after the last egg has disappeared at the time of menopause, the AMH level is undetectable.

Perimenopausal and menopausal symptoms

It would be nice if there was an orderly way our ovaries wound down in their hormone production as we approach menopause, but this just doesn't happen. Every woman goes through this transition in a different manner. After many years of a predictable cyclic rise and fall of estrogen and progesterone, during perimenopause, the hormone levels fluctuate up and down inconsistently. Beginning up to five years prior to menopause, each month can bring a different hormonal pattern. Some months consist of "normal" cycles; others are characterized by imbalanced hormone levels that surprise us with various physical and emotional symptoms that seem to come out of the blue.

As noted, the transition from the reproductive years to the postmenopausal years has historically been referred to as the climacteric. This term derives from an ancient Greek word meaning ladder. I suspect this was because in ancient times it was observed that women going through this period in their lives experienced the same ups and downs as we do today. At various points in history the climacteric was felt to cause insanity! Indeed, a passage from a medical article written in 1887 entitled *Uterine Disease as a Factor in the Production of Insanity* reads as follows:

> *"The ovaries, after long years of service, have not the ability of retiring in graceful old age, but become irritated, transmit their irritation to the abdominal ganglia, which in turn transmit the irritation to the brain, producing disturbances in the cerebral tissue exhibiting themselves in extreme nervousness or in an outbreak of actual insanity."*[10]

No one believes any longer that menopause causes insanity, but clearly, the loss of hormones affects our cognition and causes mood changes. Books on menopause talk about women being in a "brain fog." This isn't a term found in medical dictionaries but conveys an accurate picture of how some women feel during this time. Lots of things may contribute to this condition – such as lack of sleep, stress, or trying to juggle too many balls at once at home and/or at work. However, it is known that estrogen plays a major role in brain function, and loss of estrogen causes a decline in the production of a number of our brain's neurotransmitters, in particular, serotonin and acetylcholine – two important chemicals that play a role in mood and cognitive function. I will discuss more about the effects of hormones on the brain in Chapter 14.

While one positive aspect of going through menopause is not having any further menstrual periods, the havoc our uterus puts us through leading up to that final day can be downright unpleasant. Unlike most of the reproductive years, when there are monthly ovulations and predictable menstrual periods, as a woman gets closer to menopause, several things start happening. The length of time from the end of a menstrual period to ovulation decreases. Instead of a

28-day cycle, the interval gets shorter and shorter – sometimes causing menses to be separated by only a couple of weeks. At other times, we may not ovulate in a given month. This leads to a missed menstrual period (and the "OMG! Am I pregnant?" scare). When the next menstrual period finally shows up some 50 or 60 days later, it can be a doozy, with prolonged or heavy bleeding. In addition, at some point in between these cycles, it is common to experience unexpected (and often embarrassing) spotting or bleeding. This is because, without ovulation-induced progesterone production, ongoing estrogen stimulation creates a buildup of the lining of the uterus which can slough off at any time.

Besides putting up with mood changes and unpredictable menstrual bleeding during perimenopause, other symptoms develop from these hormonal imbalances. At any time, in any given month, one can encounter unexpected breast tenderness, bloating, fluid retention, sleep disturbance, or changes in appetite. To say the least, these can be annoying and can greatly interfere with one's relationships and activities. And to make it worse, within 24 hours, the hormones can readjust – and these symptoms can suddenly disappear – making a woman really wonder if she is indeed going crazy!

Dealing with these symptoms is difficult. In my practice, I have found that just explaining the hormonal changes that cause these problems helps many women cope. In addition, I encourage them to follow other healthy lifestyle measures – such as getting adequate sleep, eating healthy meals (low sugar, low salt, and low fat) and exercising regularly. Sometimes anti-anxiety and antidepressant medications are prescribed.

The only way to balance the hormone fluctuations occurring in perimenopause is to use hormone treatment. This can be accomplished in several ways. The most common method is to put a woman on low-dose birth control pills. These provide hormone levels that are slightly higher than what the body makes. The brain gets "fooled" into thinking the estrogen is coming from the ovaries – so the pituitary stops producing FSH and LH. The end result is that the ovaries shut down and don't send out erratic spurts of hormones. And because the contraceptive pills are a daily fixed dose, the estrogen and progestogen levels in the blood remain stable. The additional benefit is that this treatment also provides birth control for women who need contraception.

Hello, hot flashes!

At some point during the climacteric, hot flashes almost always materialize. Overall, 70 to 80% of women experience these unwelcome visitors during this transition. Also referred to as *hot flushes*, they usually show up with a vengeance in the year or two prior to menopause but up to 40% of women will experience them intermittently many years before that time.[11]

The typical hot flash begins with a sudden sensation of warmth – generally in the upper chest and head but can be perceived throughout the entire body. It is rapidly followed by sweating – which is the body's way of cooling off. Some women rarely get an episode; others get them throughout the day and night. A hot flash generally lasts a few minutes, but some women feel uncomfortable for up to an hour. They can be mild or severe, and wax and wane in frequency and intensity. The medical term for hot flashes is *vasomotor* symptoms. This comes from the fact that the blood vessels (or *vascular* channels) which are surrounded by muscles (*motor* units) dilate during the hot flash. The dilation increases blood flow near the surface of the skin which causes warmth and flushing.

It is amazing how many different ways these vasomotor symptoms can present. Not infrequently, heart pounding or palpitations are the prominent sensations, which have occasionally prompted a call from a patient concerned she is having a heart attack! Some women don't experience the heat, they just suddenly feel cold. Some women encounter very atypical symptoms such as feeling pressure in the head, burning or tingling sensations, nausea, shortness of breath, or suddenly having trouble concentrating.

Scientists have developed a technique where the actual physiologic changes occurring during a hot flash can be detected. Sensors are placed on the skin and measure the amount of heat and perspiration being generated. Women wear these devices and are monitored for 24 hours, and are instructed to record whenever they feel a hot flash. Surprisingly, in many of these studies, the instrument picks up vasomotor episodes not reported in the patients' diaries – indicating that the changes occurred but were not recognized by the women as hot flashes. In some subjects, this lack of awareness occurred for up to half of their daily hot flash incidents.[12] I found this information very interesting. While various studies on menopause report that up to 80% of women experience hot flashes, I wonder if it is actually much higher than this because some women probably have symptoms they may not recognize as a hot flash.

Certain things can precipitate or make hot flashes worse. Foods and beverages that can trigger them include alcohol, caffeine, and spicy dishes. Hot weather or a sudden temperature change can cause them. Feeling flustered or even being in a confined space can precipitate them. Even the well-intentioned affection of a loved one can bring one on. When you think about it, there really is nowhere we can escape these pesky rascals!

More than you may want to know about hot flashes

Hot flashes have been scientifically studied. Typically, at the start of one, the heart rate increases and there is increased blood flow to the skin. This makes the skin temperature rise slightly. The internal core temperature also goes up a tiny amount, but the subjective sensation of heat is much greater (i.e., "I feel like I'm burning up!"). To cool things off the brain directs the sweat glands to produce a thin film of perspiration over the skin. This causes an evaporative cooling effect – which actually can cause the body temperature to drop a little, and create the sensation of being chilled. When this occurs at night we get the very bothersome *night sweats*. This is what is behind the tiresome ritual of throwing blankets on and off and getting up once or twice to change nightgowns.

The exact physiology behind the hot flash is still a little uncertain but appears to have something to do with fluctuating estrogen levels. There is an area in the brain (in the hypothalamic region) that regulates temperature and acts as an internal thermostat. During the menopausal transition, it appears that this thermostat gets very sensitive – a tiny change in body temperature or other signal triggers it to rapidly correct the situation by sending chemical messengers to the arteries in the skin to dilate and cool the body off. Then the tiny drop in temperature sets it off the other way. It only takes a subtle environmental change or other stimuli to elicit a response – which is set into motion like lightning. Think about the last time you received an embarrassing compliment and your face instantly blushed. That is how fast a hot flash can be triggered.

Hot flashes can show up many years prior to the time of menopause, but most women experience them within a couple of years of their final menstrual periods. Typically they last two to ten years after that, but studies have shown that a substantial number of women (up to 20%) experience them well past age 70 and some into their 80s and 90s.

Personally, I suspect that hot flashes are more common in older postmenopausal women than we have realized. A well-known caveat in treating older patients is that they frequently don't manifest the same symptoms as younger people. For instance, geriatric patients don't always get fevers when they come down with pneumonia and doctors need to be astute – on the lookout for other subtle clues to make the diagnosis. For this reason, I have often wondered if some of the unexplained symptoms that our older female patients frequently report, such as dizziness or transient vague "spells," could be hot flash equivalents.

There is a lot we don't know about hot flashes. We don't know why some women have more problems than others. Women who are overweight tend to report more frequent hot flashes than thinner women, which is a little unexpected because the more fat cells women have, the higher their estrogen levels. We suspect genes play a role because certain ethnic groups tend to have more hot flashes than others. African American women report more frequent hot flashes than Caucasian women, and Japanese and Chinese women report less. Interestingly, the earlier the age that a woman begins experiencing hot flashes, the worse they tend to be, and they tend to last longer than average beyond menopause.

Remedies for hot flashes

Hot flashes clearly affect a woman's quality of life and are the most frequent reason that women consult their health care providers during the menopausal transition.[13,14] Just about every expert in menopause agrees that estrogen is the most effective treatment for hot flashes. It is approved by the FDA for this indication. Most women see a dramatic improvement with modest doses of estrogen. Some women get by with less; some require unusually high amounts for relief – and this is likely due to genetic factors. No one type of estrogen preparation is felt to be superior to another. Progesterone has also been shown to help hot flash symptoms, but not to the degree that estrogen does.

Some women are reluctant to take estrogen because they are concerned about potential risks. This has led to a quest for non-hormone options to calm hot flashes. There are a number of natural agents that have been studied and, while some may be helpful, none have conclusively been shown to be consistently effective.[15] These include black cohosh, dong quai, primrose oil, and the rest of the large class of phytoestrogens found in soy products, legumes, fennel, lentils, red clover, flaxseed, yams, and other fruits, vegetables, and grains. It certainly doesn't hurt to try eating more foods containing phytoestrogens, but most women can't consume enough to really help – as the potency of these natural estrogen-like products is very weak.

The other option – purchasing derivatives of these products in pill form – is not always ideal because these dietary supplements are not regulated by the FDA. Therefore there is always a concern about their actual content and purity. Buying them from a trusted and reputable source, rather than from an unknown company on the internet, is always a good idea if a woman chooses to go this route.

Another measure that has been tested to alleviate hot flashes is acupuncture. Many women have reported some success with this, but most studies show that it really isn't any more effective than a placebo intervention.[16,17]

The pharmaceutical industry has capitalized on the pursuit to find a non-hormone answer for hot flashes. The same chemical deficiency that is associated with depression, namely the lack of serotonin, is believed to play a role in the genesis of the hot flash. Antidepressant drugs designed to raise serotonin have been available for years; the most commonly prescribed ones belong to the class called *selective serotonin reuptake inhibitors, or SSRI* drugs. So it was logical to test whether these drugs might be effective in relieving hot flashes. Enough data showing benefit was presented to the FDA that *paroxetine* (Paxil) gained approval for treating hot flashes.

My personal experience treating menopausal patients with SSRI drugs has not been very successful. Some women benefited, but others had side effects – which is common with these drugs.[18] These include dry mouth, fatigue, weight gain, dizziness, and sexual dysfunction (talk about adding insult to injury!). I have also had patients complain that their night sweats worsened while taking an SSRI, which they were not very happy about. Sweating is a little known side effect of these agents but has been reported to occur in 10 to 15% of patients.[19]

Drugs approved for treating other conditions have been studied to see if they can decrease hot flashes. Since blood vessels are involved in vasomotor activity, certain blood pressure drugs, such as *clonidine*, have been employed to treat hot flashes. Drugs used to treat seizures have also been trialed – the rationale being that they target some of the chemical pathways in the brain that have a bearing on hot flashes. None of these drugs are as effective as estrogen, and they all have their own side effects (plus they are not FDA approved for treating hot flashes).

Research is progressing on a novel treatment targeting a recently appreciated neurotransmitter in the brain that plays a role in hot flashes. These agents are called *neurokinin B receptor antagonists*. I am not sure when or if these drugs may become available. I know that some experts in menopause are excited about this new option, but my approach to any brand new class of drugs is watchful waiting to make sure there are no unsuspected adverse effects that may show up after the drug has been in widespread use. In the case of this drug class, initial studies have already shown that it may cause some liver toxicity.[20]

A fairly new product, *Duavee,* was approved to treat hot flashes in 2013. This contains a low-dose conjugated estrogen product (which is not anything new), plus a second drug, *bazedoxifene,* which is a new *selective estrogen receptor modulator* (SERM). I will be discussing SERMs in great detail in the next chapter but, basically, they are designer drugs that can block some of the unwanted adverse effects of estrogen. The concept behind Duavee is that its estrogen component combats the hot flashes while the SERM blocks any negative effects that may be caused by the estrogen (such as breast or uterine stimulation). This drug is gaining popularity, but I am reluctant to prescribe it. It seems counterintuitive to me that women looking for an option to avoid estrogen would consider taking a drug that contains not only estrogen but a fairly new drug that may have unknown risks of its own. Our past experience with SERMs is that occasionally an unexpected adverse effect shows up only after they have been on the market for an extended period of time.

Other therapies and agents to help hot flashes are in development – spurred by the prevailing reluctance to prescribe HRT. During a breakfast meeting at a menopause conference that I recently attended, there was one young man amongst the rest of us mid-life women. Sensing we were curious to know why he was there, he shared with us that he did not know very much about menopause and was sent to the conference to get an education. It turns out he had recently been hired in the marketing department for a company making a wrist bracelet being designed to detect and counteract hot flashes. Intrigued, I googled this and discovered there are a number of devices being marketed to women to treat hot flashes. However, I couldn't find much evidence to support their effectiveness when I researched these further.

The bottom line is that there are many options besides estrogen that are being promoted to help menopausal symptoms. Women should be informed about the benefits and risks of other drugs or treatments and compare how they stack up to the benefits and risks of HRT.

Is there more to the hot flash than a hot flash?

Over the years hot flashes have been considered a nuisance at best and a quality of life aspect at worst. They are often dismissed as an innocuous rite of passage that women need to endure and get through. Frequently they are portrayed as comical (picture the stereotypical image of a mid-life woman desperately fanning herself at some function – to the amusement of those around her). But recent research indicates that these pesky symptoms have more medical significance than we have appreciated. It is suspected that hot flashes may be either a marker or even a cause of heart disease.[21]

The connection between hot flashes and heart disease became apparent in studies that found that women who suffer the most hot flashes, especially those experiencing them well before menopause, appear to have a higher than expected rate of cardiovascular complications.[22] It is unclear why this may be, but there are a number of potential explanations.

The vasomotor changes accompanying hot flashes can affect blood pressure and cause inflammation within the lining of the arteries.[23] These are factors that are known to promote the deposition of plaque – the cholesterol-laden gunk that builds up and eventually creates the blockages that cause heart attacks and strokes. It is speculated that severe and prolonged hot flashes may be damaging to the arteries. Research that supports this comes from an interesting study that compared MRI scans on women who had severe hot flashes with women who hadn't suffered from them.[24] The women with the most hot flashes had more *white matter hyperintensities* noted throughout their brain matter. These are tiny speckles that show up as "hot spots" on the scans. They are commonly found as people age and are believed to represent minute areas of brain damage caused by blockages in tiny arteries. This study really impressed me because it suggests that women with bad hot flashes may not only be at increased risk for heart disease, but may be at greater risk for strokes and even dementia.

Frequent and severe hot flashes may also adversely affect our cardiovascular systems through other mechanisms. The chemical messengers in the brain associated with hot flashes are involved in the autonomic nervous system, which controls our heart rhythm and vascular tone. The heart pounding and palpitations that many women experience with their hot flashes may represent a response to high levels of adrenaline, which could be detrimental to the heart in the long run.

The apparent connection between hot flashes and heart disease raises dozens of questions that need answers. Do hot flashes actually cause vascular problems, or are they just a marker alerting us to who may be at more risk for heart disease? If they are a marker for a woman at risk, should we be more aggressive in recommending other things that are known to prevent heart disease – such as prescribing statin drugs to lower cholesterol? Even more pressing, does this imply that we should be encouraging estrogen replacement as the ideal treatment for hot flashes, rather than other drugs that simply help women cope with them? And shouldn't we be using doses of estrogen that are effective in eliminating them rather than encouraging women to use the lowest doses possible to get by? It may take years before enough studies are done to answer these questions, but in the meantime, I am glad that the guidelines do allow estrogen treatment for hot flashes – even though the reasoning behind this is not for cardiovascular protection.

Other menopausal consequences

Although hot flashes are the cardinal symptom of menopause, women experience a host of other symptoms. Sleep problems are commonly reported. It goes without saying that sleep deprivation compromises daytime alertness and energy, but it also correlates with a number of adverse health problems. Lack of sleep and poor quality of sleep have been associated with higher risk of hypertension, heart disease, diabetes, obesity, and depression. How menopause affects sleep is likely multifactorial. There is no question that night sweats are very disruptive, but studies show that menopause negatively affects our sleep even in the absence of these vasomotor symptoms.[25] The loss of estrogen has also been felt to be a factor in causing sleep apnea – a common condition resulting in disturbed sleep.[26]

Another area negatively impacted by menopause is the genitourinary system. The cells lining the vagina, vulva, and opening to the bladder behave much like the cells making up our external skin – providing a barrier of protection from external insults. During our reproductive years, high estrogen levels help keep the tissues in these areas resilient to injury and infection. As the estrogen level falls, the lining of these tissues becomes thinner and fragile. Many women start to notice some changes "down there" well before

19

menopause, and symptoms gradually worsen over time. Eventually, this leads to dryness, discomfort with intercourse, and increased susceptibility to infections. This subject is covered in greater detail in Chapter 16.

In addition to the very noticeable acute symptoms of menopause, a number of other areas in our body are gradually impacted by the loss of hormones. While it is controversial whether menopause, per se, is responsible for the mid-life weight gain that occurs, there is convincing evidence that the loss of estrogen affects where fat gets deposited. After menopause women rapidly accumulate fat in and around the abdominal area. We start morphing into "apples" which is the not-so-complimentary description of having an increasingly rounded body contour with an increase in central (belly) fat. This particular pattern of fat accumulation is associated with a number of medical problems such as diabetes and heart disease – important issues that will be discussed in later chapters.

Numerous other changes occur after menopause – some obvious and some not so obvious. Estrogen loss weakens connective tissue which impacts our bones, joints, muscles, and skin. Major changes happen in our brains, our hearts, and even our livers and colons. These, as well as what we know about the effects of hormone replacement in each of these systems, are covered in detail in later chapters of this book.

Why do we go through menopause?

It may strike you that many of the changes that occur during menopause are not very desirable. You may wonder, as many of us do, why this happens to us. Men do not experience an abrupt decline in testosterone at midlife. Their male hormone levels fall slightly as they age, but basically persist at relatively high levels throughout their lives. If men do lose their hormones (such as through surgical removal of the testicles) they are subject to many of the same problems that women encounter – hot flashes, mood changes, and higher rates of osteoporosis. In addition, their cholesterol increases, they lose muscle mass, and become impotent. (In reference to this last issue, I always chuckle when I think about how men would view the controversy about whether or not they should take testosterone if they had to decide on hormone replacement!)

Furthermore, a man does not lose his reproductive capacity until practically the day he dies, whereas a woman's fertility is coupled with her loss of estrogen production. This raises an interesting question. Why does a woman lose her ability to bear offspring many years before the end of her life?

Generally, survival of a species places a high priority on successful and prolonged procreation. The very fact that women lose their reproductive ability at mid-life is somewhat against the laws of nature.

Humans are one of the few species where this occurs. Some apes do go through human-like menopause – where their hormones decline and eggs deplete – but this occurs relatively close to the end of their life expectancy. Almost all other animals continue to reproduce until shortly before the time they die. Your first thought would be that perhaps it is a matter of longevity – that species with long life spans are the ones that would be likely to quit reproducing at midlife. This doesn't seem to be the case, however, because other animals that live long lives, like elephants and blue whales, continue to bear offspring until very late in life.

Researchers interested in menopause have discovered that the only other species besides humans that live many years after losing their ability to bear offspring are orca whales and pilot whales. Pilot whales stop reproducing around age 35 and can live another 30 years. Orcas stop reproducing at age 50 and can live to age 90 or even longer.

It remains a medical mystery why humans and orcas go through menopause, but there are some theories. This research is particularly interesting to me since I was born and raised in the Pacific Northwest – home to some of the best-studied orca families in the nation. Orcas are the sleek black and white whales, also known as killer whales. You may have seen one of these magnificent creatures at SeaWorld.

Naturalists have been studying our orca populations since the 1960s and have identified several families they call pods. Each family member is named and recognized by the characteristics of his or her fins and coloring. These whales are very social and stay together for life in their pods traveling up and down the Pacific coast and inland waters feeding primarily on salmon.

The current theory proposed to explain menopause in these animals is known as the *grandmother hypothesis*.[27] Basically, the concept is that it is advantageous for the entire family if the matriarch of the pod stops having children when her children reach sexual maturity. In this way, several survival benefits for her and the pod occur. She doesn't compete with her own daughters in finding food for their offspring – thus improving her grandchildren's chances of survival. Grandmother is able to play the role of the matriarch, using her years of knowledge to lead the pod to the best fishing areas, unencumbered with a young calf. It has been estimated that for her to be able to get enough sustenance to nurse a growing calf, she would need to consume 42% more calories daily.[28] (That is a lot of salmon!) Credibility for the grandmother hypothesis has come from researchers who have observed these behaviors in our local whale populations as they make their annual treks up and down the west coast.[28]

This is of course just a theory and may not explain why humans go through menopause. Skeptics would point out that research has shown that the average age of menopause hasn't changed much since ancient times, and we have been taught that it wasn't until about a hundred years ago that women lived much past age 50. So, throughout most of human history women would not live the 20 or 30 years post menopause that would be necessary to realize a similar evolutionary change. However, there has been research that indicates that some ancient hunter-gatherer cultures may have had longer life spans than we have believed.[29] If so, it would have been advantageous for the matriarch of the group to not be encumbered with young children and be able to contribute more in collecting and sharing food; thus promoting the survival of her extended family.

We may never know the answer to why we are programmed to go through menopause once we reach our fiftieth birthday. It is difficult to imagine what type of historic evidence would give archaeologists any clues to work with. The reality is, however, that women are living longer lives and spending more and more years in a hormone-deficient state.

Chapter 3
Our Hormones, Drugs, and Menopause

Our body is full of different kinds of hormones. Over a hundred years ago scientists began extracting hormones from the glands of animals and purifying them for medicinal use. Since then we have been able to identify the exact chemical structure of our various hormones and synthesize identical products, or products with similar actions, for almost all of the ones our bodies make. In the decision about whether or not to consider HRT, it's important to be familiar with the various hormone options and treatments that are available. These will be reviewed in this chapter following an explanation of the types of hormones our bodies make and what they do.

The rise and fall of our sex hormones

Our sex hormones constitute a large group of hormones and include estrogen, progesterone, testosterone, and some of their related compounds. We call them sex hormones because they play the primary role in differentiating males from females. They accomplish this by interacting with many of our organs to create the unique features that set the sexes apart. This process starts shortly after conception. Once an egg is fertilized, the early embryo either has two **X** chromosomes (in females) or has the male configuration – which is an **X** and a **Y** chromosome. Interestingly, until about six weeks of gestation, the two sexes are identical in their development. Then, under the direction of the **Y** chromosome, the tissue destined to be a testicle starts making testosterone, which then promotes the development of the male sex organs. Without the **Y** chromosome, the fetus develops into a female and estrogen production occurs. The presence and amounts of our sex hormones impact not only how the sexual organs develop but how other systems such as the neurologic system function. (This explains why from conception some pregnant mothers seem to know whether they are carrying a boy or a girl!) The role our hormones play in the development of personality and gender identification in the fetal brain is an area of fascinating research.

During childhood, the levels of sex hormones are low but play essential roles necessary for normal growth and development of many of our organs, particularly our brains and musculoskeletal systems. Estrogen and testosterone production increases markedly at puberty and promotes the maturation of sexual organs and other changes characteristic of adolescence. The fact that they are at work in many areas of the body should be obvious when you think about the features typical of this stage of life. Hair starts appearing in new areas, fat gets deposited in new places, the skin becomes oily, breasts enlarge, voices change, and pigment changes on the skin appear – not to mention the impressive effects that hormones play in the brain. Every parent has had to tell themselves at one time or another that it is "the hormones" that must be making their adolescent behave like a moody monster.

Puberty heralds the onset of the reproductive years in women, which are characterized by the cyclic rise and fall of all of our sex hormones. During her 20s and 30s, a woman experiences the highest levels of all her sex hormones. Around age 40, however, the testosterone level drops substantially. Then as she rounds the corner to age 50, it declines further, along with the abrupt drop in estrogen and progesterone. By the time menopause rolls around, all of the sex hormones are substantially lower than they were 25 years earlier. The low levels of hormones that do persist are generated from sources other than the ovaries, primarily the adrenal glands.

The decline of estrogen, and to a lesser extent progesterone and testosterone, has a major impact on many areas of a woman's body – as you will see in the coming chapters. Whether or not women should replace those gone missing has been a controversy for decades. Choosing to take hormone replacement or one of the multitude of options prescribed for menopausal treatment is a complicated decision.

Cholesterol – the basic building block

The basic building block for all of the female and male sex hormones is the cholesterol molecule. Cholesterol gets maligned for being a bad thing, but the truth of the matter is that it is a critical element necessary for life. Besides being the core unit for many of our hormones, it is a main component of the membrane around all of our cells and also used to make bile and fat-soluble vitamins.

Although we eat foods rich in cholesterol, such as meat and eggs, over 75% of our cholesterol is actually produced from simpler elements in our body. The cholesterol molecule itself has a characteristic four-ring shape (like four hula-hoops linked together) and all of our sex hormones have this basic geometric structure. Specialized enzymes either attach or remove various atomic units, like hydrogen, onto the cholesterol base unit to create estrogen, progesterone, and testosterone. These are all remarkably similar chemically but have very different actions in the body. All of these agents stemming from the cholesterol skeleton belong to the *steroid* family. So while we generally think of steroids as the ones in cortisone creams, our sex hormones are considered steroids as well.

The estrogens our body makes

The two main estrogens in a woman's body are *estradiol* and *estrone*. Estradiol is the principal hormone present in the body during the reproductive years. It is produced by the ovarian follicle which is the tissue surrounding the egg. Estradiol is also known as **E2** and is the most potent natural female estrogen. The prescription form of this bears the generic name *17beta-estradiol*. This is the same as the natural estradiol made by the body. When a woman takes this either orally or applies it topically on the skin, her body doesn't know whether it came from an outside source or was made internally.

The other principal female hormone circulating in the blood is estrone or **E1**. This was actually the first form of estrogen used in treating hormone-deficient women back in the 1930s. Estrone is less potent than estradiol – but is readily converted into estradiol in the body. So if a woman is using an estrone product for HRT much of it will be transformed into estradiol after it gets into the circulatory system.

After menopause, when all the eggs and follicles have disappeared, very little estradiol is produced. So, most of the estrogen in the body at that point is in the form of estrone. This comes primarily from steroid precursors made in the adrenal glands but is also produced in many different tissues. Some estrone is made in the ovaries but much is produced by our fat cells. You may have heard that overweight and obese women have higher estrogen levels, and this is why. The more fat cells we have, the more estrone we generate.

Estriol or **E3** is a very weak estrogen and primarily plays a role during pregnancy. It is produced in large quantities by the placenta. Some naturopathic providers recommend estriol for postmenopausal treatment, but most menopause experts do not concur with this. It likely is of questionable benefit due to its low potency. However, researchers studying estriol have found that it may have some unique properties that may be useful in treating other conditions such as multiple sclerosis.[1]

Another less frequently mentioned natural estrogen, estetrol **(E4)**, is made by the liver of a developing fetus – so is only found in pregnant women. There has been recent interest in this form of estrogen as a possible therapy in menopause as it appears to have beneficial effects on the bone and vaginal tissue without increasing the risk of breast cancer.[2]

While estradiol and estrone are the basic human estrogens, their chemical structures are further modified by reactions in the liver and other tissues into a variety of sub-forms of estrogen which give them slightly different properties. One such process is known as *conjugation*. Almost all animals, including humans, have a variety of these conjugated estrogens in the circulation. One reason this occurs is to convert them into inactive "storage" forms of hormones, where they can be converted as needed back into active forms; another is to alter them in a way that allows them to go through the kidneys to be excreted out of the body in the urine.

After menopause the total amount of estrogen produced decreases substantially so that the amount is only about 10% of the level a woman had when she was ovulating. Estradiol production goes down by about 90% and the estrone level falls by about 30%. This results in a higher proportion of estrone to estradiol in postmenopausal women. We can measure these levels in the lab but there generally isn't much reason to do so after menopause, since we know that all women will be at comparably low levels. Some providers order hormone levels to monitor replacement therapy. This can be helpful to assess if the HRT formulation being taken is getting absorbed, but measuring estrogen levels isn't generally recommended. The levels in the blood don't always reflect how much estrogen is really getting inside our cells – so treatment is usually based on clinical measures rather than lab values.

The array of oral estrogen products

Most of our sex hormones were discovered over a century ago by scientists analyzing and purifying products from urine and testing what sort of properties they had. We've come a long way since then as pharmaceutical companies have found ways to synthesize these hormones from steroid-like substances found in nature. There are so many different hormone products that, even as a physician, it is difficult to keep track of all the brand names that have come on the market. There is a dizzying array of estrogen-containing birth control pills as well as products to treat menopausal symptoms.

Most birth control pills contain some type of estrogen along with a progesterone-like drug. Even though there are over 30 different names for the various contraceptive pills, they all contain one form of estrogen, *ethinyl estradiol*. This is a potent synthetic estrogen that creates estrogen levels higher than what the ovaries produce. This "fools" the brain into thinking a woman is pregnant, thus inhibiting ovulation.

It is not necessary to have estrogen levels this high to effectively treat hot flashes and other menopausal symptoms, so contraceptive hormones are not used for HRT in postmenopausal women. However, they often can be helpful during the perimenopausal period. During this time many women have irregular menses and using low-dose birth control pills is effective in regulating them. Treatment is continued until it can be determined that a woman has indeed gone through menopause. Then she can switch to one of the regimens used for HRT if she desires. It is important to re-emphasize that the standard doses of HRT are not sufficient to prevent pregnancy!

When it comes time to consider hormone replacement therapy, there are numerous products to choose from. They differ in their chemical structures and potencies. Some are identical to the hormones produced by the body; others have different chemical properties. Before getting into a detailed discussion, I should point out that if a woman has her uterus, most menopause experts recommend that she include a progesterone-like drug along with an estrogen drug for hormone replacement. The main reason for this is that taking estrogen alone can increase the risk of cancer of the uterus; taking both drugs has been shown to prevent this. If a woman has had a hysterectomy, then she would typically just take an estrogen drug.

The first widely prescribed estrogen for hormone replacement was Premarin. Pregnant horses, like many animals, excrete large amounts of conjugated estrogen compounds in their urine. Premarin is produced by extracting these estrogen products from their urine, purifying them, and manufacturing them into pills. (Thus the name is derived from *Pregnant Mares Urine)*. This type of hormone product is also referred to as a *conjugated equine estrogen,* or *CEE,* since the term *equine* means "horse-like." About half of the estrogen in Premarin is in the form of estrone, which is identical to the estrone circulating in women. The other half is composed of a dozen estrogens unique to horses. So while most of the estrogens in Premarin behave identically in the body as human estrogen, the unique horse products can act in slightly different ways. This likely accounts for one reason that

Premarin may show some unique benefits or side effects compared to pure estradiol or estrone.

Non-horse based estrogen formulations were subsequently formulated. Essentially all of these are derived from plants – primarily soy and yams. These plants contain steroid-like chemicals that can be modified in laboratories. The resulting products differ in the way they are chemically modified or formulated – primarily to render them in forms that can be orally absorbed. The most common product produced from plants is pure estradiol, labeled as 17beta-estradiol. It is available in a generic form (a common brand name is Estrace). Other products include an estrone drug called estropipate (brand names Ogen, Ortho-est), an esterified estrogen product (Menest), and a conjugated plant product (Cenestin). All of these products can produce comparable blood levels of estrogens although with slightly different ratios of estradiol to estrone. However, this is not that significant because the body converts one form to the other as needed, so they all produce comparable effects if given in appropriate doses.

Standard doses for these oral products have been determined – basically, doses that have been shown to control most women's hot flashes, and provide adequate doses to help women's bones from losing mass and prevent osteoporosis. The standard daily dose for the conjugated estrogen products is 0.625 mg. For estradiol, it is one mg. and for estrone, it is 0.75 mg. These strengths all provide essentially the same estrogen effects in the body and seem to work for the majority of women. However, some women require more or less and so the doses are adjusted up or down depending on a woman's response. To facilitate this, most of the products come in a number of strengths to enable a woman and her doctor to fine-tune the dose that works best for her.

Over the last ten years, we have also seen a plethora of novel, ultra-low-dose estrogen preparations come on the market. This has stemmed from the guidelines that came out after the Women's Health Initiative (WHI) study that recommended that women use the lowest dose of HRT for the shortest period of time to control symptoms. These low-dose estrogens are approved for the treatment of hot flashes. Some women find them effective, but others do not. In general terms, the lower the estrogen dose, the less effect it will have. Lower doses may carry less risk for an adverse effect but generally will not be as helpful in preventing hot flashes and bone thinning as much as the standard doses.[3] One question that comes up is whether these low-dose products can be taken without a progesterone-like drug if a woman has a uterus. Since they can stimulate the uterine lining to some degree, this would imply there could be an increased risk of uterine cancer if taken alone.[4]

The first-pass effect and ways around it

All of the oral products discussed above follow the same route – they are swallowed, dissolve in the stomach, and then enter the bloodstream. But the immediate next stop is the liver. This triggers a series of events that we refer to as *the first-pass effect.* It is beyond the scope of this book to explain this phenomenon in detail, but basically, orally administered drugs can be rapidly inactivated or converted into other forms by the liver. This usually necessitates giving higher doses of drugs than would be needed if they were administered directly into the bloodstream. The consequences of this pathway are that a number of chemical events occur. Proteins are produced that have various effects in the body – some beneficial, others detrimental.

One positive consequence of this first-pass effect is the production of more HDL cholesterol, which is our "good cholesterol." It is associated with a lower risk of heart disease. A negative consequence of the first-pass effect is that the liver makes proteins that promote blood coagulation, which increases the risk of blood clots. Other proteins that are stimulated by this phenomenon are ones that act as carriers for our hormones as they circulate in the bloodstream. High levels of these proteins bind hormones – rendering them inactive. This can also interfere with the ability to accurately measure their levels on blood tests.

To avoid these first-pass effects, estrogen would need to bypass the stomach and get directly into the circulatory system some other way. This can be accomplished through several means. In the past, estrogen was frequently given by an injection into a muscle. One advantage of this route is that the hormone is absorbed slowly over time, and need only be given every two to three weeks. However, since most people don't like shots, and they need to be administered by a health professional, this form of HRT is rarely used today.

The most convenient way to avoid the first-pass effect is to apply hormones onto the skin. When estrogen is applied topically in this manner it is absorbed by tiny vessels under the skin and enters directly into the blood circulation – much like the way the estrogen made by the ovaries is released into the bloodstream. Estrogen therapy placed on the skin is referred to as *transdermal administration.* There are a number of FDA approved transdermal estrogen products, all of which contain 17beta-estradiol. They are available in the form of patches, sprays, gels, and creams. The patches have become very popular. When they first came out they were the size of giant Band-Aids, but now they look like semi-transparent postage stamps. Products such as these include Vivelle, Climara, and Menostar, plus a number of generic patches. They come in variable strengths and are applied once or twice weekly. The dosing of these products can be confusing – since they are in different increments than the pills. Generally speaking, when we talk about dosing of an estradiol patch – the 0.05 mg patch is equivalent to one mg. of oral estradiol or 0.625 mg of Premarin. Topical forms of estradiol are also available in gels (such as EstroGel), and sprays (such as EvaMist). These products are usually applied on a daily basis.

There are also clinics whose providers insert estrogen pellets under the skin, which release estrogen slowly over time. These are not approved by the FDA. One concern about this form of administration is that once inserted, they can't readily be removed and can release estrogen for a prolonged time – sometimes up to several years.

Estrogen can also be administered *intravaginally* (via the vagina) where it seeps into the bloodstream through the vaginal wall. These products come in the form of creams or suppositories, which are inserted once or twice daily, or as rings impregnated with estrogen, which is slowly released over time. Some of these vaginal preparations provide estrogen levels comparable to oral forms; others are very low-dose products intended only to treat vaginal symptoms such as itching or dryness.

All of the transdermal, vaginal, and injectable estrogens avoid the first-pass effect. It has only been relatively recently that we are appreciating that the route of administration of a hormone can have an impact on the benefits and risks of therapy. Studies are indicating that transdermal estrogen may behave more like the natural estrogens that our body makes, which may make them less likely to cause adverse effects such as blood clots. This is primarily because they avoid the first-pass effects. Oral drugs, which necessitate the administration of higher doses, may increase the incidence of side effects, such as gallstones. The distinction between the different routes of estrogen therapy and health impacts will be addressed in the coming chapters. An awareness of this issue is important because it has a bearing on some of the discrepancies of outcomes in studies assessing the benefits and risks of HRT.

Comments on natural estrogens and bioidentical hormones

The term *natural estrogens* is often confusing. Technically this refers to those hormones produced naturally in our body, namely estradiol, estrone and the dozen other estrogen derivatives our ovaries and other cells make. Since there are no products with exactly all these ingredients, I often have an extended discussion with a patient who insists that she wants to only take natural estrogen. The conversation goes something like this. I explain:

"Well, there are no estrogen products derived from humans on the market – so your choices would be either natural estrogens from horses that we can collect through their urine, or estrogens derived from substances that occur naturally in plants, which have been chemically altered."

This usually elicits some disdain from my patient, as the idea of ingesting products from horses' urine is not appealing and taking synthetic estrogens produced in a lab doesn't seem to fit that "natural" definition. So, frequently the discussion leads to talking about *bioidentical hormones* – which is the term many women equate with natural hormones. However, this moniker is also somewhat misleading because there is no single "identical" estrogen product that contains all of our hormones (E1, E2, E3 and all of their conjugated versions).

I then explain what the generally accepted concept of bioidentical hormone treatment has come to mean. With respect to estrogen, it has come to mean a product that contains various amounts of estradiol, estrone, and sometimes estriol roughly in proportions that were present when we were in the prime of our lives, around age 35. Typically, practitioners who prescribe bioidentical therapy also dispense some progesterone and testosterone as well.

These bioidentical hormones are generally created by compounding pharmacies – which are pharmacies that specialize in formulating various preparations of medicine tailored to meet specific needs for unique situations. They utilize commercially produced generic hormone products, mix them in creams or gels, and dispense them in various proprietary applicators, which allow them to be applied to the skin, into the vagina, or onto the labia. Compounding pharmacies employ licensed pharmacists and require a prescription from a physician or other licensed provider to dispense their products.

Promoting and dispensing bioidentical hormones has become a huge business. As prescriptions written for conventional hormone therapy products plummeted after the WHI, the number of women who turned to bioidentical products soared.[5] It is estimated that nearly a third of hormone users in North America use these products – accounting for an estimated one to two million prescriptions per year.[6] Much of this is due to their supporters' claims, and users' beliefs, that these products are "natural" and therefore do not have the same risks as their commercial counterparts. Such claims are unfounded since these bioidentical products contain estrogen and behave just like all the estrogen products on the market.

Another reason that women mistakenly believe that bioidentical hormones are safer than commercial products is that compounding pharmacies are not required to provide the type of literature that comes with drugs dispensed by traditional pharmacies – those several pages of information that accompany every bottle of pills. In the case of estrogen products, like Premarin, there is an extensive list of risks and precautions, some items bolded with a black frame around them – the FDA's black box warnings designed to grab your attention. Professional societies dedicated to menopausal care are working to get the government to insist that compounded products carry the same labeling and patient education as the commercial preparations. However, despite intense efforts, they are not making much headway to get this problem corrected.

Many experts in the field, including board members of the North American Menopause Society, discourage the use of these compounded products and have many concerns regarding them. While there are many reputable and responsible compounding pharmacies, there are unscrupulous internet pharmacies that not only mislead women about the safety of bioidentical products but sell products of questionable purity. Some compounded formulations may contain unknown components, such as viruses, bacteria, or harmful contaminants. Unlike commercial pharmacies, which are under strict oversight by the FDA, compounding pharmacies are primarily regulated by state pharmacy boards where there can be minimal or inconsistent monitoring. This can lead to issues with quality control.

An issue that worries experts in menopause is that a bioidentical product may not contain the specified amounts of the hormones ordered in a prescription. For instance, if a woman is taking them with the intention to prevent osteoporosis, and they don't contain adequate amounts of estrogen, she may unknowingly not be getting protection. Of even greater concern is that if a woman still has her uterus, it is important that she gets adequate doses of progesterone to prevent uterine cancer. There have been case reports where women on compounded bioidentical hormone therapy developed uterine cancers believed to be due to an insufficient amount of progesterone in the preparations that they were taking.[7] Another reason bioidentical progesterone may be ineffective is that these formulations are frequently dispensed as topical gels or creams, and it has been shown that progesterone applied to the skin has unpredictable levels of absorption. This is a reason why many menopause experts discourage women from using this form of progesterone for hormone replacement.[8]

With all these choices, what is the best estrogen to take?

Women have different preferences and reasons why a particular alternative suits their needs. When deciding on the type of estrogen, there are many things a woman needs to consider. Should she take pure estradiol or the combination of hormones known as the conjugated estrogens? Are the ones that are produced synthetically from plants better than the ones derived from horses? Are the transdermal ones better than the oral ones? Is there ever a reason to choose something made by a compounding pharmacy?

Here are factors to take into consideration:

- Is your goal to use hormones solely to treat vaginal symptoms such as dryness? If so, opt for one of the very low-dose vaginal suppositories or creams designed specifically for that purpose.

- If your goal is to take adequate hormone doses to prevent osteoporosis or some of the other conditions associated with estrogen deficiency, then consider using the more standard oral or topical hormone preparations.

- Cost considerations – pills are generally the cheapest, but patches are becoming more affordable in generic forms.

- Tolerability issues – it is unusual, but sometimes oral products cause nausea, a side effect that would not likely occur with transdermal estrogen. On the other hand, some women find patches problematic. They may not stay affixed, or the adhesive in the patch can cause a rash or irritation. Creams and gels may also cause some skin reactions.

- Convenience and ease of use – some women prefer a daily pill; others find it easier to apply a weekly or twice-weekly patch.

- The source where the hormones come from can be an issue. The idea of using a drug derived from horses bothers some women, either based on concerns for animal rights or just on principle. Taking a product made from plants may be preferable for these patients. In addition, some women may have an allergic reaction to horse products.

- The pros and cons of the first-pass effect will help you determine whether an oral estrogen or transdermal estrogen is preferable. If raising your HDL is a priority, the oral forms may be more desirable. On the other hand, transdermal estrogen appears to carry a lower risk of blood clots and gallstones.

- Estrogen applied onto a woman's skin can rub off onto a child or pet coming into direct contact shortly after application. There have been rare instances where, after repeated contact, this caused abnormally high amounts of estrogen in a child.[9] This may be a concern for some women who care for infants.

- There are also decisions to make regarding the preferable oral agent if that is the route you choose. The products on the market can be composed of estradiol, estrone, or the conjugated equine estrogens which contain some estrogens unique to horses. As will be discussed in future chapters the subtle differences between these forms may lead to slightly different health impacts.

- If compounded bioidentical hormone therapy is chosen, there are issues regarding product quality and safety. There are over 50,000 compounding pharmacies. Choosing a reputable one is important, but can be difficult. Women need to rely on guidance from their providers and consider stores that have the best oversight, such as those certified by the independent Pharmacy Compounding Accreditation Board (PCAB). The Accreditation Commission for Health Care lists accredited compounding pharmacies on their website, www.achc.org.

What about progesterone?

Let's now turn to a discussion of the other significant female sex hormone, progesterone, sometimes referred to as **P4**. You may be interested to learn that all of our sex hormones are actually derived from the progesterone molecule. It is a crucial early component in the pathway where cholesterol is converted into other steroid hormones. During the reproductive years, the principal source of progesterone production is the corpus luteum, which is the tissue left over from the follicle after an egg is released. A primary function of progesterone is to stabilize the lining of the uterus to prepare it for implantation of the fertilized egg. If fertilization occurs, progesterone plays a vital role in maintaining a viable pregnancy.

In a typical menstrual cycle, the estrogen level rises and peaks mid-cycle and then declines. Progesterone appears mid-cycle and then remains elevated until menstruation occurs, then it decreases along with the estrogen. Progesterone affects body temperature, and this is the reason women can use a basal body temperature rise to time when they ovulate. At mid-cycle, the body temperature makes a slight upward spike of one-half degree Fahrenheit.

Once a woman's supply of eggs is depleted, there no longer is a major source of progesterone production – so after menopause, the level of progesterone declines substantially. Whereas the loss of estrogen is associated with a number of adverse events, we have long assumed that progesterone loss is not very significant. However, it has been demonstrated that there are progesterone receptors in many tissues including our breasts, bones, arteries, and nervous systems. This means that progesterone plays some role in each of these areas. How much of the postmenopausal changes that occur may be directly related to the loss of progesterone is unclear and it will be interesting to see what future research reveals.

The array of progestogen products

The term *progestogen* refers to all agents, natural or synthetic, that have progesterone-like properties. The name *progesterone* should only be used to designate the natural form of progesterone that the body produces. For years, progesterone was not available as an oral pill because it is not absorbed well through the stomach. So synthetic drugs, created to be easily absorbed, and which exert progesterone-like effects in the body, were developed. These are referred to as *progestins*. They are derived from the chemical conversion of progesterone-like compounds found in plants.

Progestins initially found their main use in birth control pills back in the 1960s and are still used in these products today. All of the combination oral contraceptive pills contain ethinyl estradiol and one of the many different types of progestins available – such as *norethindrone, levonorgestrel* or *desogestrel*. Since these different progestins have distinct chemical structures, they don't all act in identical ways in the body. Some can cause male-like side effects such as acne. Others have diuretic properties that make them act like mild water pills.

Up until the turn of the century the vast majority of women placed on HRT were given synthetic progestins. The drug Provera (*medroxyprogesterone)* has been the one most commonly prescribed in the U.S. and has been the progestogen used in most of the American studies assessing the benefits and risks of HRT, including the Women's Health Initiative Study. In Europe, other progestins have been favored, and so studies on HRT originating in these countries generally utilized drugs other than medroxyprogesterone. I mention this now because this difference in the progestogens used in studies may explain why there may be different outcomes in studies conducted in various parts of the world.

To render progesterone absorbable, the pharmacy industry came up with products that are micronized (broken down into tiny particles), which allows them to be dissolved in the stomach and then pass into the circulatory system. The first such product to appear in the U.S. was a drug called *Prometrium* which was approved for HRT treatment in the late 1990s. Widespread use was limited due to its expense, and even when generic natural progesterone became available many years later, the cost was prohibitive for many women. Fortunately, with time, it is becoming more affordable. As will be discussed in the coming chapters, research is indicating that in many respects natural progesterone may be the preferable choice of a progestogen for hormone replacement therapy.

It should be noted that commercially available progesterone capsules in the U.S. contain peanut oil, which is a clear contraindication for anyone with a peanut allergy. Other countries have begun using products using sunflower oil, but these have not yet been approved by the FDA.

Natural progesterone can also be inserted into the vagina in the form of creams and suppositories. This mode of treatment has been used commonly in Europe. In the U.S. there are commercial vaginal progesterone products being used to treat at-risk pregnancies, but these are not approved by the FDA for postmenopausal therapy. Vaginal progesterone products made by compounding pharmacies are frequently prescribed by naturopathic physicians as part of a bioidentical HRT regimen. This mode of administration is an option for some women but has obvious drawbacks – mainly the inconvenience of having to insert something in the vagina on a daily or sometimes twice daily basis. One advantage of intra-vaginal administration is that lower doses can be given. Since the primary purpose of the progestogen in hormone therapy is to protect against uterine cancer, intra-vaginal progesterone achieves this with lower doses because it is administered in close proximity to the uterus.

Topical progesterone preparations applied to the skin are also produced by compounding pharmacies and are used in some bioidentical hormone treatment regimens. There are no commercially available FDA approved progesterone creams for transdermal use (although there are two combination estrogen-progestin patches on the market). As discussed above, many experts are concerned about transdermal application of progesterone because there may be inconsistent absorption such that adequate levels may not be achieved to prevent uterine cancer.[10,11] Some prescribers advocate measuring progesterone levels in the blood. However, blood levels may not correlate well with the concentration of the progesterone at various tissue sites – which may lead to underdosing or overdosing.[12,13]

There are also IUDs (intrauterine devices) that contain a progestin. IUDs are small devices, generally made of plastic, that are inserted into the uterus that slowly release a small amount of progestogen continuously over a multi-year period. The advantage of an IUD is that it delivers a very low dose of the progestin and so very little ends up in the bloodstream, decreasing the chance of any adverse side effects. Currently, the hormone-containing IUDs, such as Mirena, are not approved for HRT treatment, but many gynecologists insert them for this purpose. There are some downsides to using an IUD, however. This includes discomfort on insertion and removal, occasionally persistent cramping, a slight predisposition to pelvic infections, and the rare risks of the device causing a uterine perforation.

The role of a progestogen in HRT

The main reason to take a progestogen for hormone replacement therapy is to counteract estrogen's effects on the uterus. How hormones affect the uterus will be presented in Chapter 9. However, whether a woman without a uterus should take a progestogen merits some discussion. Some naturopathic and longevity clinicians recommend that all women, regardless of their uterine status, take progesterone as part of their HRT regimen. They believe that it is an integral part of bioidentical hormone treatment and advise their patients that it is necessary to "balance" estrogen. This is a nebulous concept and not one that is recognized by most traditionally trained doctors as a clear medical rationalization for prescribing a progestogen. This is because it is unclear if the loss of progesterone at the time of menopause carries any negative effect, and we don't know if replacing it provides any unique benefit.

However, progesterone receptors are present in many parts of the body – probably everywhere you find the ubiquitous estrogen receptors. This implies progesterone performs some function in all of these areas – some we know much about, others we have much to learn about. This leads to the unanswered question of whether or not all women would benefit from replacing their progesterone after menopause. Would adding progesterone to estrogen replacement have benefits in other areas besides just the uterus?

One area where progesterone administration may positively contribute is bone health. Progesterone administered to animals has a beneficial effect on bone preservation.[14,15] Studies in humans have shown that women on estrogen plus a progestogen maintain better bone densities than women on estrogen alone.[16-20] Whether or not taking a progestogen alone helps prevent osteoporosis is unclear.

Progesterone receptors are present in the brain and there is considerable interest in understanding the function of progesterone in the nervous system. Research is revealing that it plays a more important role than we have appreciated in the past. Studies show that progesterone facilitates how brain cells interact with each other, decreases inflammation, and helps protect against nerve damage.[21] It also is involved in the brain pathways that deal with hot flashes and studies have shown that taking a progestogen can help relieve hot flashes.[22]

Progesterone appears to have mild sedative and possible anti-anxiety effects, and some studies have shown that it improves sleep.[22,23] There has been speculation that progesterone therapy may help some of the mood changes associated with the menopause transition. Support from this comes from studies using progesterone to help women suffering from PMS. One theory regarding the cause of this disorder is that these women have low progesterone levels – however, this hasn't been consistently demonstrated.[24]

We are a long way from understanding the many effects progesterone has on our various systems, much less how the different progestins may act. So, at this point, conventional medicine practice guidelines do not recommend that women who have had a hysterectomy take a progestogen. But much of this is based on the uncertainty of whether progestogen therapy causes adverse effects in postmenopausal women. It may come down to the particular progestogen taken.

Ways to take combined estrogen and progestogen

As noted, a woman who still has a uterus is advised to take a progestogen with her estrogen if she chooses HRT. Various regimens combining these two hormones can be used. Mimicking how our hormones fluctuated monthly during our reproductive years has seemed like a logical approach. This involves prescribing an estrogen every day, then adding the progestogen mid-cycle for ten to twelve days each month. We refer to this method as *cyclic hormone therapy*. By doing this, a woman can expect a monthly bleeding event similar to those she had during her reproductive years. I tell patients the hormones are causing a "fake" menstrual period.

Monthly withdrawal bleeding, as we call these fake periods, can continue for five to eight years on this regimen until the uterus ages to the point where it doesn't respond to hormones. The specter of having monthly periods for this long does not appeal to many women, understandably, because one of the benefits of menopause is not having to buy any more pads or tampons! Therefore another option of taking HRT that does not induce monthly bleeding became popular. This involves administering an estrogen along with a progestogen every day. Taking the hormones this way prevents uterine cancer but doesn't cause a monthly big buildup of the lining inside the uterus to create a monthly period. Initially, this regimen can cause some intermittent spotting, but that usually resolves within the first year of treatment.

A variety of combinations of the various available hormone preparations can be used in either of the regimens described above. Some type of estrogen is taken throughout the month. This can be in the form of a pill taken daily, an estrogen product applied to the skin, or an intra-vaginal preparation. Then, along with one of these forms of estrogen, some form of progestogen, either oral or vaginal, is taken daily. If a woman prefers the cyclic option, a higher dose of progestogen is added at the end of each month. Some providers advocate increasing the interval between progestogen administration to every two to three months instead of monthly. While this is likely sufficient to protect the uterus from cancer, there is a remote concern that less frequent administration is not as reliable as a monthly regimen.

While typically women are given prescriptions for both an estrogen product and a progestogen, there are several products that contain both hormones in a single pill. The drug Prempro contains Premarin and Provera in various strengths. There are several other preparations that contain estradiol and other progestins – such as Activella and Femhrt. These come in packets that look like birth control pills but are much lower in potency. Late in 2019 the FDA approved Bijuva a medication that contains estradiol (one mg) and natural progesterone (100 mg) as a single capsule to be taken once daily. While it may be convenient to take both of these hormones in one pill, it is six times more expensive than taking each component individually (approximately $200.00 per month compared to $35.00 per month).

There are two combination patch products that contain estradiol and a synthetic progestogen. As mentioned, topical progesterone appears to have unreliable absorption, but these synthetic progestogen patches have received FDA approval. In my experience, they have not been commonly used, either due to cost, or because they caused frequent episodes of vaginal bleeding or spotting.

Finally, the other regimen some women choose is to take some form of estrogen along with a progestogen-containing IUD (such as the Mirena IUD). As noted, these IUDs are not currently approved for HRT, but many reputable clinicians attest to their reliability and safety.

Do progestogens affect the risks and benefits of HRT?

Because the focus on prescribing a progestogen was primarily to make sure women did not get uterine cancer, there has been a tacit assumption that it is otherwise a fairly innocuous intervention. Perhaps this is why, for many years, in doing studies assessing the benefits and risks of HRT, we have been guilty of lumping all forms of hormone replacement therapy together. In many large observational studies women were simply asked if they were using HRT, not clearly differentiating the type and mode of hormone treatment they were taking, or even indicating whether or not they were taking a progestogen along with an estrogen. This has led to much uncertainty about the outcomes of these studies because now we can't be sure which, if any, of the hormones the women were taking may have played a role in any of the beneficial or negative events noted.

In addition, we tended to assume that all progestogens behaved the same way in the body. Only fairly recently have we been paying attention to the fact that this is not the case. When scientists first designed synthetic progestogens, the goal was to find drugs that would be readily absorbed orally and that would interact with the progesterone receptors in the uterus – just like natural progesterone. So, all progestins have the same effect in the uterus. That has been the hallmark of any drug being able to call itself a progestogen. However, it turns out that while a particular progestin may cause effects identical to natural progesterone in some tissues, it may have a different effect in other areas. This is because synthetic progestins are all structurally different. Some share overlapping features with other steroid hormones and can interact with receptors other than progesterone receptors. For instance, some progestins can fit into a testosterone receptor and cause some male-like side effects such as hair growth or acne.

A poorly appreciated finding of the WHI studies is that women who were given both estrogen and a synthetic progestin had higher rates of breast cancer than women on estrogen alone. Similar outcomes have been shown in other studies.[25] In addition, it appears that synthetic progestins have a bearing on how HRT affects the cardiovascular system. Unlike natural progesterone, the synthetic progestins may attenuate estrogen's beneficial effect on cholesterol as well as how it interacts with the lining of the arteries.[26,27,28] In later chapters, I will be going into greater detail on what we are learning about how synthetic progestins may be behind some of the undesirable effects that have been reported in women on hormone replacement.

The take-home message, and one that will be emphasized in the coming chapters, is that the type of progestogen administered clearly has an impact on the overall risks of taking HRT. Natural progesterone appears to be the safest choice but many more large-scale studies are needed to assess how it affects each and all of our body systems when given as part of an HRT regimen.

Other drugs used in menopause treatment

I am including a discussion of other drugs used to treat menopausal symptoms and conditions because it is important for women to be aware of alternatives that are frequently recommended and how they compare to HRT. All too often I have come across a patient whose doctor discouraged her from taking estrogen, and recommended some other drug, but didn't fully inform her of the risks and benefits of the alternative. When women are considering HRT, this type of information should be part of their decision-making process.

SERMs – What they are and what they do

You may have heard of *SERMs* – but what the heck are they? SERM stands for *selective estrogen receptor modulator*. These are not estrogens. They are drugs that have been fabricated to either behave in the body like estrogen or, conversely, to block estrogen from acting. We describe the latter property as having *anti-estrogen* effects.

Estrogen, as well as progesterone and testosterone, are made from the basic steroid building block cholesterol. SERMs have an entirely different molecular skeleton than a steroid. However, they have enough similarities that portions of them can hook onto an estrogen receptor and trigger an action. For instance, a SERM may attach to bone cells and prevent bone breakdown, like natural estrogen. Or conversely, SERMs have been designed to attach to breast cells and prevent the body's natural estrogen from attaching. In this way, they would negate any estrogen-induced stimulation that would promote cell growth. This is an example of an anti-estrogen effect.

Each SERM has unique properties that cause it to act in different ways at the various estrogen receptor sites. The ideal SERM would be one that promotes all of the positive effects of estrogen, but none of the negative effects. Unfortunately, the perfect SERM hasn't yet been developed. While all of the current SERMs on the market help prevent osteoporosis, two undesirable properties common to them are that they can increase the chance of a blood clot and, rather than relieve hot flashes, they can make them worse!

The first SERM widely used was tamoxifen. It was designed and continues to be a treatment for breast cancer as it strongly blocks estrogen stimulation in breast tissue. You may have heard the terms *ER (estrogen receptor) positive* or *ER (estrogen receptor) negative* in breast cancer discussions. This is because some breast cancers possess intact estrogen receptors and some do not. Those cancers that are ER-positive tend to grow faster when estrogen is present. So, a SERM that blocks estrogen would help prevent this form of cancer from growing. Estrogen receptor negative cancers aren't helped with SERM treatment. (Interestingly, even though ER-negative cancers are not stimulated by estrogen, they generally are much more aggressive and carry a worse prognosis.)

One positive estrogen-like attribute of tamoxifen is that it decreases bone turnover and helps prevent osteoporosis. However, it can stimulate the build-up of the uterine lining which increases the risk of uterine cancer. Prolonged use of tamoxifen has also been found to slightly increase the risk of another type of cancer called a sarcoma. Because of these concerns, the duration of tamoxifen treatment is generally a maximum of five years.

Raloxifene, or Evista, was the next SERM to become popular and it was designed primarily to have estrogen-like effects on our bones and was introduced as another option to prevent osteoporosis. It is approved and effective for this use, but it is not as effective as estrogen. Raloxifene does not increase the risk of uterine cancer and actually has been shown to help prevent breast cancer. While these benefits are appealing, many women, especially as they first enter menopause, find that it causes major worsening of their hot flashes.

Both of these SERMs, like estrogen, appear to have positive effects on a woman's cholesterol, heart, and blood vessels and may help prevent cardiovascular disease. But they increase the risk of blood clots, and a frequent side effect is leg cramps. They also do not have estrogen's positive impact on vaginal discomfort and dryness, and some women experience more vaginal discharge while on tamoxifen.

Bazedoxifene is another SERM that is being used in Mexico and a number of other foreign countries for either the prevention or treatment of osteoporosis. It is not approved in the U.S. as a single agent but has recently been approved in a combination product with estrogen to treat hot flashes. The brand name of this combination drug is Duavee. This type of compound is being referred to as a *tissue-selective estrogen complex.* The estrogen component leads to beneficial effects on the bones and vaginal tissue, plus it helps relieve hot flashes. The SERM portion acts as an anti-estrogen to negate the adverse effects of estrogen on the uterus and thus prevents uterine cancer. It appears to have a favorable effect on the cholesterol pattern.[29] The risk of blood clots is increased. It is unknown how Duavee affects the risk of breast cancer and, because it is relatively new, we really don't know about other long-term risks and benefits.

A fairly new SERM that appeared on the market around 2014 is Osphena or ospemifene. This agent has very weak estrogen-like effects. This SERM is approved only for treating menopausal vaginal symptoms, such as thinning and dryness. The labeling on the patient inserts reads that it *"should be used for the shortest duration possible consistent with treatment goals and risks for the individual woman."* I find this a little peculiar since the changes women experience in the vaginal area after menopause get progressively worse over time and by stopping therapy women will be right back where they started with a recurrence of their vaginal thinning. The caution regarding judicious use of this drug comes from studies that indicate it may increase the risk of stroke, and it can stimulate the lining of the uterus to a small degree, which could potentially increase the risk of uterine cancer. Women with a history of breast cancer are not advised to take this SERM. It may have some minor benefit in preventing bone loss.[30] Women taking it can get worsening of their hot flashes.[31] Like all SERMs, there is a potential increased risk of blood clots, but there is little data on this so far.[32]

SERMs may very well be one answer to treating some of the negative consequences of menopause and many clinicians are excited about them as an alternative to hormones. However, a SERM that not only treats hot flashes but has positive estrogen-like effects on the bones, vagina, and heart – without increasing the risk of blood clots, strokes, or cancer – has not yet been created. Huge amounts of money are being poured into the search for this miracle drug. One concern that arises in my mind, however, is that we are manipulating chemicals that are being designed to target estrogen receptors in parts of the body we know about. However, since there are thousands of estrogen receptors throughout the body, it is conceivable a new SERM may have some action in some receptor in some area that we didn't anticipate. If this causes a negative effect it may not be immediately obvious and may take years to become apparent.

The bottom line is that SERMs can confer many benefits, but also carry risks. Whether a SERM provides more benefits than risks than estrogen may vary from woman to woman depending on her underlying unique health situation. A woman at high risk for osteoporosis with strong risk factors for breast cancer would likely benefit more from a SERM such as Raloxifene than she would from taking hormones. However, for a woman with terrible hot flashes and a past history of blood clots, a transdermal estrogen would probably be a better choice. The decision to use HRT versus a SERM is complex and many factors need to be considered.

Drugs that may be confused with SERMs

Before leaving this section, a few comments on other drugs that may be confused with SERMs would be appropriate. Even after menopause, there is a small amount of estrogen circulating in our body – most of which comes from the transformation of male hormones made in the adrenal glands. Women who have been diagnosed with estrogen receptor-positive breast cancer benefit from drugs that can suppress the effects of this residual estrogen. You may have heard of the anti-estrogen drugs called *aromatase inhibitors* (Arimidex, Femara, and Aromasin) which are used for breast cancer treatment. These aromatase inhibitors block the conversion of male hormones into estrogen and substantially decrease the level of estrogen in the circulation. In addition, there is a relatively new class of drugs called SERDs, which are *selective estrogen receptor down-regulators*. These drugs have strong anti-estrogen effects and are being studied for breast cancer treatment. They do not play a role in menopausal hormone replacement therapy.

Another drug worth mentioning is tibolone. This drug is not available in the U.S. as of 2019 but may be approved by the FDA in the future. It is a unique synthetic steroid that has estrogen-like, progesterone-like, and testosterone-like properties. It appears to help hot flashes, although it is not as effective as estrogen. It helps protect against bone loss. It does not appear to have negative effects on the heart. And, because of the testosterone-like effects, it may have some slight benefit on sexual function and libido. A large review of many studies of this drug was published in 2016. The authors concluded that the risk of developing uterine cancer, breast cancer, or a stroke from taking tibolone would be minimal – comparable to that from taking estrogen products.[33] If tibolone does appear on the market, women should have extended discussions with their health care providers to review the benefit/risk ratio of taking this new type of drug and obtain a clear understanding of how this product compares to estrogen treatment.

Phytoestrogens and other estrogen-like products

Many women who are worried that taking estrogen is harmful have turned to phytoestrogens as an alternative to commercial hormone drugs. These products have been touted as beneficial for menopausal symptoms without any risks. Phytoestrogens really aren't estrogens because they don't come from the same molecular family as the rest of the body's sex hormones. They are compounds that occur naturally in many plants, fruits, and vegetables and have mild estrogen-like properties. One category of phytoestrogens known as *lignans* is found in flaxseed, lentils, grains, and in vegetables like kale, cabbage, and Brussels sprouts. The other major group is the *isoflavones* which are derived primarily from soybeans as well as chickpeas, lentils, and red clover. In fact, one of the first observations that these plants had estrogen effects came from farmers back in the 1940s who noticed that their sheep that grazed on fields of red clover had disorders in their reproductive systems.[34]

45

Phytoestrogens can connect to estrogen receptors and can cause some estrogen effects, but also can act like SERMs and cause anti-estrogen effects. They have been promoted to improve hot flashes and some women swear they do. However, studies have not shown that they are clearly better than a placebo.[35] It has also been controversial whether phytoestrogens help prevent bone loss as studies have shown conflicting results.[36,37]

Conceivably phytoestrogens could promote the growth of breast cancers, but because they are quite weak in their estrogen effects, this would not be expected to be very significant. However, because of the unknowns and uncertainty of how these agents work, some experts caution women with breast cancer to limit their consumption.

The other products that have estrogen-like effects attributed to them belong to a diverse group of chemicals sometimes referred to as "estrogenics." These include synthetic compounds such as BPA (bisphenol A), BPS (bisphenol S), phthalates and a dozen other products involved in manufacturing. They can also be found in consumer products – particularly in plastics, but also in herbicides, soaps, sunscreens, dyes, and cosmetics. These chemicals receive much media attention (leading to actions such as banning BPA in infants' bottles) because of concerns they are accumulating in our environment and causing adverse health effects. These agents can interact with both estrogen and testosterone receptors and trigger some hormone effects. They have been implicated as adversely affecting sexual organ development in humans and other animals, and decreasing sperm levels in men. There is heated controversy about the significance of the degree of risk from these agents and what to do about them. While research does attest to many of the adverse effects – most of which is documented in animals exposed to high doses – it is unclear if the actual amounts humans come in contact with pose as much hazard as claimed.

Unfortunately, because these chemicals have something to do with estrogen pathways, these discussions have generated negative attention on all estrogens in general. It is important to understand the differences between these "estrogenic" compounds and natural estrogens. While they may interact with estrogen receptors in the way SERMs do, their chemical structure differs substantially from estrogen. Their predominant action appears to be mainly due to their interaction with male hormone receptors, and through this and other mechanisms may decrease the amount of testosterone available for its biologic effects. For all of these reasons, these agents should not be regarded as estrogens, but rather as "hormone disrupters."

Testosterone and other male hormones

This brings us to a discussion of the third major category of sex hormones, which are androgens – the term encompassing all of the male hormones. Like estrogens, androgens are normally present in both sexes. When you hear the words "testosterone treatment" you may immediately visualize an athlete with bulky muscles, who likely has been using these agents illicitly. Male hormones clearly increase muscular growth and strength and so have been coveted by many a bodybuilder. Testosterone and its chemical cousins are the drivers of male sexual development and function – so we tend to think of them as not being that important in women's health. However, they play an essential role in many areas in a woman's body – including maintaining normal ovarian function, bone metabolism, cognition, and sexual function. Of course, women have much lower levels of male hormones than men do.

You may be surprised to learn that all of our estrogen is actually made from the conversion of the same male hormone that makes testosterone – and that this occurs inside the ovaries! The amount of testosterone in our bodies varies depending upon our stage in life. Like estrogen, the testosterone level in little girls is quite low, but its production ramps up along with our other hormones as we enter puberty (thus accounting for some of the undesirable attributes such as acne and oily skin). Then, throughout our reproductive years, the level of testosterone fluctuates up and down during the menstrual cycle, peaking mid-month when we ovulate. (That makes sense, doesn't it?)

Many women may be surprised to learn that their testosterone levels peak in their mid-thirties and then start declining gradually. By the time they reach menopause, their testosterone levels are already quite low and don't change much after that for the rest of their lives. However, at the time of menopause, when estrogen levels drop, the testosterone present in the body is able to exert more pronounced male-like effects. This includes some physical changes such as the appearance of facial hair but also can affect the way sugar and fat are metabolized by postmenopausal women. These changes, which increase the risk of heart disease and diabetes, are discussed in later chapters.

As you likely know, men don't go through menopause. Their hormone levels decline gradually with age but don't drop dramatically like ours. However, some men truly do develop abrupt testosterone deficiency due to surgery or a disease involving the testicles (a common one in days past was mumps). If this occurs these men are confronted with hot flashes, muscle weakness, and impotence, among other things. Not surprisingly, most men opt for testosterone replacement in these circumstances. Treatment is accomplished either by administering a testosterone shot every two to three weeks, or via gels applied to the skin daily. The doses recommended involve a fairly liberal amount of gel that needs to be applied. These products have warnings with them that caution men not to come into close contact (such as skin-to-skin) with their partners or children shortly after application – because they could be exposed to the male hormone inadvertently. (I actually thought this warning was a little overkill until I had a patient with unexplained hair growth and high testosterone levels – that eventually we traced to the topical testosterone product being used by her newlywed husband!)

The big question women have is whether testosterone replacement should be something postmenopausal women should consider. Many naturopathic and longevity clinics strongly endorse this. Unfortunately, there is a paucity of research in this area, and the traditional medical community tends to feel it is not necessary and possibly associated with potential adverse effects, such as cardiovascular complications. In addition, while testosterone is beneficial for the bones, other treatments (including estrogen) are available. The one area where testosterone may have a unique indication would be its benefit in improving libido, an interest in having sex. I discuss the subject of testosterone treatment for menopause in Chapter 16.

Besides testosterone, the other major androgens circulating in women, in descending order of serum concentration, are *dehydroepiandrosterone sulfate* (DHEAS), *dehydroepiandrosterone* (DHEA), *androstenedione*, and *dihydrotestosterone* (DHT). The adrenal glands and the ovaries are the main sites of production of these hormones. The levels of DHEA and DHEAS also peak in our mid-30s and decline gradually with age so that by age 70 to 80 the levels are about 20% of their previous highs. DHEA is converted into testosterone and estrogen in the body. DHEAS is DHEA that has a sulfur compound attached to it and this prevents the DHEA from being broken down too quickly.

DHEA is available over the counter in pills ranging from 10 to 50 mg. They are sold and labeled as a dietary supplement so there is little regulatory oversight by the FDA. Therefore, the quality, purity, and strength of each pill cannot be assumed to be reliable. DHEA supplementation has been touted to increase energy and improve women's sexual function and interest. Some studies support this, but a large review published in 2014 found no benefit of oral DHEA in postmenopausal women with normal adrenal function.[38] The role of DHEA in menopause treatment is discussed in more detail in Chapter 16.

Decision Making Helper

Key Considerations

The two major estrogens produced in women are estradiol and estrone, and the body converts these back and forth into each other. Commercial products containing these estrogens are available. Estradiol is available as an oral pill, injectable shot, topical patch, gel, spray, and in intra-vaginal forms. Estradiol administered on the skin, through the vagina, or into the muscle gets into the circulation directly, and most closely approximates how estradiol produced in the ovary behaves. Estradiol in these forms may be preferable to oral estradiol because oral estradiol triggers reactions in the liver that may cause negative effects.

Other drugs are used in menopause management. They have many of the same actions as estradiol, but can also have other effects. They all have their unique attributes which are summarized below. Additional detail on the role these drugs play in menopausal management will appear in later chapters.

- Premarin contains estrone plus some estrogens unique to horses. Premarin improves the cholesterol more than transdermal estradiol. Premarin may be less likely to cause breast cancer than estradiol.

- SERMs have estrogen-like effects, but also some anti-estrogen effects. They help prevent bone loss and some SERMs decrease the risk of breast cancer and improve menopausal vaginal thinning. They do not improve hot flashes. All of them increase the risk of blood clots. Some SERMs can increase the risk of uterine cancer.

- Phytoestrogens are substances in plants that have weak estrogen-like effects and are not really estrogens. They also can cause anti-estrogen effects. They are not generally effective for hot flashes, although some women find them helpful. They are not very effective in preventing osteoporosis.

- Progestogens are used in combination with an estrogen in women who have a uterus. Taking a progestogen is not felt to be necessary if a woman has had a hysterectomy. Progestogens may decrease some of the beneficial effects of estrogen. Synthetic progestogens may cause more negative effects than natural progesterone and may contribute to a higher risk of breast cancer, and may have a negative effect on the cardiovascular system. Natural oral or vaginal progesterone appears to be the preferred choice in HRT. Currently, all U.S. oral preparations of progesterone contain peanut oil which must be avoided by women allergic to peanuts. Progesterone cream applied to the skin may be absorbed inconsistently and is discouraged by most experts. Taking a progestogen alone without estrogen is not encouraged for HRT – but studies are limited. Progesterone may help hot flashes, stabilize mood, and prevent bone loss to a degree.

- Bioidentical compounded hormone preparations prepared by compounding pharmacies are made from commercial generic estrogen and progesterone products, typically derived from plant sources. They, therefore, will have all of the properties as the commercial products. Since compounded drugs are not closely regulated by the FDA, many experts have concerns about how reliable these products are with respect to their dosage levels and purity.

- Testosterone at low doses may help libido but may cause adverse effects such as acne and male-like hair growth. There are no commercially available topical testosterone products approved for women in the U.S. Compounding pharmacies formulate topical testosterone in low doses designed for menopausal women but many experts are concerned about the reliability of these products.

In deciding on drug therapy to treat symptoms and conditions associated with menopause, women should be aware of the various hormone preparations available and differences in how they behave in the body. Any decision to use non-hormone treatments should also involve consideration of the benefits and risks of these alternatives.

Current guidelines regarding hormone replacement therapy

Since the 2002 publication of the WHI study, most doctors have followed the guidelines generated from its findings. So as of 2019, most doctors recommend that women use the lowest dose of HRT for the shortest period of time to control symptoms. The guidelines do not specifically recommend one form of estrogen or progestogen over another. Many guidelines encourage providers to treat women with non-hormone preparations before resorting to hormones. When initiating HRT it has been recommended that health care providers initially prescribe a low dose, increase the dose as needed, periodically monitor response to treatment, and then discontinue hormones when symptoms abate. Current guidelines do not recommend male hormones for menopausal treatment.

For women complaining only of vaginal symptoms such as dryness, topical lubricants, such as Replens, are recommended, and then if further therapy is needed, low-dose vaginally-applied estrogens are considered the first-line treatment. The oral SERM Osphena has also been approved for this indication. A new DHEA product, prasterone, has also been approved to treat vaginal symptoms.

What the guidelines don't acknowledge

Many menopause experts disagree with using the lowest dose of hormones for the shortest period of time and recommend that women use doses effective to control symptoms, and for the duration needed consistent with their treatment goals. This is based on abundant data that indicates the benefits of HRT outweigh the risks for most women who initiate HRT before the age of 60.

The risk and benefits of HRT may not only depend on the age of initiation but on the type and mode of hormone therapy. Evidence is accumulating that indicates that transdermal estrogen and natural progesterone may be much less likely to cause adverse effects than oral estrogen preparations and synthetic progestogens when used in HRT regimens.

Chapter 4
Medical Studies 101

Understanding the way studies are done and interpreted will better help you appreciate the current controversies in menopausal treatment. It is incredible how much knowledge we have accumulated about our world since ancient times. Scientists are forever making observations, posing questions, and then attempting to prove or disprove theories ranging from how gravity works to why bugs become resistant to antibiotics. Studies are conducted and their findings are presented. The results are then reviewed by other experts in the field. The conclusions may be criticized, applauded, or even rejected due to apparent flaws in the study (or worse – deliberate dishonesty for financial gain!). Further studies are done to test the findings. If enough data is generated to pass certain mathematical tests, it is considered reliable scientific evidence. In the medical field, this translates to treatment recommendations and health care guidelines.

Not uncommonly two studies on the same subject may reach different conclusions. Why does this occur? The answer can usually be found by carefully analyzing the studies and discovering that they varied in their design. The specific characteristics of the patients in the study can make a difference in the outcomes. For instance, one study may involve patients within a wide age range, whereas another may not include anyone over age 65. One study may exclude patients who have a particular diagnosis, such as diabetes; another may include such patients. One study may have spanned over ten years, and another just five years. So while the results of one study may apply to its given population over a given time frame, a comparable study involving a different set of participants or parameters may come up with different conclusions.

To illustrate this, an article appeared recently in our local Sunday paper with the headline "*Calcium and Vitamin D Do Not Prevent Fractures.*" Many readers might simply note the headline and assume this applies to everybody and throw out their bottles of vitamin D. But if you read the details of the study, it involved a group of generally healthy older adults in China who were living independently. This is a fairly limited population whose culture, lifestyle, diet, and genetic makeup are quite unique. So you should not generalize the findings and assume they would apply to other populations, such as a group of nursing home patients living in Norway. Because the latter group would be more frail and inactive and receive much less exposure to sunshine, they would be at a higher risk of osteoporosis. A comparable study on them would likely reveal that the addition of vitamin D to their diets would make a difference in decreasing the risk of a fracture.

Other factors in the way studies are designed need to be scrutinized – such as how data was collected. For instance, in studying how hormones affect blood pressure, one study may have relied on a patient's self-reporting of the readings whereas another study may have required the patient to come into the clinic to be tested. The latter method would tend to give more reliable readings. Another factor to look at when comparing studies is to note the specific types of treatment given. This is an issue that has clouded our understanding of the benefits and risks of hormone replacement therapy. Many early studies that set out to determine if HRT caused any adverse effects simply asked women if they took menopausal hormones. Since there are different regimens and types of estrogens and progestogens, lumping them all together and concluding that women on HRT had higher risks of a particular problem may have led to misleading results.

To help reconcile the differences between a large number of studies on the same issue, researchers perform a process called a meta-analysis. This type of study pools the results of multiple studies. It attempts to make an overall assessment of whether there are more positive findings or more negative findings regarding a particular treatment, or whether there is no significant difference. Theoretically, by summarizing numerous studies involving thousands of people, bias is reduced – studies that deviate one way or the other would tend to cancel each other out. So, the conclusions of this type of study are very helpful in assessing whether a treatment carries more benefits than risks. Throughout this book I reference a number of meta-analyses that address various aspects of hormone use.

New research findings are frequently presented at medical conferences, and a press release to the media may ensue – sometimes before the study appears in medical journals. I can't tell you how many times a patient would see me for a routine appointment, morning newspaper in hand, and ask me about some new headline, such as *"Caffeine Causes Cancer"* or *"Autism Linked to Childhood Vaccines."* Or, in the case of hormone replacement therapy, *"New Study Shows Doctors Have Been Harming Patients Prescribing HRT."* I would often be in the frustrating position of informing a patient that I hadn't read the details of the study – and couldn't really weigh in on it. I also would try to diplomatically let him or her know that I usually don't rely on the daily news for my continuing medical education! Too often articles in the press are incomplete and misleading and may even reflect some bias.

Even when the full article is available in a professional journal, to fully digest the contents can be time-consuming. Busy doctors frequently just manage to read an abstract or the concluding paragraph. They may not be able to assess the many factors that need to be considered in deciding the merits of the study. What exactly was the goal of the study? Who performed it? How many patients were enrolled? How long were they followed? And probably most important of all: what type of study was performed? This makes a difference as to how reliable the results may be. I hope you continue to read this chapter as I would like to spend a little time discussing this subject. Understanding the way studies are done and interpreted will better help you appreciate the current controversies in menopausal treatment.

Types of studies

There are many types of studies. They range from simple case reports, which describe an unusual finding or rare disease, to studies that mine massive amounts of information from huge databases. Collectively the knowledge from these efforts furthers our understanding of diseases and best treatments.

A tremendous amount of medical knowledge comes from basic research in the lab. These studies use microbiological and biochemical techniques. An example of this would be the development of a new antibiotic and placing it on a culture plate covered with bacteria to see if it is effective in killing the organisms. This was how the great scientist Dr. Alexander Fleming accidentally discovered penicillin in 1928. Rumor has it that he did not keep his lab meticulously clean. Apparently, some mold spores came in through a window landing on one of his petri dishes growing bacteria. To his surprise, this produced a liquid that killed the bacteria. This substance, which he originally dubbed "mould juice," was isolated and purified. Years later he received the Noble Prize for discovering the antibiotic that has saved millions of lives.

A great deal of what we are learning about menopause treatment involves research in the lab. Scientists have been able to identify the biochemical reactions that control many of the processes in our body where our hormones play a role. For instance, they have discovered precisely how estrogen keeps our bone remodeling cells in balance to prevent osteoporosis. Similarly, there has been much research into how estrogen interacts with the cells lining our blood vessels to help retard the buildup of plaque.

An area where we are gaining a great deal of knowledge about how our hormones work comes from the development of SERMs. By analyzing estrogen receptors and then developing drugs that interact with them, we are learning how estrogen causes changes in the chemical processes in the body's cells.

There also are many studies using animals and, as much as we don't like to think about this type of research, without it we wouldn't be where we are today – not only in understanding biological functions but in finding life-saving drugs and treatments. Usually, rats and mice are the initial subjects and rodents have been used in many experiments regarding hormone treatment. Removing an animal's ovaries induces menopause. Scientists assess how these animals age compared to their cage mates that didn't have the surgery, and evaluate how each group responds to hormone replacement. More detail on some of this research will be presented in the chapters discussing the effects of hormones on our various bodily systems.

Basic research gives much valuable information, but as far as arriving at optimal treatment recommendations for humans, studies must be done on real people. Besides the meta-analyses mentioned above, there are two major types of studies done in medicine to evaluate a medical intervention or treatment. One type is referred to as an *observational study* and the other is an experimental or *clinical* trial. It is extremely important to recognize the difference between these two basic types of studies.

Observational studies – retrospective and prospective

Observational studies are studies where researchers observe and gather data on some phenomena but don't intervene or change anything in the patients' lives. This can either be done retrospectively (studying events that have already occurred) or prospectively (gathering data going forward).

One type of a retrospective study would be one where researchers comb through databases and assess how many patients taking a certain medication had a particular disease. An example of this was a study that was published a few years ago that concluded that drugs commonly prescribed for heartburn, such as Nexium or Prilosec, caused osteoporosis. This was alarming news and a number of my patients independently quit their drugs when they read this in the newspaper. They told me that did not want to take something that would damage their bones. However, we later learned that this study misled us because, like all observational studies, this only showed there was an association between osteoporosis and these drugs – not cause and effect. It turned out that, because these drugs suppress acid and because acid is needed to absorb calcium and vitamin D, taking acid-suppressing drugs led to low calcium and vitamin D levels which increase the chance of osteoporosis.[1] Administering extra doses of these supplements would have overcome the problem.

Although studies of this nature need to be interpreted with caution, they do give us valuable information. There have been many retrospective studies dealing with menopause and hormone issues. Studying women who have had their ovaries removed prior to natural menopause has been revealing. Over the years it has been noted that these women appeared to have higher risk of several problems and this has prompted further study. For instance, it was suspected that premature menopause increased the risk of developing diabetes. To assess this, researchers have searched through institutional databases and compiled a list of women with a diagnosis of diabetes. Of these, they tabulated how many had had ovarian surgery. They then assessed whether there were more cases of diabetes in the surgical group compared to the women who retained their ovaries. Finding that this was the case has led to an awareness that estrogen plays a role in preventing diabetes.

A *prospective* observational study is where researchers recruit women for a study and record a number of characteristics such as their ages, weights, medications, smoking history, exercise, etc. The women are then followed over time, and information about health outcomes is compiled to determine if there are any correlations. This particular type of study, where a group of individuals who share certain characteristics is followed over time, is also referred to as a *cohort* study.

An example of this type of study is one known as the Nurses Study, which will be referred to at various points in this book. In this study, thousands of nurses were followed over two decades tracking their hormone use and medical status. One of the findings that resulted from this study was that women who used HRT had a 50% reduction in heart attacks compared to women who had not taken hormones. When this study was published in the 1990s it was reassuring to those of us who had been prescribing hormones for our patients. However, we had to keep in mind that this was an observational study – so there was always the background awareness that the results should be interpreted with a degree of caution. This is because observational studies cannot control what is called *confounding factors* – meaning unknown factors that could have affected the results. In the Nurses Study, it is possible that there was something about nurses' lifestyles that affected the results. Perhaps their diets were healthier making them less prone to heart disease than women in other occupations.

Observational studies, both retrospective and prospective, have been extremely important in shaping medical care. They have aided us in advising patients on healthy choices and have been the springboard for more advanced investigations. However, because of the issues I have presented, they are not considered as definitive as the other major category of studies, known as *clinical trials*.

Clinical trials

In this type of study, patients are enrolled, some treatment is given, and the participants are followed over time to study the effects of the treatment. This is in contrast to observational studies, which don't involve administering any kind of treatment. The goal of a clinical trial is to eliminate confounding factors that may affect the credibility of the results.

The most rigorous type of study in this category is a *randomized, controlled, double-blind study*. In this type of study, volunteers are recruited and randomly assigned to be in one or more treatment groups, or in a placebo group. A placebo is basically a sugar pill or a "sham" procedure. In these clinical trials, neither the patient nor the researcher knows whether the actual treatment or placebo is being administered. (This is where the term *blind* fits in.) Both groups are followed over a period of time and the outcomes in each group, good and bad, are tabulated and analyzed.

It is important to have a placebo group because it has been shown that a large percentage of people (20% to 60% or more depending on the treatment or condition) actually respond to a placebo. In order to demonstrate that an intervention is effective, it must demonstrate results that are beyond any achieved by a placebo. The other value of having a placebo group is that it helps clarify whether side effects that occur are due to the treatment or just by chance. If participants in the placebo group share the same percentage of any given side effect, such as dizziness or cold symptoms, you can generally assume that the issue wasn't due to the treatment.

A critical feature of a clinical trial is that each group has comparable numbers of patients with like characteristics such as gender, age, weight, smoking status, and pertinent medical conditions. In this way, the groups are as similar as possible so that the only difference between them is the intervention being studied. This type of study is considered the most reliable way to determine the efficacy of a given treatment and tends to become the gold standard for guiding patient care. When a large-scale clinical trial is performed, its results carry much more weight in making health policy than observational studies.[2] The Women's Health Initiative Study (WHI) is an example of such a randomized, double-blind study. So, as you will see throughout this book, the WHI has left an indelible mark on menopause management.

Clinical studies are difficult to perform since a great deal of effort needs to go into the design, recruitment, data collection, and the final evaluation of the results. They require a considerable amount of funding. Some analysts estimate a good study can cost up to $35,000 per enrollee.[3] The WHI study, one of the most expensive studies ever funded by the National Institute of Health, cost about 260 million dollars.[4] That was in "1990 dollars" and you can expect it would cost way more today.

While the randomized clinical trials are the gold standard, it is important that their conclusions are accurately applied. One error that can occur is studying a limited group of individuals and then generalizing conclusions to apply to a wide range of people. For instance, there have been many studies involving patients in the VA (Veterans Administration) system. Results from these studies may apply to this group, which includes predominantly men who have served in the armed services, but may not be applicable to other segments of the population.

Another shortcoming of large randomized clinical trials is they tend to be relatively short in duration, usually less than ten years. This may not be enough time to capture potential long-term benefits or risks. For example, suppose the health department secured funding to evaluate the dangers of smoking by enrolling two comparable groups of patients in a six-year-long study where the participants in one group were told to smoke a pack of cigarettes a day and the other told to not smoke (of course, this would not be an ethical study today!). A short study like this could conclude that smoking is *not* harmful to your health! This would be because the long-term adverse health impacts from smoking, such as emphysema and lung cancer, would not show up until decades later. This situation is one where observational data on the long-term risks of smoking actually gives us better information.

How we learn from different types of studies

The different types of studies contribute to building our knowledge each in their own way. Observational studies initially show some correlations; clinical studies attempt to confirm cause and effect. Then studies in the lab try to explain the reasons for the findings. History is replete with examples of this process. For instance, malaria has been a devastating illness since ancient times. Because it was observed that people frequently became ill around marshes, it was thought the toxic vapors from swamps caused the illness – thus the name *mal aria*, Italian for *bad air*. It was then suspected that mosquitoes, rather than the vapors, were the cause. In the 1800s researchers subjected volunteers to mosquitoes that had been feeding on patients infected with malaria and found that they developed the disease (not a study that would ever be allowed today!). Eventually, a parasite residing in the mosquitoes was identified as the culprit.[5]

In some cases, we need to rely heavily on observational studies because it would be impractical or unethical to do a randomized trial. For instance, let's say researchers wanted to determine if removing a woman's ovaries increases her risk of heart disease. They obviously are not going to ask women to sign up to have their ovaries removed in the name of science! Observational studies would be necessary to obtain this type of information. Researchers could cull through hospital databases and tabulate the number of women diagnosed with a heart attack who also have had ovarian surgery. Or, they could design a study where women admitted for this surgery could agree to participate in a study where they would be followed over a period of years to assess the development of heart disease.

Observational studies would also be necessary in situations where researchers wanted to study an alternative treatment that would deviate from accepted practices. If some measure has been accepted as the standard of care, you are not going to deliberately withhold some treatment from a patient to test a theory. An example of this would be a proposal to test if vaccines cause autism. It would be malpractice to randomly enroll children into two study groups – one that is given their polio, measles, mumps, and other vaccines and another group that is not given any of these life-saving immunizations.

Fortunately, for the most part, the results of large observational trials and large clinical trials tend to be in agreement. It is when they come up with clear discrepancies that eyebrows get raised. This is the situation that we are dealing with today regarding hormone replacement therapy. For most of the twentieth century, hormone replacement therapy for menopausal women was considered beneficial and, in fact, encouraged not only to treat hot flashes, but to prevent a number of chronic diseases, such as osteoporosis, heart disease, and even dementia. This recommendation was based on a large number of observational studies that showed the benefits substantially outweighed the risks.

Then, in 2002 the conclusions of the WHI study were published – announcing that HRT carried more risks than benefits. This not only upset the apple cart regarding menopausal management, it destroyed it. Because the WHI was a huge, double-blind, randomized study, it became the gold standard and has been a force to be reckoned with. Its qualifications established it as the basis for the way to manage menopausal women with hormones. No longer were hormones recommended as a standard treatment for most women entering menopause. Doctors were advised to reserve them only to treat extremely symptomatic women with the lowest dose for the shortest period of time.

Why the conclusions of the WHI were so disparate from earlier studies has caused much scrutiny. A number of interesting findings have emerged which will be addressed in subsequent sections of this book. The dilemma that confronts us, however, is that high-quality studies will be needed to rectify the shortcomings that have been identified in the WHI. Whether these studies will occur is unclear. For me, this is troubling because thousands of women are being discouraged from taking hormone replacement and there is an upwelling of evidence that this may have a negative impact on their future health. As you continue reading this book, you will understand why we should be concerned.

Decision Making Helper

The purpose in presenting the information in this chapter is to introduce you to the types of studies that determine effective medical treatments and help you understand why some studies carry more weight than others in creating guidelines. A number of studies regarding HRT will be presented in this book. Having this background will help you appreciate why there is so much controversy regarding the benefits and risks of HRT. The following are factors to consider.

In assessing the merits of a study, it is important to keep in mind the manner in which the study was performed. Although randomized, controlled studies, like the WHI, carry a huge amount of weight, other studies give us meaningful information, especially those that involve thousands of women followed over many years.

When you hear about a new medical study, make an effort to learn more about it. Was it performed by a reputable institution such as a university and written by experts in the field? Was it published in a respected magazine such as the *Journal of the American Medical Association*, or did it appear in some very obscure, small newsletter? Were just a few patients studied or a large group? If you are assessing whether a particular outcome may apply to you, did the study include patients comparable to your age group, ethnicity, sex or other specific characteristics?

Was it a meta-analysis? Recall that this type of study compiles a large group of studies. Its conclusions tend to be more meaningful than the results of a single, small study.

If not a meta-analysis, was this an observational study or an actual clinical trial? Observational studies do not carry the same weight as clinical trials.

Where did the funding for the study come from? Large studies from the National Institute of Health (NIH) or other objective sources are generally free from bias, as opposed to those sponsored by pharmaceutical companies or some other group that is promoting a product for sale.

If you have concerns after reading a study that may affect you – don't panic and stop or adjust your medications. Set up a visit to discuss the study with your health care provider.

Chapter 5
Estrogen Therapy – A Brief History

If you're wondering whether or not you should take hormone replacement medications when you reach menopause, you're not alone. Thousands of women reach this life milestone every day and until it actually occurs, most probably haven't thought too much about it. Then, suddenly, with the onset of hot flashes and sleep problems, they are confronted with a very difficult decision. Is it a good idea to take estrogen or is it better to just tough things out? Do the benefits outweigh the risks? The goal of this book is to help you answer these questions. Having an overview of the history of hormone therapy will help you better understand why women struggle with this decision and why HRT has been so controversial.

Estrogen therapy – the early years and early controversies

Estrone was the first type of estrogen discovered. It was recovered from the urine of pregnant women in the 1920s and initially was given as an injection to treat women with premature estrogen deficiency. Oral sources of hormones were not readily available for another 25 years, and for the most part, weren't considered a treatment for menopause. The prevailing attitude at that time was that menopause was simply a phase of a woman's life to be accepted – like puberty and pregnancy. There's no doubt that women were having troubling symptoms, but I imagine that not many felt comfortable complaining to a predominantly male physician community about hot flashes, much less confiding about their vaginal dryness and discomfort with intercourse!

By the 1950s, however, estrogen became commercially available and many women found it a welcome antidote for their uncomfortable symptoms. Estrogen's popularity skyrocketed with the appearance of the book, *Feminine Forever,* written by gynecologist Dr. Robert Wilson.[1] Published in 1966, the book promoted the use of estrogen not only to treat hot flashes but as a way to maintain sexuality and youthful vigor. Dr. Wilson urged women to abandon the notion that they dutifully accept their symptoms without complaint.

Thousands of women eagerly jumped on the estrogen bandwagon and articles on the miracles of estrogen dominated women's magazines across the country.

However, even among women, controversy roiled. A very vocal faction of women activists denounced HRT – scorning the notion that male doctors should be venerated for "medicalizing" a normal female physiological process. And, they were likewise indignant that pharmaceutical companies should profit by selling products claiming to restore a woman's femininity. Conversely, other feminine activists urged women to claim autonomy for their bodies – and that it was a woman's choice whether or not to embrace estrogen therapy.

Even within the medical ranks, there was conflict about the wisdom of treating menopause with estrogen. Many prominent gynecologists disagreed with Dr. Wilson and stood firm in their opinion that women should not rely on hormones to get them through a natural life transition that didn't constitute an illness. A textbook in the early 1970s offered the following recommendations for treatment:

> *"At times sympathetic explanation and reassurance must be fortified by judicious and temporary use of sedatives and tranquilizers, but these should be discontinued as soon as fears and anxieties are allayed and the patient has been encouraged to meet and adjust realistically to her changing environment by finding new interests and activities."*[2]

This paternalistic approach must have frustrated many women. Perhaps that was a reason Dr. Wilson's book continued to be a big hit for years. Premarin, the principal form of estrogen available commercially, became one of the most frequently prescribed drugs in the country over the next decade.

The risks and benefits of estrogen therapy become apparent

As more women took HRT for extended periods of time, adverse effects began to appear. Women taking hormones were developing more blood clots. Although the risk was very low, these clots were associated with a potentially fatal outcome if one dislodged and traveled to the lungs. In addition, an unusually high number of women were being diagnosed with uterine cancer. This revelation darkened the popularity of menopausal hormones until, in the mid-1970s, medical investigators determined that women taking estrogen required concurrent treatment with a progestogen. I will explain more about how estrogen affects the uterus in Chapter 9, but it was quickly discovered that combined therapy with both hormones eliminated the risk of uterine cancer.

However, women and their health care providers became increasingly alarmed when it appeared that women on long-term hormones were developing breast cancer at rising rates – regardless of whether they took both hormones. This perceived danger of hormone therapy fueled a growing anti-estrogen sentiment among some women – raising fears that estrogen was carcinogenic.

Despite these issues, during this same period it was coming to light that taking HRT was associated with some significant health benefits – one being its powerful bone-preserving property. At the time there was no effective treatment for osteoporosis, the condition where bones become so fragile a simple misstep leads to a fracture. The consequences of a hip fracture were associated with major complications, including pneumonia and even death – at rates comparable to dying from breast cancer.

In addition, it appeared that women treated with HRT were much less likely to die from a heart attack than women not on therapy. A number of studies published in the 1990s brought this to our attention.[3] I was in medical school when the Nurses Study embarked – enrolling over 48,000 women and following them for the next ten years. The investigators found that women on HRT had a 50% lower risk of having a major coronary event, including fatal and non-fatal heart attacks, when compared to women who had not taken them.[4]

Another major study, known as the Leisure World Study, involved 8,800 women ages 40 through 101 who lived in a retirement community (you guessed it – Leisure World in California).[5] They were sent detailed questionnaires in 1981 about hormone use and other health items. Ten years later it was reported that taking estrogen decreased mortality by 20%, primarily due to a decrease in heart-related fatalities.

It wasn't clear exactly why hormone replacement made such a big difference in preventing heart disease, but it was suspected that its beneficial effects on cholesterol were a major reason. It had long been appreciated that women tend to have higher HDL (the "good" cholesterol) levels and lower LDL (the "bad" cholesterol) levels than men and it was believed that estrogen was the magic factor. Clinical studies subsequently demonstrated that HRT treatment improved cholesterol profiles.[6] As well, other research indicated that estrogen had properties that played roles in preventing the buildup of plaque on the arteries.[7]

The benefits of HRT prevail

From 1970 to 2000 the bulk of evidence indicated that the benefits of HRT outweighed the risks and during this time estrogen therapy was considered to be very appropriate for most women entering menopause and beyond. Sales for Premarin topped the charts once again. I and most of my colleagues who practiced medicine during this period felt comfortable prescribing them – not just for relieving hot flashes but with the belief that treatment would prevent future complications. Textbooks during this time had conclusions such as the following:

> *"Estrogen replacement therapy (ERT) is the most effective treatment for vasomotor hot flushes and urethrovaginal atrophy in postmenopausal women. Evidence also suggests that ERT delays osteoporosis and may even reduce the risk of atherosclerosis. Despite continuing controversy, the risks of ERT are now considered minimal. With individualized therapy and appropriate monitoring, ERT with progestin supplements appears to be safe and effective for the great majority of postmenopausal women."* [8]

As noted, the above statement has the phrase "*may even reduce the risk of atherosclerosis.*" The author implies that while there was much evidence to support this, the studies were primarily observational – and, as discussed in Chapter 4, couldn't be regarded as definitive.

Since cardiovascular disease was the number one cause of death in both men and women, there was considerable interest in determining if HRT should be adopted as the standard of care as an intervention to prevent heart disease. To accomplish this, what was needed were clinical studies to clear the path to encourage HRT for essentially all menopausal women. This quest spurred two major studies, the Heart and Estrogen/Progestin Replacement Study (HERS) and the Women's Health Initiative Study (WHI).

The benefits of HRT come into question

The HERS study was an attempt to determine if women with pre-existing heart disease would benefit from HRT.[9] Women who had been diagnosed with a previous heart attack or confirmed coronary artery disease were placed on

Premarin and Provera and compared to women given a placebo. Their ages ranged from 60 to 73. It was expected that hormones would prevent further heart problems in these women but, unexpectedly, this was not the case. Published in 1998, the study concluded that women taking hormones fared no better than women on a placebo with respect to the progression of their heart disease.

During this same time frame, the National Institute of Health launched the Women's Health Initiative Study (WHI).[10] Unlike the HERS study, which involved women with known heart disease, the goal of the WHI study was to establish the heart-protective benefits of HRT, as well as other benefits and risks, in *healthy* menopausal women. The WHI was a mammoth undertaking and encompassed all the qualities of a good study. It was a large, prospective, double-blinded, randomized clinical trial, run by respected academic researchers.

Although the HERS study failed to show that HRT helped women who had heart disease, those of us in the medical community were expecting the WHI to confirm what was believed – that treating *healthy* women with hormones would prevent heart attacks. Unfortunately, as noted previously, the results of the WHI study ended up being a bombshell in the field of menopausal hormone treatment. Published in 2002, the investigators found that, instead of a lower risk of vascular complications, such as heart attacks and strokes, there was a higher risk! The conclusions of the WHI were totally unexpected. Virtually overnight, things changed. Thousands of women stopped their hormones.[11]

Because the characteristics of the WHI qualified it to be a gold standard type of study, its results dictated a change in the way menopause was managed. Instead of encouraging women to use hormones, physicians were obligated to steer women away from them. Guidelines quickly came out that switched off the green light for prescribing hormones for almost every menopausal woman, reserving them only for limited situations. In essence, estrogen was indicated only for women with extreme symptoms and was not to be used for the prevention of any chronic medical condition.

Little did the medical community realize that the conclusions of the WHI would have long-lasting implications and be the foundation behind the guidelines for years to come. Physicians entering practice after 2002 have received very little training regarding HRT and, as a consequence, have little knowledge and experience prescribing hormone drugs. Funding for new research into HRT has been almost non-existent. The impression that hormone therapy was dangerous was embedded in an entire generation of women approaching menopause. Ten years after the WHI only a fraction of women entering menopause were placed on hormones compared to ten years prior to the study's publication.

Will HRT ever regain popularity?

The disparity between the conclusions of the WHI and our previous belief that the benefits of HRT outweighed the risks has been perplexing. Not surprisingly, the details of the WHI have been meticulously scrutinized over the last decade, and a number of developments have unfolded that may tip the scales back to favoring hormone replacement. This information will be presented in the following chapters along with a more detailed look at the WHI and why it has misled us.

Chapter 6
The WHI – The Good, the Bad, and the Ugly

There is no doubt that in the last century one of the most significant events impacting how we treat menopausal women was the National Institute of Health's massive endeavor – the Women's Health Initiative. This landmark study, known as the WHI, reversed decades' long endorsement of the benefits of hormone replacement therapy and cast doubt about the overall safety of giving estrogen to menopausal women. The WHI remains the cornerstone of today's guidelines. Unfortunately, rather than becoming the pillar of clarity for guiding the optimal approach for women as they entered menopause, it has turned out to be an anchor weighing down and holding back women and their providers from opportunities to reap significant health benefits. This is because, despite being a solidly organized and orchestrated study, some of its conclusions are being inappropriately applied. In this chapter, I describe the aspects of the study in detail – what was good, what was bad, and what has turned ugly!

Pre-WHI

As introduced in the previous chapters, it has long been appreciated that taking hormones after menopause has many benefits. And, like most medical treatments, it was also acknowledged there were some risks. For many years it was known that HRT use increased the risk of blood clots and seemed to promote breast cancers – which, although not trivial issues, were more than counterbalanced by its effectiveness in preventing the deadly consequences of osteoporosis-related fractures. There was also considerable evidence that hormones decreased the risk of dementia and other age-related changes.

However, the pivotal benefit of taking HRT that tipped the scales to its being a strongly recommended therapy was its beneficial effect on the cardiovascular system. Prior to the WHI, a number of observations and studies had convinced the medical community that there was something about estrogen that protected the heart. It was known that women had better cholesterol profiles than men – a trait attributed to estrogen. And, throughout their reproductive years, women were noted to have far fewer heart attacks than men of comparable ages. However, after menopause the rate of heart attacks in women rose steadily. Replacing those hormones by taking HRT seemed like a logical intervention to keep this from happening, and many early studies supported this. But, to solidify that HRT should officially be a recommended intervention to prevent heart disease, a definitive large-scale study was needed.

The birth of the WHI

In 1991 the U.S. National Institute of Health launched the Women's Health Initiative – one of the largest studies of its kind ever undertaken in the United States. A number of academic centers and a Who's Who list of respected menopause experts across the country were involved in this endeavor. The WHI had two major parts – an observational study and a clinical study. Approximately 168,000 women between the ages of 50 and 79 were recruited from 1993 to 1998. Of those, approximately 100,000 women, who were either unwilling or ineligible to participate in the clinical part of the study (meaning that they could not or did not want to go on any medication), agreed to be in the observational study. The women in the observational WHI study have been followed over many years and researchers have been periodically collecting data on their medical status as they progress beyond menopause. Since these women were not treated with hormones, I am not delving into any aspects of the observational study in this book.

The remaining 68,000 who signed up to be part of the clinical trial could choose to participate in several study groups – one of which was to assess the effects of HRT. This is the aspect of the WHI which is addressed in this book. This segment of the WHI enrolled approximately 28,000 women. Half of the women were placed on hormones and the other half on a placebo (recall that a placebo is basically a sugar pill with no active ingredients in it). Since women who had had a hysterectomy needed only to take estrogen, one branch (the *estrogen-only arm*) consisted of women either on estrogen alone or on a placebo. The other branch (referred to as the *estrogen-progestogen arm*) consisted of women who still had a uterus. They received either combined therapy with estrogen and a progestogen or a placebo. The estrogen-progestogen arm of the WHI Study consisted of 16,608 women and it started two years prior to the estrogen-only arm which consisted of 10,739 women. The hormones used in both branches were given on a daily basis and were the common preparations and doses prescribed in the U.S. in that era – Premarin 0.625 mg. in the estrogen-only arm; Premarin 0.625mg plus Provera (medroxyprogesterone) 2.5 mg. in the estrogen-progestogen arm.

This WHI clinical study was designed to be the ultimate prospective, double-blind, randomized trial to determine the beneficial effects of HRT on the heart, as well as to evaluate the safety and efficacy of hormone therapy on other menopausal issues. The intention of the WHI was to recruit a large number of "generally healthy" (more on this later) participants. As is required in this type of study, the women in the treatment groups and the placebo groups were to be comparable. This meant that there had to be equal numbers of women in each group with similar characteristics such as their age, weight, smoking history, blood pressure status, or presence of diabetes and other health conditions. Neither the investigators nor the women knew who was taking the actual hormones or placebo pills.

Over the course of the study, the women were seen regularly in clinics where they were evaluated. A huge amount of data was gathered including lab tests, weight and blood pressure measurements, and documentation of any symptoms or other medical issues.[1] Over the ensuing years, thousands of articles on various aspects of the WHI have been published.

The premature termination of the WHI

One of the issues about the WHI that generated a lot of press attention was the fact that the study was "halted prematurely." When this was announced, it heightened concern that estrogen therapy might pose hidden dangers and added fuel to the campaigns of anti-hormone groups and individuals. The reality, however, is that the decision to potentially terminate early was built into the design of the study as a cautionary measure. This was because it was believed that estrogen treatment could promote breast cancer and it was decided ahead of time to stop the study if a certain number of breast cancers developed. The study was planned to go for seven years but the estrogen-progestogen arm was halted shortly after five years due to the fact that the number of new breast cancers exceeded the number predetermined to be the threshold for stopping the study. Upon hearing this, you likely assume this must have been a pretty substantial number. However, this is not the case. Of the 8,000 plus women taking both Premarin and Provera, there were approximately 206 new cases of breast cancer diagnosed. In the placebo group, there were approximately 155 cases of breast cancer. What this boils down to was that there were only about ten more cases per year of breast cancer developing in the women taking hormones compared to women not taking them.

The other arm of the WHI, where women were taking estrogen alone without a progestogen, ended in 2004.[2] It also was halted a little earlier than planned. However, this was not because of a breast cancer issue. In fact, in this arm, there actually were more breast cancers in the women taking a placebo than in women on estrogen! (I will be going into much more detail on this important piece of information in Chapter 10). The reason this segment of the study was stopped was that a higher rate of strokes appeared in the women on estrogen – something that was unexpected. Not to dismiss the seriousness of this complication, the risk was very low with roughly six more cases per year in the women taking estrogen. In addition, the criteria used to define a "stroke" were considered fairly broad. Some of the women had neurologic symptoms that did not cause permanent damage.

So both of these studies were terminated early, which is really not that unusual and was based on the premise of being cautious. And, certainly, in the first arm, an increase of breast cancer diagnoses was anticipated. Details of the number of negative outcomes observed in this study, as well as the positive outcomes, will be presented later in this chapter.

What was and wasn't expected

As expected, the WHI study confirmed that women taking hormones were at a higher risk for blood clots but at a lower risk for fractures – findings that correlated with earlier observational studies. However, the shocking news that wasn't anticipated as an outcome was a higher risk of heart attacks in the women taking hormone replacement therapy. This was unsettling because a major purpose of the study was to confirm what everyone had assumed – that HRT prevented heart disease. The results of the estrogen-progestogen arm of the study were announced in a press release in 2002 (well before many of us even received our medical journals that reported the study!). We were blindsided as we opened our morning papers to read headlines such as what appeared in the *New York Times*:

> *"Red Flag on Hormone Replacement"* *". . . there are serious risks to using the hormones for years, risks that far outweigh the few benefits, the National Institutes of Health announced Tuesday."* [3]

Other articles came out with headings such as:

> *Study is Cancelled Due To Rise Seen In Cancer Risk!*

Hormone Replacement Therapy – A Shock to the Medical System!

What appeared on front pages across the country were proclamations that taking HRT causes a 26% higher risk of a heart attack, a 26% increased risk of breast cancer, and that it doubles the risk of getting a blood clot. These were very alarming statistics. And, on top of this, the media jumped on the fact the study was halted prematurely – which made things sound even more dire. There ensued a flurry of articles implying that drug companies had been preying on vulnerable menopausal women and that doctors had been misleading their patients, as well as other disparaging editorials that made me cringe. What happened next bordered on widespread panic. Providers everywhere were inundated with frantic phone calls from patients. Many women simply stopped their hormones.

Providers, unsure of what to make of the findings, held back on prescribing any form of HRT. Subsequent reports highlighted the effect the WHI study had on hormone use. By the end of 2003, the number of prescriptions filled for HRT plummeted and continued to spiral downward. Over the next ten years, there was about an 80% reduction in claims for hormone prescriptions reported by the insurance industry.[4] Prior to the WHI, it has been estimated that up to 33% of women ages 50 to 74 were taking hormones.[4] Ten years later less than 5% of the more than 47 million menopausal women were taking them.[5,6]

The WHI study clearly impacted most of us who were in practice in 2002. It caused considerable confusion and some disbelief. Up until that time most of my patients had not been particularly worried about taking their hormones. In fact, they were delighted that one or two little pills each day eliminated their terrible hot flashes, improved their sleep, and cleared up their vaginal and bladder complaints. And, I was pleased with their good bone density reports and cholesterol readings. But following the barrage of coverage in the press about the damaging effects of HRT, many of my patients were leery of taking them even before coming in for an appointment to discuss what they should do. They were getting the message that it was better to buckle up and tough out their symptoms rather than take something as risky as HRT. In addition, they were reading article after article appearing weekly in the media revealing "new, previously unappreciated dangers" of HRT discovered by the WHI study.

One such report examining the effects of HRT on mental function concluded that women on estrogen and a progestogen had twice the rate of dementia, including Alzheimer's disease! Another told women that the WHI found that hormone treatment worsened urinary incontinence. I remember one very indignant patient telling me that the HRT I had been prescribing caused her urinary problems and why hadn't I known better! (As I will discuss in Chapter 16, other studies on the effects of hormones and the bladder have not come to this same conclusion.)

Rather than encouraging HRT, the WHI conclusions led to new guidelines discouraging HRT. Providers were advised to treat only very symptomatic women with the lowest dose of hormones for the shortest period of time. HRT was no longer felt to be an acceptable treatment for the long-term benefits that we used to believe they conferred and, although they could be considered for prevention of osteoporosis, they were not the treatment of choice and advisable only in limited situations. The WHI was and continues to be the ultimate gold standard study. Its qualifications have made it the Holy Grail on which treatment guidelines for HRT are based.

As physicians, we were put in a difficult position. It has been hard for many of us to simply accept the findings of the WHI and change our attitude about HRT without some degree of skepticism. For me, the icing on the cake that made me really question the creditability of the study was the conclusion that hormone therapy *did nothing to improve a woman's overall quality of life.* I read that part of the study several times in disbelief. Were years of watching my patients responding so favorably to HRT just a figment of my imagination!? I don't know how many times patients let me know how much better their lives were on HRT. Estrogen cured their hot flashes, cleared their brain fogginess, and helped them sleep. Their sex lives improved, their moods were calmer, and they "felt back to their old selves again." It was very difficult for me to believe that the women in the WHI did not report similar benefits.

Not surprisingly, as the dust settled many healthcare providers and academicians started looking closely at the study. It was a mystery why the WHI came up with findings that were so opposite to the many earlier studies and our personal observations about HRT. To better help you understand why we should question this study, let's review some important aspects of it in more detail.

Dissecting the WHI – relative risk vs. absolute risk

The first thing to critically examine is the actual number of adverse events that occurred. There are many ways that study results can be reported, and this can greatly affect how one views the significance of the findings. When the media reported that HRT increased the risks of breast cancer and heart attacks on the order of 26% each, this sounds very scary. But is it? Many of my patients thought so. A typical conversation discussing HRT frequently went like this:

"I decided to stop my hormones when I read that one out of four women taking them will get breast cancer and that scares me."

My response, "No, a 26% increased risk in breast cancer doesn't mean one out of four women will have this risk. The study actually showed that only about one in one thousand women would be at increased risk by taking HRT."

Then I would explain how these seemingly contradictory numbers could be obtained from the same data.

"At the end of the study, the investigators tabulated the number of women who had some event, such as breast cancer, in each group. To arrive at the 26% increase risk number, they compared the results from each group side-by-side and presented the percentage difference between the treatment and placebo groups. This was the *relative risk*. This is different than the *absolute risk*, which would be obtained by presenting the number of breast cancers that occurred out of the total number of women. Doing it this way would come up with a much smaller number."

Recognizing that it was difficult for my patients to grasp the difference between these types of risk measurements, I would present things in another way. Frequently, outcomes are reported in a standardized way, such as so many events per 10,000 patient-years – extrapolating the number of events that would occur if you had exactly 10,000 patients. Then you can say that for every 10,000 people treated for one year there would be "**x**" number of events. Reporting data in this way makes a side-by-side comparison of the results understandable. (I hope you are still with me. If not re-read this paragraph as it is important!)

Here are the adjusted results found in the estrogen-progestogen arm of the WHI.[1,7] For every 10,000 women taking HRT each year there were:

8 *more* breast cancers than in the placebo group
8 *more* strokes than in the placebo group
7 *more* heart attacks than in the placebo group
18 *more* blood clots than in the placebo group

and

6 *fewer* cases of colon cancer than in the placebo group
5 *fewer* hip fractures than in the placebo group

As you can see, reporting the results in terms of absolute risk is a more meaningful way for women to understand the risks of a given therapy. This is how women should look at the overall risk for an adverse event when considering whether to take HRT. While eight women may face an increased risk of breast cancer by taking both hormones, the other 9,992 taking hormones would not increase their risk of breast cancer. When viewed in this manner, the overall risk of taking HRT appears pretty minimal.

When you read these numbers, you may wonder why the WHI investigators could report that the conclusions of the study were meaningful. As it turns out the numbers reached a threshold that made them statistically significant. If you were a governmental health care official and applied these results to a large population, then these numbers carry more impact. That is how guidelines get developed and justified. However, from the perspective of a single individual, the risk numbers quoted above are actually considered rare. In fact, in medical reporting circles, the following grading system is used to designate how common or how rare a medical event is.[8]

Very common...greater than or equal to 1/10
Common..........greater than or equal to 1/100 but less than 1/10
Uncommon......greater than or equal to 1/1000 but less than 1/100
Rare..............greater than or equal to 1/10,000 but less than 10/10000
Very rare.........less than 1/10,000

Based on these numbers, the actual chance of having any single adverse event taking HRT is considered to be **rare** (other than blood clots which would be classified as being uncommon).

Now, let's look at the results of the estrogen-only arm of the study where women taking estrogen were compared to women on a placebo.[6] Recall that women in this branch of the study all had hysterectomies and did not need to take a progestogen.

For every 10,000 women taking estrogen each year there would be:

> 12 *more* strokes than in the placebo group
> 6 *more* blood clots than in the placebo group
> One *more* case of colon cancer than in the placebo group

and

> 5 *fewer* heart attacks than in the placebo group
> 7 *fewer* breast cancers than in the placebo group
> 6 *fewer* hip fractures than in the placebo group

Dissecting the WHI – different outcomes between the study arms

You will note that there are some surprising differences in the outcomes between these two arms. Notably, women treated with estrogen plus progestogen had higher rates of heart attacks and breast cancer than women on estrogen alone. In fact, women on estrogen alone not only had lower rates of heart attacks compared to women taking a placebo but also had lower rates of breast cancer. What?! This was quite amazing, yet, when the estrogen-only study results came out in 2004, I don't recall any big fanfare in the media retracting what they so notoriously claimed a couple of years earlier. We didn't see headlines proclaiming that *"Estrogen doesn't increase heart attacks and breast cancer after all."*

In addition, there did not seem to be much attention in the medical literature regarding the major differences in outcomes of the two branches of the study – particularly the observation that the women in the second arm, who were on estrogen alone, appeared to have fewer adverse events. Furthermore, from my perspective, there was little discussion that perhaps it was the progestogen administered in the earlier arm of the WHI that accounted for the differences in outcomes. You would think people would question right away that there might be something about medroxyprogesterone that may have caused some problems. Unfortunately, I think that the damage had already been done from the earlier WHI study as far as the shift in opinion about estrogen safety. In most people's minds, HRT was bad for the heart and the breasts regardless of the type or mode of hormone treatment.

Dissecting the WHI – characteristics of the women enrolled

The next very important aspect of the WHI study to examine carefully is the composition of the women enrolled in the study. The intent of the investigators of the WHI was to enroll "generally healthy" women and study the effects of hormone treatment on, well, generally healthy women. This is in contrast to the previous big clinical study, the HERS study, that specifically recruited women who had pre-existing heart disease.

However, if you look at the characteristics of the women enrolled in the WHI, you will note that a large proportion of them had health issues.[9,10]

In fact:

- Only 21% of the women in the estrogen and progestogen arm were of normal weight. 45% were obese, which means they were roughly 30 or more pounds overweight. In the estrogen-only arm of the study, 31% of the women were normal weight and 35% were obese.

- 48% of the women in the combined therapy arm had high blood pressure. In the estrogen-only group, 36% had high blood pressure.

- 48% in the combined group had a history of smoking and 10% still smoked at enrollment. In the second arm, 40% had a history of smoking and 11% were current smokers.

What this means is that many of the women in this study were already at fairly high risk for heart disease due to their obesity, high blood pressure, and smoking. Whether this group truly can be construed as a "generally healthy" population is questionable.

In addition, it should be noted that women who were experiencing severe hot flashes were excluded from the study (perhaps because of concern that they would drop out if their symptoms did not respond to a placebo). Whether the exclusion of women with severe hot flashes affected the results of the study is of interest. There is considerable research into the significance of hot flashes and whether women with severe hot flashes have different propensities for heart disease and other complications. Could it be that women with hot flashes would have the most to gain from HRT? Certainly, at a minimum, by excluding these women, concluding that HRT has no impact on the quality of a woman's life cannot be fairly assessed.

However, the most noteworthy issue to point out, and what is turning out to be of huge significance, is that the average age of the women recruited for both arms of the WHI study was *63 years old.* 67% of the women were between ages 60 to 79 years old, and 26% were over age 70! What should be obvious is that, clearly the women in the WHI were not representative of the typical menopausal woman debating whether or not to take hormones – whose average age is 52 (and more likely than not having hot flashes). Only 3.5% of WHI participants were 50 to 54 years of age – the age when women typically start HRT. So, the majority of women had already completed their transition through menopause and were many years into postmenopause before being placed on hormone therapy.

In summary: the good, the bad, and the ugly

The good

A good aspect of the WHI study is that it was a prospective, randomized, double-blind type of study, which is considered to be the gold standard of clinical studies. It was performed by a large cadre of respected menopause experts, was huge in its scope and magnitude, and supposedly free of bias. An exhaustive amount of data was generated which has greatly furthered our understanding of many aspects of menopause.

The bad

The study has a major drawback in that there were only two drugs used – Premarin and medroxyprogesterone. These were the drugs commonly used in the U.S. for HRT at the time – so it does make sense to have settled on this combination. The generic progestogen was inexpensive and readily available. Premarin, on the other hand, was a brand name product. The manufacturer played a role in providing this for the study. This aspect has drawn criticism.

The ugly

Here is what I, and many others, find particularly upsetting about the WHI study. The conclusions of the study:

- *have been extrapolated to include all forms of HRT*

- *have been applied to all menopausal women, regardless of age*

Somehow, that only one type of estrogen and one type of progestogen were used, and that the women in the study were primarily older, were glossed over when it came to developing guidelines. Although the WHI was a high-quality study, these particular details were dismissed and its findings have been applied in a blanket fashion to all menopausal women on any type of hormone treatment. There is good reason to believe that this is inappropriate.

Whether using other hormones in the study would have changed the outcomes is not just a matter of speculation. Premarin clearly differs in many respects from the estrogens naturally present in a woman's body and, as described earlier, synthetic progestins are chemically very different than natural progesterone. A great deal of evidence is accumulating that indicates that transdermal estradiol and natural progesterone have significantly different, and probably less adverse, effects in many areas of the body. Much more on how the type of HRT affects specific health issues will be presented in the coming chapters.

In addition, the women in the study were not truly representative of the typical women going through menopause. They were considerably older and most had not taken any sort of hormones when they went through menopause. So, for many of these women, years had elapsed with hardly any estrogen or progesterone circulating in their bodies.

This is turning out to be a very important issue. It has sparked the million-dollar question: *Does taking HRT early, at the time of the menopausal transition, behave differently in the body than taking it ten or more years later?* If so, then the results of the WHI should only apply to this latter subset of older women. This would explain a major reason why the WHI results contrasted to the earlier studies – which primarily included younger, recently menopausal women. This very interesting revelation is becoming a hot topic in menopausal hormone therapy today and is being referred to as the *Timing Hypothesis.* We are now asking the question: *Does HRT provide more benefits than risks . . . depending on your age?* The answer to this very key question carries tremendous significance and will be explored in much more detail in subsequent chapters.

The WHI – 15 years later

It has now been over 15 years since the WHI studies were published. Remarkably, a number of women from the original WHI study groups have continued to be followed by the investigators. An article on their status was published in 2017 in the well-respected *Journal of the American Medical Association.*[11] The authors reported that, despite the noted increase in heart attacks and breast cancer diagnoses that occurred during the study period, the women who had been on HRT *had no higher rates of death from heart disease or cancer than the women who had taken a placebo*!

Furthermore, the subset of women who were between the ages of 50 to 59 when they entered the study and started hormones had *fewer* adverse health effects and *fewer* deaths than their counterparts who had taken a placebo. Does this mean that taking HRT actually improved their long-term health? What would have happened if they had taken them longer? These and so many other questions remain unanswered.

New studies and re-analyses of old data have been affirming the observation that initiating HRT in younger women may indeed offer more benefits than risks. Yet, despite this rising tide of awareness, women entering menopause are not being encouraged to initiate HRT because the guidelines continue to rely heavily on the WHI. Whether a study of its caliber will ever be forthcoming is doubtful. For some reason, it seems that the original message about the dangers of hormones persists unyieldingly in the minds of policymakers.

However, as more data accumulates, we may see some changes in attitudes. Many experts already are encouraging a more liberal approach to initiating HRT – particularly for women having hot flashes.[12,13] They are advocating that providers consider prescribing adequate doses of hormones to control symptoms and continue therapy as long as needed to achieve treatment goals.

Whether there will ever be encouragement for women to use HRT for preventative therapy for other conditions such as heart disease remains dubious. My concern is that there appears to be a window of opportunity that many women will miss as we debate these issues. The purpose of this book is to educate women so they can better decide what is best for them and not simply sit on the sidelines waiting for changes in the guidelines to appear that better address the risks and benefits for younger women just entering menopause.

Decision Making Helper

Key Considerations

The WHI study is considered the best source of evidence we have regarding the benefits and risks of menopausal hormone therapy. Articles in both scientific and lay publications refer to this study when recommendations are made regarding menopausal hormone treatment. Women should be aware of the shortcomings of the study – regarding the ages of the participants, their baseline health status, and the particular hormones that were administered. Therefore, the findings of the WHI may not apply to younger women and those on other hormone regimens.

The key features to be aware of regarding the WHI are that:

- The majority of the women were considerably older than the age at which most women would normally start taking HRT.

- Many had underlying risk factors for heart disease such as high blood pressure.

- Women who were having hot flashes were excluded from the study.

- Only one type of estrogen was used which was oral Premarin; only one type of progestogen was used which was medroxyprogesterone.

- The study demonstrated an increase in breast cancer and heart attacks only in the women who took estrogen plus a progestogen. Women who took estrogen-only had a decreased risk of breast cancer and heart attacks compared to women taking a placebo.

- Long-term follow-up studies of the WHI participants have revealed that the women who took HRT did not die any earlier than the women on a placebo.

- Women on HRT had fewer fractures and lower rates of colon cancer.

Chapter 7
Estrogen Receptors and the Timing Hypothesis

Ever since the WHI study came out, the medical community has grappled with why its findings were so unexpected and disparate from earlier studies that examined the risks and benefits of HRT. We are starting to unravel much of this mystery, and a key issue has to do with the age a woman is when she starts HRT.

Most of the studies done before the arrival of the WHI involved women who were between the ages of 45 and 55 – the typical age when menopausal symptoms appear. This is in contrast to the WHI study where HRT was given to women who were considerably older – some whose bodies had not seen estrogen for up to 25 years! This big difference in ages has not gone unnoticed. The discrepancy has raised the question of whether studies comprised predominately of younger women have different outcomes than studies that include a large proportion of older women. This has led to a concept referred to as the *Timing Hypothesis.*

A hypothesis is defined as a *supposition or proposed explanation made on the basis of limited evidence as a starting point for further investigation.* This is where we are regarding the timing issue. We have accumulated a substantial amount of data sufficient to put forth the proposal that hormones behave differently in the bodies of younger women going through menopause than they do in older women who have been deprived of hormones for a number of years. This very well may explain why the same therapy, i.e., hormone administration, leads to different outcomes in different studies. Initiating HRT in younger women may provide more benefit than risk; initiating hormones in older women may carry more risk than benefit. However, there isn't universal acceptance of this concept. We lack large clinical studies to validate this theory. So I think it is instructive to review how the Timing Hypothesis has evolved and the evidence we have that supports it.

The studies leading to the Timing Hypothesis

As discussed previously, one of the major early observational studies that indicated HRT prevented heart disease was the large Nurses Study which took place a decade prior to the WHI. The nurses in that study were predominantly women who started hormones when they initially entered the menopausal transition – so most of them were younger than the age of 55. At the end of this study, women taking HRT had a nearly 50% decreased risk of having a heart attack compared to women not taking them. These impressive findings, on top of a number of other earlier studies showing the cardiac benefits of taking estrogen, made most clinicians back in the 1990s fairly confident that prescribing HRT for hot flashes would also be good for their patients from a cardiovascular perspective. Although most of the participants in the Nurses Study were generally healthy, approximately 2,500 women entering the study did have a diagnosis of heart disease. But even in this group of women, hormone treatment appeared to lower the rates of heart attacks and death compared to women not taking hormones.[1]

However, a number of subsequent studies, including the HERS study, did not show that giving hormones to women with established heart disease was beneficial.[2-6] These findings were somewhat puzzling because it was known that estrogen improved cholesterol and this should help prevent not only the onset of heart disease but also slow down the progression of existing heart disease. As researchers pondered this issue a very obvious revelation presented itself – and that was that heart disease typically doesn't occur until late in a woman's life. It is rare to have hardening of the arteries at age 50 but becomes increasingly likely after the age of 65. So it is not surprising that studies designed to assess the effects of HRT on cardiac disease recruited women who were older. This was certainly the case in the HERS study where the average age of the women was 65. The end result of this study was that taking HRT for four years was no better than a placebo in preventing cardiac complications.

Although this lack of benefit was unexpected, it was not as shocking as the results of the WHI study published a couple of years later when it was concluded that hormone replacement actually *increased* the risk of heart attacks. The findings were published in the *Journal of the American Medical Association* (JAMA) in 2002. The concluding paragraph read:

> *"CONCLUSIONS Overall health risks exceeded benefits from use of combined estrogen plus progestin for an average 5.2-year*

*follow-up among healthy postmenopausal US women. All-cause
mortality was not affected during the trial. The risk-benefit
profile found in this trial is not consistent with the requirements
for a viable intervention for primary prevention of chronic
diseases, and the results indicate that this regimen should not be
initiated or continued for primary prevention of coronary heart
disease."*[7]

The bottom line of this study was interpreted by the medical community, as well as the general public, to conclude that HRT carries more risks than benefits. Furthermore, it left the impression that hormones are of questionable value and possibly even dangerous. The fact that the average age of the women in the WHI was 63 and that very few of them were in the 50 to 55 year age group was not mentioned in the concluding statement quoted above. These details did not seem to get widely disseminated and, even more disturbingly, this information did not get addressed in the new guidelines, which essentially discouraged HRT for all women, regardless of age.

Does age make a difference?

However, many menopause experts noted that age may be an issue and at some point there appeared to be a collective "aha" moment when it was realized that outcomes might depend on the time when HRT is initiated. A number of researchers began looking at the earlier observational studies to dissect any differences that occurred in women starting HRT earlier vs. later. The data from the Nurses Study was re-examined. Although most of the women enrolled were treated with HRT shortly after the onset of menopause, there were some women who started them later in life. When these two groups were compared it was found that it was the younger women who benefited substantially from being on HRT whereas women who were older actually had a slight increase in cardiac risk.[8]

What about the younger women in the WHI? Although the majority of women were older, there were a little over a thousand women between the ages of 50 and 59 at the time they enrolled in the study. But it wasn't until 2007 (and then later in 2011) that we saw articles appearing in the *Journal of the American Medical Association* specifically reporting on this group.[9,10] What was found was that younger women who had taken estrogen therapy alone not only had a decreased risk of heart disease but also a decreased risk of strokes as well as lower rates of diabetes and breast cancer. Younger women taking both estrogen and progestogen also had lower risks of these complications, although not as substantial as in the estrogen-only group. So eyebrows were being raised – the timing when hormones were initiated appeared to make a major difference.

The next step was to design randomized clinical trials looking exclusively at treating younger women. The first study in this vein was the Kronos Early Estrogen Prevention Study (KEEPS).[11] Over 700 women within three years of menopause, without heart disease, were enrolled and placed in three different groups. One group of women was given 0.45 mg of Premarin daily plus 200 mg of micronized progesterone for the last 12 days each month. A second group was treated with a 0.05 mg transdermal estradiol patch plus 200 mg of micronized progesterone for 12 days each month. The third group was a placebo group.

Before discussing the outcomes of this study, I would like to point out several things. This study also sought to address whether the type of HRT would make a difference – so two forms of estrogen preparations were used – Premarin (but at a lower dose than in the WHI) and a transdermal estradiol patch. In addition, natural progesterone rather than a synthetic progestin was chosen. Also, instead of taking estrogen and progestogen daily (as in the WHI), a cyclic protocol was used (meaning that the estrogen was given throughout the month and the progesterone was given for the last 12 days of each month).

Because the study period was short, less than five years, and the women were relatively young, it was unlikely that many, if any, of the women would experience a heart attack during the time the study was ongoing. So the investigators used other means to assess for the development of heart disease. This was done by doing CAT scans of the heart and ultrasound studies of the carotid arteries in the neck, both which indirectly assess for the presence of plaque – the precursor to a heart attack and stroke. The women entering the study received these tests to make sure they were free of unsuspected atherosclerosis or heart disease at the beginning of the study. The scans were then repeated during and at the end of the study to look for any changes.

Many of us anxiously waited for this study to be finalized – hoping it would show that hormones really did help prevent heart disease in young women. Unfortunately, this wasn't what the study concluded. After four years, the investigators reported that there were no significant differences in any of the groups. None of the hormone regimens led to lower rates of plaque development in the carotid arteries. And, while the women on hormones had less calcium buildup on the heart arteries compared to the women on a placebo, the authors acknowledged that the differences between the two groups were extremely minor.

There ensued quite a bit of discourse about the significance of this study. Because the authors could not demonstrate that hormones significantly decreased plaque build-up, many prominent menopause experts put the kibosh on the credibility of the Timing Hypothesis. Articles with titles such as *"KRONOS Study Ends the Debate on HRT"* appeared claiming that this study invalidated assertions that hormones prevented heart disease in young, healthy women.

However, others interpreted the results differently – noting that this study didn't assess real endpoints, like heart attacks. And the fact that the women on hormones did not show a *progression* of hardening of the arteries was in itself reassuring. Had the study gone on for a longer period of time, a benefit in plaque reduction might have been demonstrated.

Fortunately, other clinical studies using other endpoints were underway. In 1999, several years prior to the conclusion of the WHI study, a study in Europe had begun – the Danish Osteoporosis Prevention Study (DOPS).[12] Approximately 1,000 women, with a mean age of 50, were recruited and randomized into two groups – treated with either hormone therapy or a placebo. The aim was to evaluate the major risks and benefits of HRT therapy. The study was published in 2012. At the end of ten years, women treated with hormones had a 52% reduction in heart attacks, heart failure, or death. Subsequent follow-up data continued to show these benefits.[13] It was also noted that the younger a woman was when starting HRT, the more benefit she received. This study gave more support to the assertion that hormones, taken at the time of menopause, decrease cardiac risk.

A year after this, the results of a major study from Finland appeared. The Finnish government keeps a nationwide registry on the health status of its citizens. Using this data, researchers undertook a massive effort to assess the effects of hormone treatment on a number of outcomes.[14] Beginning in 1994 and going forward, the records of over 480,000 women were scrutinized. The authors found that women who had been on HRT for at least three years had a 38% decrease in cardiovascular death. The greatest benefit was seen for women who had started HRT prior to the age of 60.

In 2015 there was a Cochrane report regarding HRT.[15] The Cochrane organization is a respected international group that formulates evidence-based reports on important health care practices. Independent experts analyze the major and reputable studies on a subject and provide a summary of the findings. This paper reported that, based on their analysis, women who started taking HRT within ten years of menopause had a 48% lower risk of coronary heart disease and a 30% lower mortality rate than women not taking HRT. In addition, HRT did not increase the risk of a stroke relative to treatment with a placebo.

Cumulatively these studies added credibility to the Timing Hypothesis in that they at least support the presumption that treating younger women with HRT was beneficial from a cardiac standpoint. However, what was needed was some way to test this theory more directly by comparing younger women and older women side-by-side.

The Timing Hypothesis gains momentum

Such an effort came in the form of the ELITE study. ELITE is the acronym for the Early versus Late Intervention Trial with Estradiol. This study enrolled 643 healthy postmenopausal women and divided them into two groups based on when they went through menopause. If women were within six years of menopause they were named the *early group* (average age 55.4 years). The other group, the *late group*, were women who had gone more than ten years beyond menopause (average age 65.4 years).[16]

The women were treated either with oral estradiol (one mg.) or a placebo. Women with a uterus also took natural progesterone suppositories inserted vaginally ten days each month. The study went on for about seven years. Similar to the KEEPS study, the researchers used the ultrasound technique to assess how much plaque developed on the carotid arteries. They obtained these measurements on the enrollees every six months.

What was found was that in the early group, the women taking estrogen had *less* progression of artery thickening than the women on a placebo. For the women who were more than ten years beyond menopause, the degree of hardening of the arteries progressed similarly in both the treatment and placebo groups. What this study tells us is that starting HRT early prevents plaque development, but starting it late does not. This study gives further support to the Timing Hypothesis – demonstrating that the initiation of hormones is helpful if started early, but not later.

Other avenues of research have been done that support the Timing Hypothesis. A number of animal studies in the lab have been carried out.[17] Mice can be made menopausal by removing their ovaries. These mice develop diseases such as atherosclerosis and diabetes – just as in humans. Studies similar to the ELITE study have been carried out. These have shown that estrogen given to newly menopausal mice prevents atherosclerosis from forming. However, administering estrogen to older, menopausal mice that had already developed plaque did not prevent it from worsening.

A similar study was performed in female monkeys that had their ovaries removed.[18] One group was given estrogen shortly after their surgery, and in another group, estrogen was not given for two years (which would be the equivalent of six human years). The researchers then evaluated the degree of hardening of the arteries. They found that estrogen treatment prevented plaque development in the younger monkeys, but did not benefit the older menopausal monkeys.

Does the Timing Hypothesis apply to other health conditions?

While much of the data supporting the Timing Hypothesis has been derived from studying how HRT affects the cardiovascular system, other health conditions are also influenced by the timing of when hormone therapy is initiated. The effects of estrogen on the brain have been extensively studied. In animal research, mice that were placed on estrogen shortly after becoming menopausal had less inflammatory responses to brain injury than mice that did not receive treatment.[19] Since much of the cellular injury from strokes, as well as from the processes that lead to Alzheimer's Disease, is due to inflammation, this suggests that the presence of estrogen helps mitigate the severity of these disorders – but possibly only if initiated soon after women go through menopause. This would explain why a sub-study of the WHI did not find that hormone treatment was beneficial for dementia. The women in that sub-study were all over the age of 65.[20]

Other studies have demonstrated that early estrogen administration helps prevent diabetes. A risk factor for diabetes is a condition known as insulin resistance. Estrogen administration helps prevent this from developing both in animal and human studies.[21] Furthermore, it has been shown that this protective effect only occurs when women take estrogen shortly after becoming menopausal. Administering estrogen ten years past menopause does not appear to improve insulin resistance.[22]

All of this data indicates that estrogen plays a positive role in various areas of the body when administered early – but not when given later. So the big question that remains is what causes estrogen replacement to behave so differently in younger women compared to women ten years or so beyond menopause? This is an area of fascinating and relatively new research.

Introducing hormone receptors

To better understand why this might occur we need to delve deeper into how hormones, such as estrogen and progesterone, do the things they do in the body. What is going on at a cellular level? This brings us to a more detailed discussion of hormone receptors. I would like to spend some time making sure you thoroughly understand how hormone receptors function since they play a key role in explaining the Timing Hypothesis, as well as how hormone replacement therapy exerts its various effects in the body.

I often recall those days back in medical school, when, while talking to a patient in her hospital room, a nurse would appear with a cupful of pills. *"Time for your morning medication,"* she would cheerfully announce. I remember staring at the assortment of tablets and capsules being presented and wondering how it was that each one could find its way inside her body to accomplish its intended mission. The Tylenol needed to find the pain center in her brain to relieve her headache, the Prilosec had to locate and block the acid-producing cells in her stomach, and the antibiotic needed to seek and destroy the bacteria causing her pneumonia.

After watching my patient dutifully swallow her meds, I visualized them dissolving in her stomach and then entering her circulatory system. There they would be pumped throughout her body along with a myriad of other chemical compounds swirling in her bloodstream – electrolytes, proteins, enzymes, and, of course, hormones.

How do these thousands of unique elements know where to go and cause things to happen? We can give the credit to the millions of receptors that coat all of our cells. Receptors are complex protein-based compounds attached to the surface of the cell, which act like microscopic catchers' mitts. They will only interact with certain elements of a specific size and shape – much like a lock and key. As our hormones, drugs, and other molecules race throughout our circulatory system, they eventually connect with their specific receptors. When this marriage occurs, a physiologic event is triggered. For instance, when insulin attaches to its receptor, it causes "doors" on the cell to open, allowing the entry of blood sugar. This lowers the blood sugar level in the bloodstream.

Sometimes an interaction with a receptor initiates an immediate event. Other times it sets off a cascade of molecular reactions inside the cell that ultimately affect the DNA. Hormones, in particular, have this ability. They can instruct DNA to activate certain genes, such as the ones that lead to the formation of proteins that become the building blocks for our breasts and sexual organs.

The events orchestrated by hormones that transform a young girl into a woman are pretty obvious, but most of us are not really aware of what our hormones are doing in other areas. We know that there are thousands of estrogen and progesterone receptors throughout the body. These are present not only in the uterus, breast, and ovaries, but in the brain, bones, connective tissue, skin, muscles, gut, and the cells lining the arteries. What this means is that our hormones play significant roles in all these areas.

More on hormone and receptor interactions

The way receptors work is extremely complex. Different cells can have different combinations of receptors. In the case of estrogen receptors, we know that there are at least two major forms, *alpha* and *beta*. When estrogen hooks onto one type, a certain action occurs and when it hooks onto another type, a different action occurs. Some tissues have mostly alpha receptors and others mostly beta. Not all estrogen preparations hook onto both. Some of the estrogens in Premarin, for example, interact with some receptors and not others. This may explain why outcomes in studies using horse-derived estrogens may have different outcomes than studies using pure estradiol. Similarly, the differences in the various synthetic progestins cause them to attach preferentially to one type of progesterone receptor or another.

The pharmaceutical industry capitalizes on knowing the structure of our hormone receptors. They have been able to synthesize lookalike products in the lab that will fit into them. In simple terms, think of a section of a jigsaw puzzle missing one piece. The hole in the puzzle would be the receptor. You look for a piece (or in the case of the biochemist in the lab, create a molecule) that will fit into that slot. In the drug-making business, it doesn't have to be an exact fit, just have enough matching characteristics that it can partially fit into a receptor where it can promote an action. That is how the various synthetic progestins have come into existence. They resemble natural progesterone in many respects but can have very different chemical structures.

Similarly, this is how drug companies have developed SERMs. Because they are not exact replicas of our natural hormones, SERMs can either cause estrogen-like effects or in some cases anti-estrogen effects. SERMs with anti-estrogen effects are created by making a drug that hooks onto the receptor and, rather than triggering any reaction, it simply blocks natural estrogen from attaching. This is how some of the breast cancer drugs work. They prevent any circulating estrogen made in our bodies post menopause from being able to stimulate breast cancer cells.

The hormone-receptor interaction is actually even more complex than I have thus far described, and a scientist could devote his or her whole career to studying how just one type of hormone receptor works. It is actually not just a matter of an estrogen molecule finding its receptor. There is a host of ancillary molecular elements and chemical reactions that ultimately have to proceed in an orderly manner to make a successful hormone-receptor marriage work. A minor abnormality anywhere in this cascade could affect this process.

Genetics play a huge role in how efficiently our hormones work, particularly if there are defects affecting the structure and function of our hormone receptors. For instance, an abnormal gene could be responsible for a minor alteration in the shape of the estrogen receptors in the bones. This may interfere with how well estrogen can bind to the receptor and thus attenuate its ability to slow down bone loss. This could account for why some women or ethnic groups have more osteoporosis than others.[23] A more drastic deformation in a receptor can create infertility in a woman, or birth defects in a developing fetus. Other receptor defects may account for the variability among women when it comes to the severity of their menopause symptoms, or how their bodies respond to hormone replacement.

A great deal of our understanding of what estrogen does in our bodies has come from animal studies. Mice can be genetically altered to eliminate the gene that is responsible for making the estrogen receptor – so no receptors are present on any of their cells. Therefore, even if there is estrogen circulating in the bloodstream it can't exert any effects. These mice develop premature osteoporosis, hardening of their arteries, and diabetes – all consequences of the absent estrogen effect. This type of research contributes to our understanding of how estrogen deficiency increases these risks.

I came across a particularly interesting case report that further illustrates the adverse consequences of not having estrogen receptors.[24] While the dominant male sex hormone is testosterone, men rely on having small amounts of estrogen to enable a number of vital functions in their bodies. This particular case was about a 28-year male who was born with a genetic defect that affected his body's ability to make estrogen receptors, so his cells essentially were devoid of them. One of the main reasons this happened was because his parents were second cousins and both, unfortunately, had this genetic defect (which is why marrying relatives is not a good idea). In this situation, this patient's cells were not able to respond to the estrogen present in his body. The consequences were that he was infertile, obese, and developed osteoporosis and premature hardening of the arteries – which led to a heart attack at the age of 31. This was an informative example highlighting the important role that estrogen plays in preventing these conditions not only in women but in men!

As with estrogen receptors, we have progesterone receptors just about everywhere in our body. We know some of the roles that progesterone plays in our various systems, but we still have much to learn. The organ most extensively studied is the uterus. Natural progesterone plays a major role in creating the monthly menstrual cycle, as well as counteracting any estrogen-induced cancer-causing effects. All of the synthetic progestins exert the same effect on the uterus – although most are quite a bit more potent than natural progesterone. In fact medroxyprogesterone (Provera) is 100 times stronger than natural progesterone in the way it acts on the uterus.

We are realizing that because synthetic progestins have different chemical structures, they can act differently than natural progesterone in some areas of the body. They may not be able to trigger progesterone-like actions at all receptor sites and potentially could cause an undesirable action in some cases. This is one reason why there has been so much variability in the studies on the outcomes of HRT. More about how different HRT combinations appear to have different effects in the body will be discussed in subsequent chapters.

Estrogen receptors and the Timing Hypothesis

I've spent a great deal of this chapter educating you about receptors and now it is time to use this background to explain how estrogen receptors fit into the Timing Hypothesis. The key to understanding this theory are the following premises:

A. Hormone receptors in women who initiate HRT at the time of menopause continue to function just as they did prior to menopause.

B. If women do not take HRT when they first go through menopause, their hormone receptors either disappear or don't interact with hormones normally and, after a prolonged period of estrogen deprivation, they possibly cannot be reactivated.

In other words, if a woman is not given HRT at about the time when her own estrogen levels go down, she loses the ability to respond to estrogen. So even if she takes HRT when she is older, it will not have the same effects as it would have had when she was younger because her estrogen receptors are not functional.

The fact that we can lose receptor function is not just conjecture. Receptors are not permanent fixtures. They are created inside a cell under the direction of DNA and after they are formed, position themselves on the cell membrane. But, the cell can also withdraw them back inside the cell where they can be destroyed or repurposed. They can appear and/or disappear under certain conditions.

We know that with aging our cells lose receptors. This has been demonstrated in the brain. The receptors for our neurotransmitters, such as adrenaline, acetylcholine, and dopamine diminish with age.[25] A loss of estrogen receptors in the walls of the arteries and the muscles of postmenopausal women has also been documented.[27-28]

From research studies we have learned that blood levels of estrogen and progesterone can have a bearing on how many receptors appear on certain cells. The Timing Hypothesis is based on the assumption that exposing women to a continuous and uninterrupted supply of estrogen (by having them start HRT at the time of menopause) keeps their receptors intact. However, by delaying HRT and depriving the receptors of estrogen for a prolonged period, the receptors decline and no longer can be "rekindled."

A study published in 2017 supported this theory.[27] Researchers enrolled two groups of women – one group consisted of younger women who were within six years of menopause and the second group were women ten or more years beyond menopause. The design of the study was to take a small muscle sample from each participant, treat each woman with a short course of estrogen, and then take another muscle sample following this treatment. The number of estrogen receptors was determined in the samples. The researchers found the younger women were able to retain abundant levels of estrogen receptors. The older women (those ten or more years beyond menopause) had fewer estrogen receptors and a decreased level of muscle activity compared to the younger group. So even though both groups were treated with estrogen, this did not lead to the reappearance of estrogen receptors in the older group of women.

Animal studies have also lent support to this proposition. Rats deprived of estrogen for an extended duration of time lost receptors on their arteries. Treating them with estrogen did not cause the number of receptors to increase.[28]

Research such as this, plus the clinical studies that demonstrate how HRT outcomes are affected by the age at initiation of therapy, make the Timing Hypothesis very credible. However, we don't have robust clinical studies to confirm this theory. Until (and, even if) these happen, it is unlikely there will be any change in the guidelines. So, for now, I believe it is important for women entering menopause to be aware of what we know about the Timing Hypothesis because if they are considering HRT there is a window after which starting HRT may not be advisable.

Decision Making Helper

Key Considerations

Numerous studies have suggested that taking hormones at the time of menopause decreases a woman's risk of many health disorders such as osteoporosis, heart disease, and diabetes. However, women who initiate hormone treatment late in life do not appear to achieve these benefits and may have adverse outcomes. This has led to the concept of the Timing Hypothesis. This proposes that the time a woman starts hormone replacement has a bearing on the risks and benefits of taking them.

This hypothesis may explain why studies on HRT come up with divergent results. The age of the women recruited for studies is likely a factor that affects the study outcomes.

It remains unclear why older women respond differently to HRT, but research suggests that prolonged estrogen deprivation leads to a loss of estrogen receptor function and this explains why estrogen may not be able to exert the same effects that it did when a woman was younger.

Current HRT guidelines and the Timing Hypothesis

The guidelines for initiating and taking HRT do not specifically address a woman's age with respect to the benefits and risks of hormone use.

What the guidelines don't acknowledge

The guidelines for HRT are heavily based on the WHI study, which primarily evaluated the effects of HRT on older women who initiated hormone treatment many years after the typical age of menopause. A substantial amount of data indicates that the timing of initiation of HRT is critical and the benefits of HRT outweigh the risks if they are initiated at the time of menopause. This opinion is reflected in the 2017 position statement of the North American Menopause Society which comprises thousands of menopause experts.[29]

Chapter 8
HRT and the Guidelines

Before embarking on a more detailed discussion of how hormones affect our various organ systems, I want to make certain you have a clear understanding of the current (2019) guidelines that address hormone replacement therapy.   But first, it is useful to have some background information about guidelines and how they are used in the practice of medicine.

It takes four years of college and four years of medical school to earn an MD degree. But virtually no one today starts a medical practice at that point. Most physicians spend another three to seven years doing an internship and residency program – which provides additional clinical training. In the case of subspecialists like gynecologists or cardiologists, the focus is almost exclusively in their chosen specialty fields. Internal medicine specialists (like me), family practice doctors, and geriatricians, whose jobs are to provide primary care, receive training in many diverse areas.

When physicians finally begin their practices, the learning doesn't stop. Every year new studies, new drugs, and new technologies appear on the scene. Keeping abreast of all this requires a diligent commitment to reading journals, going to continuing education programs, and learning from peers. This can be overwhelming on top of all the patient care and other administrative duties doctors have to deal with.

To help primary care physicians follow the best practices for patient care, guidelines are developed. These are usually written by a panel of experts in a particular field who review hundreds of studies published on a subject and analyze what treatments and procedures offer the best outcomes.

For instance, guidelines have been developed regarding the benefits of aspirin. It has been found that for patients who are at high risk for a stroke or heart attack, taking a daily aspirin can help prevent one of these from occurring. But for a generally healthy person, taking aspirin is either not beneficial or can cause complications such as a bleeding ulcer.   Other guidelines address when screening tests such as mammograms, colonoscopies, or PSA tests should be performed. These recommendations come from studies that have shown which of these interventions are the most effective at reducing the chances of dying from a particular cancer.

We physicians rely on guidelines because, quite frankly, it simplifies the process of knowing how to best manage patients. New studies and treatments appear every year and it is next to impossible to review all the updated research on every medical development to make these determinations on our own. Even keeping abreast of the guidelines, which change over time, can be challenging.

Guidelines – Where do they come from?

Guidelines on a particular subject can be generated by several different organizations and this is true when it comes to hormone replacement therapy. Many specialty groups such as the American College of Obstetrics and Gynecology and the American Academy of Family Physicians put out their own set of guidelines regarding menopausal management. There are also multi-disciplinary groups such as the North American Menopause Society (NAMS) and the International Menopause Society (IMS) that publish their position statements on the appropriate use of hormones.

In the U.S., there is a governmental agency called the United States Preventative Services Task Force or USPSTF. This body carries tremendous weight and is charged with analyzing data on a wide variety of preventative services and rating them as being supported by good evidence or not. For instance, they have had their say on such topics as how often we should have screening procedures, who should be tested for diabetes, and which vaccinations should be given. And, while the USPSTF was not established to determine whether insurance companies should pay for particular services, its findings are frequently used to justify coverage (or denial) of many procedures.

The Task Force assigns each recommendation a letter grade (**A**, **B**, **C**, **D**, **I**) based on the strength of the evidence and the balance of benefits and harms of a preventive service. An **A** indicates that there is high evidence to support the benefit of a service and therefore it should be offered to patients. Services that receive a **B** or a **C** are generally recommended, but the reviewers note that the evidence is not as robust and the services may not be appropriate for everyone. A **D** grade means that the USPSTF does not recommend the treatment as there appears to be no net benefit, or the harms outweigh the benefits. An **I** means there is insufficient evidence to assess the balance of the benefits and harms. It is important to be aware that the Task Force is not charged with factoring in a cost analysis in determining a recommendation grade.

The Food and Drug Administration (FDA) is a federal agency of the United States Department of Health and Human Services, one of the United States federal executive departments. It doesn't publish guidelines per se but exerts a powerful influence on how we practice medicine. The FDA's role is to protect the public health by assuring the safety, effectiveness, and quality of drugs and services available to citizens. Any prescription drug on the market has to meet not only FDA approval but this agency also must approve the content of the product labeling – those package inserts that come with your medication. Manufacturers are required to list essentially every potential side effect and risk, as well as the indications for use of the product.

Why follow the guidelines?

While physicians aren't bound by guidelines or other recommendations outlined by the USPSTF or FDA, it is prudent to follow them for a number of reasons. First of all, patients expect their providers to look out for their best interests and give advice based not just on a personal viewpoint but on the studies and expert opinions that justify the most appropriate course of treatment. For instance, there are guidelines that recommend the best choices of antibiotics for sinus infections. Unless there is a specific reason not to use the recommended antibiotics, the physician should follow the guidelines to assure the best chance of a good response.

Secondly, by following the guidelines, a physician is generally protected against an adverse judgment in a lawsuit if there is a negative outcome. For instance, patients with a heart irregularity called atrial fibrillation are generally advised to be on a strong blood thinner to prevent a stroke. However, thinning the blood carries some risk – such as causing internal bleeding. Should a serious consequence like this occur, it would be difficult to successfully sue a physician for malpractice, since he or she followed the standard of care, as outlined in the guidelines.

Payment for procedures by Medicare and other insurance companies is frequently tied to guidelines. If a guideline recommends that a particular patient should only have a colonoscopy every ten years, then getting one sooner generally won't be reimbursed unless there is a clinical reason to obtain one.

Some physicians follow guidelines "to a T" because they believe that is the best way to practice medicine. However, this can be problematic because there are many circumstances where a particular guideline may not be appropriate for a given patient or situation. After all, a guideline is intended to be a *guideline*, not something set in stone. Physicians need to weigh many factors in deciding the best course for each patient. Physicians who are very rigid in the way they follow guidelines can frequently aggravate patients who, based on their situation and preferences, request an alternative drug or treatment not recommended in the guidelines.

I often tell patients that practicing medicine is sometimes like baking a cake. Some ingredients can be substituted by other options and, even though the exact recipe isn't followed, the end result can still be a tasty dessert. The same holds true for managing a particular medical problem. Deviation from the guidelines is acceptable as long as there is a good reason to do so and the patient understands the rationale and the risks and benefits.

HRT guidelines – 2003 to 2019

As noted in previous chapters, the conclusions of the WHI led to major changes in the guidelines for hormone replacement therapy. These have persisted, and have remained essentially unchanged at the time of the writing of this book. They can be summarized by reviewing the 2019 FDA literature which reads:

> *"Indications for hormone therapy approved by the US Food and Drug Administration (FDA) in menopausal women are limited to the treatment of menopausal symptoms and the prevention of postmenopausal osteoporosis. An FDA-issued black box warning indicates that estrogen therapy, with or without progestin, should be prescribed at the lowest effective dose and for the shortest duration consistent with the patient's treatment goals and risk."*[1]

A number of points should be emphasized. This statement is basically saying that HRT is primarily approved only for current or *acute* symptoms and not for *prevention* of other conditions except for osteoporosis (which carries caveats as discussed below). So it is important to understand the difference between *acute treatment* versus *preventative treatment*. Acute treatment

100

means we are treating active symptoms – such as prescribing antibiotics for an infection, performing surgery to take out an inflamed appendix, or giving a steroid injection to calm down an inflamed joint. With respect to HRT, acute treatment means prescribing hormones for hot flashes and night sweats, and vaginal problems such as dryness.

The guidelines basically do not recommend HRT for preventative therapy, which means doing something now to prevent a problem down the line. A great deal of what we do in primary care medicine is preventative care. Most people with high blood pressure or high cholesterol do not have any acute symptoms whatsoever, and yet in many cases we strongly recommend medications, despite the fact that many of the drugs used can cause side effects or carry possible risks. The justification for doing this is that large studies have shown that over time the benefits outweigh the risks.

The FDA statement above limits the use of HRT to prevent only one condition – postmenopausal osteoporosis. This is a little misleading because this isn't a recommendation that healthy women with normal bone densities take HRT to prevent osteoporosis. When you drill down in the guidelines, estrogen is only recommended for a woman determined to be a high-risk candidate. The majority of 50-something-year-old women entering menopause do not fulfill the criteria for being high-risk and would not be candidates to take HRT to prevent osteoporosis. In addition, the guidelines recommend prescribing only the lowest dose of hormones for the shortest duration. This would hardly be the optimal treatment for preventing osteoporosis since low doses are not very effective for preserving bone density, and estrogen needs to be continued on an ongoing basis to remain effective.

What does the USPSTF have to say?

Here is where my blood starts to boil. In December 2017 the USPSTF came out with its latest recommendations regarding HRT. Prescribing hormones for menopausal women received a "**D**" rating. Recall this means that there is moderate or high certainty that there is *no net benefit to this therapy or that the harms outweigh the benefits*. The task force, therefore, discourages the use of hormonal treatment for preventative therapy.

Wow! Things have really changed since I started practicing medicine in 1981 when hormones were prescribed frequently and liberally for not only hot flashes but for preventative treatment of a number of diseases that would greatly impair a woman's later years. These included osteoporosis, heart disease, and even dementia. The results of many studies back then supported the beneficial role hormones played in warding off these conditions. Quoting excerpts from a respected textbook on menopause, *Treatment of the Postmenopausal Woman* published in 1994:

> *"Hormone replacement therapy should be viewed as specific treatment for symptoms in the short term and preventative pharmacology in the long term."* [2]

> *"Estrogen replacement therapy (ERT) can alleviate hot flashes and night sweats, relieve vaginal atrophy, prevent bone loss and osteoporotic fractures, reduce the risk of cardiovascular disease and decrease overall mortality in postmenopausal women."* [3]

The current USPSTF position is essentially a complete reversal of the advice found in this textbook and has not helped promote the use of HRT. In fact, it has tarnished its reputation further. While the task force is charged with addressing only the *preventative* indications for HRT, the conclusion of their recent statement left many women, as well as their health care providers, with the impression that estrogen therapy is inappropriate under any circumstances.

This is unfortunate and has frustrated me and other health care providers who feel that the task force relied too heavily on the WHI to come to its conclusions. This sentiment was reflected in an article that appeared in the *Climacteric* magazine, a respected menopause journal. The article was entitled, *Why The USPSTF Got it Wrong*.[4]

The impact of the post-WHI guidelines

Many of us who take care of menopausal women are uncomfortable with the current guidelines for HRT. Those of us who were in practice years ago when HRT was popular had a chance to personally follow and observe our patients over many years while they were on treatment. We were pleased to see they maintained strong bones and were mentally sharp and vibrant. They had excellent cholesterol levels and rarely seemed to develop heart disease. They looked good, and they felt good. So making an abrupt turn in the way we were told to manage menopause has been difficult to accept.

Younger physicians graduating from medical school after 2002 have a much different attitude about hormones. They have grown up with the current guidelines and don't have the historical perspective of the doctors of my generation. Very few of the new doctors that I have encountered encourage HRT, and in fact, have systematically been taking their patients off HRT if they aren't having any symptoms (and sometimes even if they are!)

The current guidelines make writing prescriptions for hormones much more problematic than in the past. While it is always prudent for physicians to document that they discussed benefits and risks of any treatment, doing so for HRT requires much more detailed charting. And not infrequently there is push back from insurance companies. I've lost count of the numerous letters I have received from some quality assurance department at Medicare or Blue Cross gently reminding me that I should re-evaluate whether a patient should continue on HRT. In some cases, a patient's insurance company would not authorize payment for her estrogen refill until I made phone calls and filled out a lengthy form to justify my prescription. All of this extra effort has been frustrating and time-consuming, and it all stems from these institutions reacting to the guidelines.

However, there may be light at the end of the tunnel. The pendulum regarding prescribing HRT may be starting to swing in another direction. The 2017 position statement from the respected North American Menopause Society has modified its position from the original post-WHI guidelines to suggest that doctors consider prescribing estrogen in *"adequate doses to control symptoms"* and *"for as long as necessary."* [5]

However, even this more liberal endorsement falls short of encouraging HRT for preventing chronic diseases, and limits treatment primarily to women having symptoms. We likely are a long way from getting back to where we were with respect to recommending hormone treatment for preventing chronic conditions. To me, this is unfortunate. Concerns stemming from the WHI about the safety of estrogen have overshadowed the many other studies that have attested to the preventative benefits of HRT.

In the following chapters of this book, I describe each organ system and review how hormone replacement therapy may play a role, not only for treating acute symptoms, but in preventing complications in each of these systems. The goal is to give you enough background information to help you decide if taking HRT will not only improve your life now but for many years to come.

Decision Making Helper

<u>Key considerations</u>

Current (2019) guidelines are based heavily on the 2002 WHI study. Its conclusions have led to the recommendations that HRT should be limited to women having hot flashes and that the lowest dose of hormones be prescribed for the shortest duration of time to control symptoms.

Guidelines are formulated by experts in a given field and are intended to reflect best practices – meaning that by following these recommendations, studies have shown that patients will receive the best results, with the most benefit and least risk. Most guidelines rely heavily on studies considered to be the most definitive, which are randomized, controlled studies.

Guidelines change over time as new information is acquired.

Guidelines are meant to be *guidelines* and in some circumstances may not be the best course for every patient depending on that patient's unique medical situation and preferences.

Regarding the guidelines for HRT, women should be aware of the distinction between taking HRT to treat symptoms, such as hot flashes, versus taking them to prevent long-term consequences.

Chapter 9
Estrogen and Your Uterus and Ovaries

You would be surprised how many older women are unclear about what organs they had removed when they had a *hysterectomy*. In their defense, most were raised during the days when women tended not to ask too many questions or even remotely challenge their physician's advice. And the internet wasn't at their fingertips – like today when in an instant you can find the nearest open pharmacy or check out which neurosurgeon should repair your aneurysm! It was also a time when uteruses and ovaries were removed much more readily than they are today.[1]

A hysterectomy refers to the surgical removal of the uterus. In the past, when women required a hysterectomy, surgeons would frequently remove most of the uterus, leaving the *cervix* (the bottom tip of the uterus) in place – believing that it played a role in achieving sexual satisfaction. However, this is no longer felt to be true,[2,3] and removing the entire uterus is now the generally accepted procedure. During my career, I occasionally came across one of these retained cervical stubs while doing a pelvic exam. It was always somewhat of a surprise to me, and frequently to the patient as well! (Note: since the primary purpose of a PAP smear is to detect cancer of the cervix, after a hysterectomy, a PAP smear is no longer needed unless the surgeon left the cervix in place.)

Hysterectomies are still one of the most frequently performed surgeries in the U.S. Approximately one in nine women eventually have one – generally to treat benign diseases – the most frequent problem being fibroids (discussed below). During a hysterectomy, the uterus is removed either through an open incision on the tummy, or it can be taken out through the vagina. Some surgeons even perform this procedure using a laparoscope. Laparoscopy is the technique where surgery is performed using tiny surgical instruments and a video camera inserted through slender tubes poked into the abdominal wall. When I heard about removing the uterus with this technique, the first question that came to mind was how an organ the size of a small pear gets pulled out of an incision less than an inch long! The answer is that the uterus is cut up or pulverized and placed into a "baggy" which can then be squeezed out through the hole. This procedure is being performed more commonly, especially as more surgeons are being trained in robotic surgery.[4] Robotic surgery is the most recent refinement of laparoscopic surgery – where instead of manipulating the little instruments directly, hand controls similar to the ones used to play video games are used. The surgeon can even be sitting across the room from the patient while performing an operation. This technology is truly amazing and you can appreciate why young doctors trained today are very good at this – since many had extensive gaming experience growing up!

Recently, the FDA has expressed concern about removing the uterus in this manner because of the rare chance that chopping it up could allow cells from an unsuspected cancer to escape and spread.[5] Most surgeons feel this would be extremely unlikely, as the diagnosis of cancer would almost always be known prior to surgery and in that case, this type of procedure would not be used. At any rate, laparoscopic or robotic surgeries are commonly performed for other gynecologic conditions such as tubal ligations and treating endometriosis.

If a premenopausal woman has had her uterus removed, her ovaries will continue to produce hormones. She will no longer have monthly menstrual periods, but she still may have symptoms, such as breast tenderness, caused by her hormones as their levels fluctuate throughout the month. In addition, she will also experience typical menopausal symptoms, such as hot flashes and mood swings, when her ovaries do eventually quit functioning.

If an ovary is removed, either separately or along with the uterus, the term for this is an *oophorectomy*. If a fallopian tube is removed, the term for this is a *salpingectomy*. There are a number of reasons why a woman may need to have her tubes or ovaries removed, including tumors, large cysts, infections, or endometriosis. If all of the female organs are taken out in one procedure, the appropriate term is a *hysterosalpingo-oophorectomy*. (You can see why it's just easier for a woman to say she had a complete hysterectomy!)

In the past, if a woman nearing menopause needed to have a hysterectomy for a benign condition, the surgeon frequently recommended that she also have an oophorectomy. The rationale behind this was that, since she was already going to have surgery, she might as well have her ovaries removed at the same time since they would be shutting down soon anyway. By doing so, she wouldn't need to worry about getting ovarian cancer in the future. (I have to admit that earlier in my career I was guilty of using this reasoning in discussions with my patients.)

We now know that this is not good advice. Besides the fact that abruptly removing the ovaries and throwing a woman into menopause overnight is associated with much more dramatic symptoms, there are other downsides. Studies have revealed that women who go through menopause earlier than expected have an increased risk of future health problems, including osteoporosis, heart disease, diabetes, and even premature death.[6,7] An awareness of this information has made many gynecologists more cautious about performing bilateral oophorectomies. Furthermore, more attention is being paid to thinking twice about performing other surgeries that may cause an earlier than normal menopause. It has been shown that removing just one ovary can cause an earlier menopause.[8] Even a simple hysterectomy can push a woman into menopause sooner than would be expected – by as much as five years![5] It is presumed that this occurs because by removing the uterus the blood supply to the ovaries gets compromised which can affect the health of the ovary. But other factors may be involved.

Hormones and the uterus and cancer

At the time of menopause, the ovaries are depleted of eggs and no longer produce estrogen and progesterone. Without ongoing stimulation from these hormones, the lining of the uterus no longer undergoes the cyclic changes that produce the menstrual flow. These are the hallmarks of menopause – the loss of fertility and the end of monthly periods. After menopause, the uterus no longer has any real function. If a woman initiates HRT at the time of menopause, however, the uterus will respond to these hormones. The uterine lining will build up and slough off in the same manner as it did during the reproductive years.

I was visiting with some of my old high school friends recently and we ended up sharing menopause stories. One of them reported that she didn't go through menopause until she was 63! I had to inform her that this was impossible. It turned out that she had been taking HRT and didn't really understand that these hormones were simply creating the menstrual flow artificially. The estrogen caused the lining inside the uterus to build up, and when she took the progesterone during the last half of the cycle (which is a common way of administering HRT) – the lining would slough off. So in essence, she was basically having "fake" periods. She didn't realize that she had actually lost her eggs years earlier and was already way past menopause.

When women like my friend take HRT in this manner, they will continue to see some monthly bleeding for a number of years until the uterus ages and no longer responds to the hormonal stimulation. At that point, no further bleeding will occur. As time goes on, both the uterus and ovaries shrink in size. In many older women, radiologists can't even see the ovaries on ultrasounds as they are so small.

The chance of developing uterine cancer for women not on HRT is about two to three per 10,000.[10] Most of these cancers originate within the internal lining of the uterus, the endometrium, and thus are referred to as *endometrial cancers*. Taking estrogen by itself, without a progestogen, increases the risk of endometrial cancer up to four to ten times the normal rate. This became apparent when doctors first started treating menopause with estrogen alone. It was then established in the early 1970s that adding a progestogen to estrogen would prevent these cancers from developing. In fact, combined treatment dramatically reduces the risk and may even decrease it below expected rates. In the WHI study, women who took combined Premarin and Provera had a lower incidence of uterine cancer than women on a placebo not only during the five years of the study when they were on the hormones but had lower rates of cancer some 13 years later in the long-term follow-up study.[11]

All forms of estrogen (except extremely low doses and the low-dose vaginal preparations designed exclusively to treat vaginal dryness), if taken without a progestogen, can increase the risk of endometrial cancer. Any type of progestogen reduces this risk – as long as an adequate amount is given. In the U.S. medroxyprogesterone (Provera) was the drug commonly used in early HRT formulations. It is very effective at protecting the uterus and is about 100 times more potent than natural progesterone. Although natural progesterone is weaker in its actions, taking the standard dose of 100 mg daily appears to adequately protect the uterus. This daily regimen may be slightly more effective than taking 200 mg for the last 12 to 14 days of each month, although there are few studies comparing these two options. Many providers believe it is acceptable for women to take 200 mg progesterone cyclically every two to three months, instead of on a monthly basis. This likely will also protect the uterus, but experts acknowledge we don't have large studies to assess this. Some gynecologists advocate that if progesterone is given less frequently than monthly, women should be screened periodically with an ultrasound to make sure there is no buildup of the endometrial lining.

As noted in Chapter 3, progesterone applied topically to the skin is poorly absorbed – so many experts discourage this mode of treatment because of concerns that adequate amounts may not reach the uterus to protect women from cancer. However, vaginally inserted progesterone 45 to 50 mg daily administered 12 to 14 days per month appears to be highly protective.[12] These doses are lower than what is given orally because the progesterone presumably only has to travel a short distance to get to the uterus to be effective.

Vaginal progesterone products are available in some European countries. In the U.S. there are commercial vaginal progesterone products designated for use in infertility treatments and managing certain pregnancy complications, but these are not approved for HRT use.[13] Women can obtain intravaginal progesterone from compounding pharmacies and many naturopathic physicians and longevity clinics treat women with these products – but as has been noted previously, these pharmacies do not receive strict FDA oversight.

Another way of counteracting the estrogen effects on the uterus is to insert a progestogen directly into the uterus by means of an IUD containing a progestin. One such IUD, the Mirena device, is being used by gynecologists in HRT regimens, but these devices are currently approved by the FDA only for use as a contraceptive and treating abnormal menstrual bleeding.

Other non-progestogen options are also being evaluated as a means to prevent estrogen-induced uterine cancer. There has been research into developing SERMs that would be effective in protecting the uterus. We may be seeing more of these in the future, but so far the only SERM on the market that counteracts estrogen effects in the uterus is Bazedoxifene. In the U.S. this drug is only available in a product containing a low dose of conjugated estrogens.

One thing to mention again is that there are a number of very low-dose estrogen products designed to be inserted in the vagina to specifically treat vaginal dryness. Most experts feel that the dose of estrogen in these agents is so small that it is not necessary to take a progestogen along with these preparations.

A few comments on uterine cancer

Any kind of cancer is scary, but endometrial cancer generally carries a fairly good prognosis – in that most women who develop it don't die from it and live full lives. This is because these cancers are usually slow-growing and are typically found at a curable stage. Unlike some cancers that can grow quite large before causing symptoms, very small uterine cancers tend to disrupt the blood vessels lining the endometrium and cause vaginal bleeding, which can be an early warning sign that cancer is developing inside the uterus. Whether a woman is on HRT or not, any abnormal bleeding should be reported to a health care provider and be investigated with further tests.

Once a woman has been diagnosed and treated for uterine cancer, the question may arise as to whether she would ever be a candidate for HRT. This has been studied. A large review showed that women who have been cured or treated for small, low-grade, endometrial cancers are not at a higher risk for recurrence or death if they take HRT.[14] However, it is not advisable for women with more advanced uterine cancer to take estrogen.

Hormones and other uterine conditions

I remember an encounter during medical school when I interviewed an elderly patient admitted for a hysterectomy. She had a thick southern accent and wasn't at all bashful about educating me, a naïve second-year medical student, about her condition. She had come down with "fireballs in the Eucharist" (or at least that's what it sounded like to me). It wasn't until years later that I learned that this term was used commonly in the south to describe uterine fibroids!

Fibroids are benign growths that develop within the wall of the uterus, much like a burl in a tree. They are extremely common. Approximately one out of three women have symptoms from them at some point in their lives, and up to 80% of hysterectomy specimens contain them.[15] When fibroids are located close to the inside surface of the uterus, they disrupt blood vessels and cause abnormal bleeding, especially around the time of menopause. This is how they generally are discovered. Although they tend to grow (even to the size of a pumpkin!), it is extremely rare for one ever to become malignant. Fibroids are stimulated by hormones and so they tend to shrink once a woman goes through menopause. Because the hormone levels achieved with HRT are lower than during the reproductive years, HRT doesn't affect fibroids in most cases. But sometimes they can enlarge, which could cause symptoms such as bleeding or discomfort. While historically we have assumed that it is estrogen that has the most effect, it may be that the synthetic progestins, such as medroxyprogesterone, are the real culprits promoting the growth of these fibroids.[16]

110

Hormones and the cervix

The cervix is the only part of the uterus that we can see directly. When we insert a speculum to do a PAP smear we look right at it. The cervix has a different type of cell covering it than exists inside the uterus. For this reason, it behaves differently than the endometrium in response to HRT. Almost all cases of cervical cancer are caused by the HPV (human papillomavirus), which causes genital warts. HRT does not appear to increase a woman's risk of cervical cancer.[17]

HRT and the ovaries

One day I overheard a woman say to a friend that she was glad to find out that her recent PAP smear came back normal – and relieved to know that she didn't have ovarian cancer. Like many women I have encountered over the years, she was not aware that a PAP smear is used to detect cervical cancer and has nothing to do with ovarian cancer. In fact, even doing a thorough pelvic exam doesn't help us diagnose this dreaded malignancy. The ovaries are so small and so deep inside the lower abdomen that it is almost impossible to feel them even in the most slender of women. So trying to detect a cancer growing inside this already diminutive organ is highly improbable until it starts causing symptoms. By that time, the cancer has usually spread outside of the ovary into the abdominal cavity. Even at this point, the symptoms may be subtle – such as mild bloating. This is why this is such a bad disease. By the time it gets diagnosed, it is already at an advanced stage.

The jury is out on how HRT affects the risk of ovarian cancer. Many women assume that hormones increase the risk but there are no convincing studies to support this. Some studies have shown a slightly increased risk and some a decreased risk.[18] In the WHI study, there was no increased risk in women on Premarin and Provera, and only one more case of ovarian cancer (four cases instead of three) in women taking estrogen alone.

As far as whether HRT is safe for women who have been treated for ovarian cancer, there is no evidence that taking hormones worsens outcomes. A large review of many studies did not find that these women developed a higher risk of recurrent ovarian cancer or death.[19]

A related question that has arisen is whether women known to have a genetic defect that increases the risk of ovarian cancer should consider HRT. A well-known example of this would be the BRCA gene abnormality which significantly increases a woman's chance of breast cancer as well as ovarian cancer. Although there is limited data regarding this, taking HRT has not been shown to increase the risk of cancer in these patients.[20] Most experts agree, however, that women with any genetic disorder of this nature should thoroughly discuss their options with their health care team, especially their oncologists.

Estrogen exerts effects on other areas of the female genitourinary system – such as the vagina and urinary tract. These areas will be covered in Chapter 16.

Decision Making Helper

Key considerations

Women with an intact uterus who wish to take estrogen should also take a progestogen to prevent uterine cancer. Any type of a progestogen taken in adequate doses will be protective. Progesterone creams applied to the skin, however, may not be reliably absorbed and therefore may not lead to adequate levels in the uterine tissue to counteract the estrogen effects. Vaginal progesterone, usually in doses half that recommended for oral use, appears to be effective, but more studies are needed, and there are no FDA approved vaginal progesterone products for HRT use. Progestogen-containing IUDs, which are on the market as contraceptives, appear to be effective for use in HRT, but are not approved by the FDA for this purpose.

Fibroids are very common and tend to shrink in size after menopause. HRT does not usually cause them to enlarge.

Taking HRT is generally safe in women who have been treated for low-grade uterine cancer, but is not advisable for women with active uterine cancer or women with a history of advanced cancer.

HRT does not increase the risk of cervical cancer.

Studies have not shown conclusively if taking HRT has an effect on the risk of developing ovarian cancer. Whether women with a history of ovarian cancer or a genetic risk for ovarian cancer are at higher risk if they take HRT is also unclear.

Any abnormal vaginal bleeding or unexplained abdominal symptoms such as bloating or pain should be promptly evaluated by a medical provider.

112

Current guidelines regarding HRT and the uterus and ovaries

The FDA requires that all commercial products for estrogen carry a warning that taking estrogen without a progestogen may increase the risk of uterine cancer.

What the guidelines don't acknowledge

Taking estrogen along with a progestogen may decrease a woman's chance of uterine cancer. Although more definitive studies are needed, HRT appears to pose a very low risk for promoting any other type of gynecological cancers.

Chapter 10
Estrogen and Your Breasts

Does estrogen cause breast cancer? I bet most women automatically assume that it does. This is because, over the years, various medical studies as well as experts in the field have been telling us that there is an association between estrogen use and breast cancer. The minute a woman gets diagnosed with breast cancer, or even has a suspicious mammogram, one of the first things a doctor (including me) tells her to do is to stop her hormones.

As I reflect back on my many years of practice, I wish that I had spent more time talking to my patients who had been newly diagnosed with breast cancer to see what was going through their minds. Did they assume that taking estrogen caused their cancers? Did they wish they had never taken it? Did they worry that their decision to take HRT shortened their lives? Would putting up with hot flashes have been a small price to pay for avoiding cancer?

It would be a shame if women agonized too much over these questions because the truth of the matter is that taking estrogen likely had nothing to do with their cancers – and what's more, their prognoses may actually turn out better because they had taken them! I know this sounds incredible, but there is considerable research showing that women who have never taken hormones who develop breast cancer don't fare as well as women who have taken them.

Women need to know this type of information because the fear of breast cancer is one of the top reasons why women shy away from HRT. In this chapter, I will review the curious relationship between hormones and breast cancer, and I suspect you will be very surprised to read what we have learned.

What is cancer?

Before moving on, it is helpful to better understand what cancer is and how it develops. So, let's start at the very beginning – from the moment of conception. After an egg and sperm unite, cell division begins – transforming an embryo into a fetus. The cells divide at an exponential rate as tiny organs are formed and quickly enlarge. Rapid cell replication continues after birth as the newborn progresses through childhood, adolescence, and then finally into an adult. But even when we are fully grown, our cells don't remain static. They continue to actively multiply, replacing themselves as needed and repairing aged and damaged tissue.

In the process of replication, a cell's DNA separates into two strands which then go on to create two identical cells. This process, occurring millions of times per day in millions of cells is subject to an "error" which can lead to a defective cell. Most of these "errors" don't cause obvious problems, and in fact, some are beneficial – which is the basis of the theory of evolution. However, some of these genetic accidents involve the cell's ability to regulate its own replication – ignoring signals to stop reproducing. This is the underlying issue with cancer. I often describe cancer as misguided cells gone wild. These cells divide unchecked, and then can invade a lymph or blood vessel where they can spread via the circulatory system to destinations throughout the body. These deposits, known as *metastases*, settle in their new locations, multiply unfettered, and grow into tumors.

Fortunately, in most cases our own immune systems can detect these deranged cells early and eradicate them before they grow unbridled and turn into a full-blown case of cancer. Patients with an immune deficiency such as AIDS or patients taking immune-suppressing drugs such as those for rheumatoid arthritis and other autoimmune diseases have an increased risk of cancer. Their bodies' immune systems are being suppressed by these drugs and cannot effectively fight defective cells that can turn into cancer.

In many cases, it is difficult to know if a small cancer has sent out "daughter" cancer cells to other parts of the body, as these tiny malignant deposits cannot be detected by even the best MRI scans until they grow to a certain size. That is why cancer may suddenly pop up five or more years later at a remote site after the original tumor was removed. In most of these cases, the cancer had already spread at the initial time of diagnosis; we just didn't have the tools to detect it.

This is a very important concept to realize when reading the studies on hormones and breast cancer. If a woman is enrolled in a study and then develops breast cancer within a year (or even up to five or more years later!), her cancer most likely was pre-existing and not caused by the treatment being studied.

Some cells in our body hardly divide at all – such as our nerve cells. Others, such as our red and white blood cells, divide frequently. When any tissue in our body gets injured for some reason, such as from a severe sunburn, the cells multiply rapidly to repair the damage. The more frequently a cell divides the more chance an error can occur. *Anything that makes cells turn over faster increases this risk.* This is another important concept to grasp because it has a lot to do with how hormones relate to breast cancer. Breast cells exposed to hormones will be stimulated to divide.

Many factors increase a person's risk of developing cancer. We know that cancer tends to run in certain families. This is because there are inherited defects that interfere with normal DNA replication and the body's ability to fight cancer cells. Such is the case in patients carrying a mutation in the **BRCA,** or **Breast Cancer,** gene. The BRCA gene is responsible for making a protein that acts to suppress or decrease tumors. Patients whose bodies can't make this protein because they have a dysfunctional BRCA gene are at risk for several types of cancers. There are two types of these breast cancer susceptibility genes, called BRCA1 and BRCA2. If a woman carries one of these abnormal genes her future risk of developing breast cancer at some point in her lifetime is on the order of 60% to 75%. However, most women (nearly 95%) who do develop breast cancer do not have a defective BRCA gene.

Is estrogen a carcinogen?

Is estrogen a carcinogen? A carcinogen is defined as *an agent that leads to cancer.* Intuitively, it doesn't seem logical that a substance naturally present in our body such as estrogen would be a carcinogen. But according to the *American Cancer Society (*ACS*)*, all estrogen and progestogen drugs are considered carcinogenic (this would include birth control pills and bioidentical hormones). They are listed on the ACS website alongside asbestos, arsenic, benzene, mustard gas, and a number of other overtly toxic substances. Certainly, landing this categorization is worrisome – so no wonder people fear that hormones cause breast cancer. However, the keywords to focus on in the definition of a carcinogen are in the phrase – *an agent* that *leads to cancer.* There is no distinction between something actually *initiating* cancer versus something *promoting* cancer. This is where the murkiness about HRT comes in.

We know that female hormones stimulate breast cells to divide. This occurs during puberty, pregnancy, in women on HRT, or in a transsexual woman treated with hormones to promote female characteristics. Both estrogen and progesterone stimulate cell division. They act on different areas of the breast. Estrogen primarily stimulates the milk ducts and progesterone stimulates the milk glands. Under the influence of these hormones, the breast develops the infrastructure to prepare it for milk production in the event of pregnancy.

After menopause, when the hormone levels go down, cell division slows down. The ducts and glands shrink and most of the breast tissue is replaced with fat. However, if HRT is administered, cell division continues. The fact that the breast cells in women taking hormones divide more frequently than women not taking hormones theoretically could put them at more risk for a random error that may produce cancer. So technically this could be construed to mean that hormones *promote* cancer and this may be why the American Cancer Society feels justified in listing hormones on their site. However, this is much different than the way other carcinogens act, such as radiation which is directly toxic to DNA.

The puzzling part about this, however, is that if it is a matter of high hormone levels stimulating breast cells, why don't we see more breast cancer in younger women whose ovaries produce much higher levels of estrogen and progesterone than we see in women on HRT; or in pregnancy where the hormone levels are astronomical? There have been some interesting thoughts and developments that may help us better understand these issues, which I will present later in this chapter.

Studies linking hormones to breast cancer

It is not surprising that, over the years, estrogen was suspected as a cause of breast cancer. It has been observed that the shorter the duration that a woman's body is exposed to estrogen, the less likely it is that she will develop breast cancer. Women who started having menstrual periods late, or women going through menopause early, appeared to have lower risks of breast cancer.[1] Conversely, the longer the exposure – by going through menarche early or by having menopause late in life – the higher the risk. These observations, as well as animal studies in the early 1900s that demonstrated that estrogen administration increased breast cancer in rats,[2] led to the assumption that estrogen therapy increased the risk of breast cancer.

Therefore, it is not surprising that as HRT became increasingly popular in the mid-1900s, the number of women being diagnosed with breast cancer started climbing. Data from the Nurses Study was published in 1993 and reported that women taking HRT experienced higher rates of breast cancer.[3] Following this, a review of 50 studies conducted prior to 1997 concluded that postmenopausal HRT increased the risk of developing breast cancer by 2.3% per year of use.[4]

Essentially, ever since doctors started treating women with hormones, there has been an assumption that they would increase the risk of breast cancer. However, because it was believed that the benefits of HRT in preventing heart attacks and fractures outweighed the risk of breast cancer, treating women with hormones was accepted as the standard of care. More women were dying of heart disease than from all forms of cancer. In addition, prior to widespread hormone use, thousands of women were compressing their spines, fracturing their hips, and facing postoperative complications or languishing in nursing homes. However, while those of us in practice routinely prescribed the commonly available HRT products, what wasn't appreciated was whether the type of hormones used would be a factor in the risks and benefits.

The progestogen breast cancer connection

As noted, since the 1970s, it has been standard practice to prescribe a progestogen along with estrogen as a necessary measure to prevent uterine cancer. There was not much concern about any downsides to doing this. In fact, there was a tacit assumption that since a progestogen counteracted the negative effects of estrogen on the uterus, it should be doing the same in the breasts. And along with that, any progestogen would do. We did not pay much attention to whether the specific progestogen made a difference. We generally assumed that it was estrogen that was the culprit in regards to breast cancer – somewhat dismissing the role of the progestogen. We now know this was shortsighted.

A few early medical studies did allude to the possibility that progestogens may increase the risk of breast cancer, but it has only been in the last 10 to 15 years that the issue has become increasingly apparent. The results of a very large study from the United Kingdom, the Million Woman Study, were published in 2003. The investigators followed a large group of women ages 50 to 64 for about 6 years.[5] Women on combination therapy (meaning they were taking a progestogen along with an estrogen) were found to have a higher rate of breast cancer and breast cancer deaths than women on estrogen alone. Another large study that enrolled 54,548 women found similar results – women using combination therapy demonstrated an increased risk of breast cancer compared to non-users, but women on estrogen alone showed no increased risk.[6] Other studies have shown similar results.[7,8]

These were large observational studies and, as discussed previously in this book, randomized clinical trials are generally necessary to confirm the findings from these types of studies. So even though the investigators in charge of the WHI suspected that they would find that women treated with combined estrogen-progestogen therapy would have higher rates of breast cancer, the way the results were publicized and disseminated gave many women the impression that this was shockingly new information. The actual press release from the sponsors of the study, the National Institute of Health, read:

> *"NHLBI Stops Trial of Estrogen Plus Progestin Due to Increased Breast Cancer Risk, Lack of Overall Benefit"* [9]

The press picked this up and had a field day with it. Never mind that an increase in breast cancer diagnoses was anticipated to occur, and that these numbers were actually quite small, and that it really wasn't the breast cancer issue but the cardiovascular results that were unexpected. What seemed to be indelibly instilled in everyone's mind going forward was the impression that HRT causes breast cancer – so much so that the results of the second branch of the WHI study which came out two years later seemed to go unnoticed by the general population. This was the branch of the WHI where women were treated only with estrogen. The conclusions of this arm of the study were that *women taking estrogen alone had a **decrease** in the incidence of breast cancer compared to women on a placebo.*

This striking outcome did not get anywhere near the fanfare from the media that was elicited by the earlier study. The findings were either ignored or dismissed by many health care providers and certainly did not prompt the guideline writers to change their recommendations on hormone replacement therapy. Needless to say, by that time the fallout from the earlier branch of the WHI had caused immediate and long-lasting reluctance in both women and their providers to embrace any form of HRT.

Fortunately, the puzzling differences in the results of the two branches of the WHI study spurred further investigation and commentary by the experts. Why would combination therapy put women at a higher risk of breast cancer? And why, for heaven's sake, did the women taking estrogen alone have a *decreased* risk of breast cancer? We will tackle the first issue, and then move on to the second.

More insights on progestogen – the elephant in the room

As noted, both estrogen and progesterone stimulate breast tissue. During a woman's reproductive years, her mammogram reflects this. The myriad ducts and glands show up on the mammogram images as whitish lines and speckles scattered across a grey background – the grey representing fat tissue. After menopause, the breasts are composed mainly of fat so the mammograms of postmenopausal women who are not on HRT look like big (or little, for some of us) homogenous grey blobs. If women take HRT, however, the mammograms have more lines and speckles and appear more like those of premenopausal women. Radiologists frequently describe their breasts as being dense and note in their comments that the findings likely are due to HRT.

I received many such reports on my patients and always reviewed their charts to confirm they were on HRT as an explanation for the findings. However, I admit that for many years I did not give much further thought on whether they were on estrogen alone versus estrogen plus a progestogen. However, we now realize that the mammograms of women on estrogen alone don't show nearly the degree of these white densities that appear on the mammograms of women taking both hormones.[10,11] It takes estrogen combined with a progestogen to cause these changes – which basically are due to a greater degree of breast cell proliferation. This observation has also been apparent when biopsies of breast tissue are examined microscopically. Women on combined HRT have higher concentrations of breast cells compared to women on estrogen alone.[11]

The fact that combined hormone therapy promotes cell division more than estrogen alone might explain why combined therapy would be more likely to promote breast cancer. However, the puzzling part about this is why, during our reproductive years (and especially with pregnancy), do we not see more breast cancer? You would expect that since the breast cells in young women are being stimulated by their high levels of hormones, there would be a high risk of a malignant error. This doesn't occur and while there is ongoing research investigating this, one interesting issue is emerging. The elephant in the room, so to speak, is turning out to be something about the *synthetic* progestogens.

Natural progesterone for HRT treatment wasn't approved until 1998 and affordable generic versions did not become available for widespread use until almost ten years later. So, much of the data we have accumulated over the years on the risks and benefits of HRT have come from women treated with synthetic versions. Medroxyprogesterone (Provera) has historically been the most common progestogen used in the U.S. Other synthetic progestins have been used in other countries.

What has become apparent is that different progestogens have different effects on the breasts, which in turn can impact a tendency to developing breast cancer.[12] A French study of 3,175 postmenopausal women followed over nine years found that women on estradiol plus medroxyprogesterone had an increased rate of breast cancer, but women on other synthetic progestogens did not.[13] A recent meta-analysis reviewed 14 studies that included women on a number of different progestogens (along with an estrogen). This analysis revealed that two particular progestogens, *levonorgestrel* (this is one found in many birth control pills) and *norethisterone*, were associated with higher rates of breast cancer than the rates associated with *dydrogesterone* (a synthetic progestin used commonly in Europe).[14] A few of the studies in this review included women treated with natural progesterone, and these women did not demonstrate a higher rate of cancer. This study and other research alerted us that not only do some progestogens cause more adverse effects than others but natural progesterone may have a greater safety profile with respect to breast cancer risk than synthetics.[15]

Why would this be? In some respects, it is not surprising because synthetics differ structurally in their molecular configurations not only from progesterone but also from each other. As noted in Chapter 7, for any hormone to cause an effect it first must attach to its receptor. This union leads to changes in the cell including signals to the DNA. Progesterone fits into the progesterone receptor like a glove, but the synthetics may only partially fit, and therefore may not trigger the same reactions as natural progesterone. In addition, they may elicit some untoward effects. Research has shown that medroxyprogesterone and some of the other synthetic forms can actually lead to the production of certain proteins that may promote cancer![16] Other undesirable cellular processes may be affected by synthetic progestins – such as pathways involving the immune system that play an essential role in guarding against cancer.

Even though it appears that some synthetic progestogens may be the real culprits behind an increased breast cancer risk, it is important to emphasize that the risk attributable to taking a synthetic progestin is very low. Millions of women have been treated with them without developing cancer. Recall that in the five-year-long WHI study there were only about 50 more cases of breast cancer in the 8,000 women taking combined Premarin and Provera.[17] This roughly equates to one additional case of breast cancer per 1,000 users annually. Many menopause experts point out that this is the same degree of risk of breast cancer attributable to drinking one glass of wine daily.[18] In fact, drinking two glasses of wine daily increases your risk of breast cancer more than taking combination HRT! Similarly, being obese, taking a statin drug like Lipitor for high cholesterol, and not exercising regularly all pose about the same risk as taking hormone therapy with an estrogen plus a synthetic progestogen.[18]

Is there a distinction between causing cancer and promoting cancer?

The other issue to revisit is the subtle but significant question of whether combined HRT actually *causes* breast cancer, or merely *promotes* it. Recall that the WHI study only went on for about five years. Breast cancer doesn't just pop up out of the blue – in most cases, it takes years (even up to 15 years!) before it is large enough to show up on a mammogram. There is an interesting analysis where experts ran calculations on the expected growth rates of typical breast cancers and applied this to the women in the WHI.[19,20] It was estimated that 94% of the cancers diagnosed during the WHI study *were already present* before the women enrolled in the study. *Therefore, most of those cancers that became apparent during that five-year period were pre-existing!* The presumption from this is that there may have been the same number of early cancers in both groups of women, but the tumors in the women taking HRT were stimulated to divide faster, and so showed up earlier on their mammograms. This suggests that HRT promoted cancer, rather than actually causing it.

This information and analysis may not be very reassuring. The distinction between promoting cancer versus causing cancer may seem like inconsequential semantics to most women. Why even consider taking something that might make a small cancer grow faster? You would think that this would increase your chances of dying sooner.

Interestingly, this is not the case. A number of studies have shown that women who take HRT actually have a lower rate of dying from their breast cancer than women who do not. Two studies by Danish researchers published in 2012 and 2014 reported this observation.[21,22] Shortly after this, researchers in Finland analyzed data from almost 490,000 women regarding their cancer and death statistics.[23] Over the period studied, one out of ten women died from breast cancer. But when they looked at how many women died from breast cancer who had taken HRT, the rate was much lower – one out of 20. This indicates that taking hormones substantially (50%!) decreased one's risk of dying from breast cancer. It was also noted that this benefit was greater the younger a woman was when starting HRT and persisted even if women continued on hormones for over ten years.

Another interesting piece of information relating to this subject comes from a long-term follow-up study of the WHI participants. Appearing in the *Journal of the American Medical Association* in 2017, the article provided an update on the status of a number of women from the original groups.[24] The conclusion of the report was that *"neither the women who had been on estrogen alone nor those in the estrogen-progestogen arm that developed breast cancer died from this disease any earlier than women who had been on placebo."* I think the findings are quite significant and remarkable, but this study only generated a blip of attention from the media.

Since the women in the WHI study were on HRT for only five years, we don't know what the outcome would have been if they had been on them longer. While this is a matter of speculation, one thing that this information should do is give women some reassurance that taking either of these HRT regimens for up to five years is not going to increase their risk of dying from breast cancer.

No doubt, this is perplexing. Taking estrogen combined with a synthetic progestogen may increase breast cancer, but it doesn't necessarily increase your risk from dying from it. More research is needed to explain why this occurs. One possibility that has been proposed is that women on hormones visit their providers more frequently and may have mammograms performed more regularly – thus their cancers get diagnosed and treated earlier resulting in better outcomes. To me, this seems unlikely. While this theory may explain the findings in observational studies, women enrolled in clinical studies are followed very closely regardless of whether they are on a placebo or on HRT.

The more likely explanation is that somehow taking HRT may predispose women to more favorable, less aggressive types of cancer. It is conceivable that the hormones somehow modify the nature of the cancer so that it behaves differently – perhaps making it less likely to spread or to be more amenable to treatment. There has been some research to support this possibility, but more data is needed to be able to know with any certainty.[25] Perhaps, by being exposed to HRT, cancer retains its estrogen and progesterone receptors to a greater degree – which portends a more favorable prognosis.

Coming full circle - does estrogen <u>decrease</u> the risk of breast cancer?

It still astounds me that very few people realize that the women in the WHI who were taking estrogen alone had a *lower risk* of breast cancer than the women on a placebo. This is perplexing and has invited much speculation. An important aspect of the WHI that likely has a bearing on this issue is the age of the women in the study. The majority of women were older and most had gone ten to twenty years beyond menopause before being placed on HRT.

A fascinating area of research has emerged that may explain why these older women may have experienced lower rates of cancer. Studies have shown that breast cells that have not been exposed to estrogen for a long period of time may change in character and respond differently to estrogen. Rather than being stimulated to grow, which we normally expect, it has been demonstrated that when these estrogen-deprived cells are subjected to estrogen they can go into *apoptosis*.[27] This is a technical word but is a good one. It is the term used to designate the natural end of a cell's life. It is possible that in the WHI study, the hormones administered to this group of older women actually forced many of their breast cells into an early death. The result would be that the treated women would have fewer actively dividing cells, which would decrease the onset and growth of breast cancer. This theory would explain why the women in the second arm of the WHI had less breast cancer than women on a placebo. It is conceivable that taking estrogen either prevented or may actually have "cured" some very early cancers in these older women!

The notion that taking estrogen could possibly have a positive effect in women with breast cancer may seem inconceivable. I recently received a phone call from a neighbor who was extremely concerned that her aunt, who had advanced breast cancer, was being treated with estrogen therapy. My neighbor was dumbfounded and wanted to know if I had ever heard such a thing. I explained to her that, yes, this is an established form of therapy in some cases and can be very effective. As far back as 1966 researchers noted that high potency estrogen treatment prevented the spread of breast cancer in rats. Subsequent studies over the years found this to be an option for some women. Although I think my neighbor was initially skeptical, she realized the doctors made the right choice because her aunt responded favorably within a number of weeks.

Another aspect of the estrogen-only arm of the WHI to discuss is the type of estrogen used in the study, which was Premarin. An interesting question to ponder is whether there is something unique about this particular formulation that may have contributed to the decreased rate of breast cancer. Recall that Premarin consists of estrone along with a mix of horse-derived estrogens. So compared to straight estradiol, it has some unique properties due to its origins from a non-human source. There has been speculation that some of these equilin (horse-derived) components may have some anti-estrogen, SERM-like properties.[28] Like Tamoxifen and other SERMs, these agents may block the estrogen effects on breast cell growth. This would effectively decrease the growth of cancer cells.

We don't have much data from clinical studies to help us decide if forms of estrogen other than Premarin have differential effects on breast cancer. Results of studies are mixed.[28,29,30] A meta-analysis published in 2017 reviewing 14 studies concluded that women on estradiol had no greater or lesser risk of breast cancer than untreated women.[14] A more recent review published in 2019 assessing over 100,000 women with breast cancer concluded that women who had used any form of estrogen for at least five years had an increased risk of developing breast cancer.[31]

What about women with known breast cancer?

This brings us to a discussion of HRT in women with current or a history of breast cancer. Most menopause experts do not advise these women to take HRT. Just like normal breast cells, most cancerous breast cells will be stimulated to divide when exposed to estrogen. Even the small levels of estrogen that persist in a woman's body after menopause (which comes from fat cells and the adrenal glands) are believed to stimulate cancerous breast cells.

Breast cancer drugs have been developed that prevent this residual estrogen from feeding cancer cells. Tamoxifen and similar SERM drugs hook onto the estrogen receptors in breast cells, blocking the attachment of estrogen and thus preventing it from exerting any effect. Another class of breast cancer drugs includes Arimidex (brand name for anastrozole) and Femara (brand name for letrozole). These drugs lower the estrogen level in the body by blocking the conversion of precursor steroids into estrogen. All of these drugs are effective for breast cancer cells that have intact estrogen receptors and studies have shown that breast cancer treatments utilizing these drugs prolong survival. So, you can see why most oncologists strongly discourage or actually outright forbid women with a history of breast cancer from considering hormone treatment. If a woman has breast cancer and takes hormones, it is logical to expect that they will make her cancer grow.

In addition, after a woman has completed treatment for breast cancer, HRT is believed to be risky. This is because hormones may stimulate a dormant nest of cancer cells that evaded eradication. Although these cells would likely grow into a detectable tumor eventually, HRT treatment may make this occur sooner.

Almost all guidelines specify that women with a history of breast cancer are not candidates for HRT. To emphasize this concern, all the inserts accompanying estrogen prescriptions carry FDA admonitions warning that women with a history of breast cancer should not take hormones. However, this is an area where there is some controversy. A number of studies have shown that HRT does not increase mortality or the risk of recurrent disease in breast cancer survivors.[32-36] Furthermore, a book published in 2018 appeared – written by a noted oncologist, Dr. Avrum Bluming and psychologist Carol Tavris PhD entitled, *Estrogen Matters, Why Taking Hormones in Menopause Improves Women's Well-Being and Lengthens Their Lives – Without Raising the Risk of Breast Cancer* presents a compelling 286 pages challenging the prevailing opinion about how we manage menopausal women with a known history of breast cancer.[37]

Because there are so many uncertainties, and due to the strongly polarized opinions about the safety of HRT in these situations, it is doubtful there will be any move to change the current guidelines. Future studies are unlikely to occur because of ethical considerations about recruiting women to enter a trial that would put them on a therapy that many experts consider dangerous.

Women with a family history of breast cancer or women with genetic markers for cancer are frequently discouraged from taking HRT but there are no definitive studies to indicate that taking hormones, particularly unopposed estrogen, would negatively affect them. In fact, in the 2017 position statement of the North American Menopause Society, it is noted that BRCA positive women are not at increased risk from taking HRT.[18]

One point to clarify, however, is that low-dose vaginal estrogens designed to treat vaginal symptoms have not been shown to affect the risk of breast cancer and carry negligible risk even among breast cancer survivors. However, if a woman is being treated for cancer, especially with the class of drugs known as aromatase inhibitors, many experts are leery of treating her with these vaginal forms of estrogen.

Putting it all together

In summary, we have reviewed the pertinent data about how HRT affects breast cancer. Whether or not estrogen *causes* breast cancer remains controversial. It is more likely that it may *promote* breast cancer by stimulating its growth. It is also unclear whether or not natural progesterone increases the risk of breast cancer, but may also be a promoter, like estrogen. Synthetic progestins have other effects that may increase the development of breast cancer, but only after long-term use. Most experts agree that taking HRT for up to five years carries negligible risk, so the fear of breast cancer should not dissuade women who are having hot flashes from considering hormone treatment.

Decision Making Helper

Key Considerations

There is strong data that indicates that taking estrogen alone for up to five years has a negligible risk of breast cancer. Taking estrogen alone for longer periods of time may promote breast cancer, but the absolute risk is small. It is unclear if one form of estrogen is preferable to another. The horse-derived estrogen compounds may have properties that decrease the risk of breast cancer.

The addition of a synthetic progestogen slightly increases the risk. It is likely that natural progesterone has less risk. A progestogen-containing IUD likely has negligible effects on breast cancer but there is little data on this.

It is unclear if taking a progestogen daily or cyclically is preferable, and there may be little difference. Some schools of thought advocate that taking the lowest amount of a progestogen is desirable, but the dose should be adequate to prevent uterine cancer.

Taking HRT using either estrogen alone or estrogen with a progestogen does not appear to increase the risk of dying from breast cancer if taken for less than 10 years, and probably even if taken for longer durations.

HRT may stimulate an existing breast cancer to grow so it is prudent to have a mammogram prior to initiating treatment and be screened regularly.

Women with a family history of breast cancer or a known genetic predisposition are not at further risk for developing breast cancer if they take HRT for treatment of hot flashes (for up to five years at least).

It is not advisable for women being treated for breast cancer to take HRT. It is also not advisable for women with a past history of breast cancer to take HRT because of concerns that hormones will stimulate residual breast cancer cells to grow. However, there is some controversy in this area – particularly because HRT may provide other benefits that may outweigh this risk.

Low-dose topical vaginal estrogens used to treat vaginal symptoms pose a negligible risk for breast cancer – even in patients with a history of breast cancer. However, consultation with an oncologist is advisable.

Current guidelines for HRT with respect to breast cancer

HRT is indicated only for short-term treatment of symptoms, primarily hot flashes. FDA warnings note that combined hormone therapy may increase the risk of developing breast cancer. Drug labeling inserts warn that estrogen and progestogens are contraindicated in women with a personal history of breast cancer.

What the guidelines don't acknowledge

Taking estrogen for up to five years carries a negligible risk of breast cancer. Adding a progestogen may slightly increase this risk. Natural progesterone appears to have less risk than a synthetic progestin.

There is considerable evidence that taking HRT does not increase a woman's risk of dying from breast cancer, and taking estrogen alone may even decrease her risk.

Chapter 11
Estrogen and Your Bones

As a medical student, when I wasn't feverishly attempting to memorize the name of every microbe, muscle group, and malady that has ever afflicted mankind, I made rounds. Rounding consisted of following knowledgeable attending physicians from bedside to bedside absorbing as much information as I could handle while trying not to get too emotionally distracted by the plights of the many unfortunate patients we saw during each shift.

I vividly remember how sad I felt caring for women who had suffered hip fractures. It seemed like every week an elderly lady was brought to the hospital by ambulance, disheveled and confused after lying helplessly on the floor for hours after a fall until a family member or neighbor had come to her aid. She would be rushed off to surgery, then endure a difficult recovery – generally in a nursing home. Frequently she would suffer some complication such as pneumonia, a blood clot, or a major decline in her ability to remain independent. The outcome was rarely a positive one.

For women born before the turn of the last century, there really was no medication available to prevent osteoporosis and its inevitable outcome. So when estrogen therapy became widely available and was shown to prevent fractures, physicians embraced what was a much-needed option for women to improve their prospects for long and independent lives. Despite the fact that estrogen use appeared to increase breast malignancies, the truth of the matter was that a woman was more likely to die from the consequences of a hip fracture than succumb to breast cancer attributed to HRT. Millions of women benefited immensely from taking hormones. By the 1990s, a couple of decades after the advent and widespread use of HRT, the incidence of hip fractures markedly declined. Those of us in practice during those times encouraged women to take HRT, not only to treat their hot flashes but to preserve their bone health.

But in 2002, when the WHI study concluded that HRT increased heart disease, enthusiasm for prescribing hormones plummeted. As women across the country abandoned their estrogens, it is not surprising that there was an upward trend in the incidence of hip fractures.[1] Although other drugs for treating osteoporosis had been developed, for a number of reasons they haven't been successful in curbing this rise in fractures. For one thing, studies have indicated that many women who went off HRT did not end up on alternative therapies to protect their bones.[1]

The magnitude of the consequences of fragile bones is alarming. Over five million people will sustain some type of osteoporosis-related fracture each year.[2] Every year, one in 30 elderly women fracture a hip – an event that can dramatically alter the course of their lives. Half will require long-term nursing care.[3] To me, it is truly disheartening that thousands of women suffer preventable fractures every year.

This chapter delves into the vital role that estrogen plays in maintaining healthy bones and preventing osteoporosis. You will learn why menopause heralds the onset of rapid bone deterioration that may not be recoverable. I'll discuss the options that have been approved for preventing and treating osteoporosis, along with the merits and risks of these alternatives. This information should be considered when deciding if HRT is the right choice for you.

Bone basics and fractures

Every year after the age of 50 the total number of cells that make up all of our bodily systems drops steadily. With this comes a decline in our neurologic and muscular functioning – which in turn leads to problems with balance, reaction time, vision, and strength. This increases the risk of falls, and coupled with the inevitable loss of bone mass, increases the risk of fractures. Whereas it takes a major insult like being thrown from a horse to break a young bone, older bones can't withstand a fall off a chair or a minor trip in the hallway during a nighttime visit to the bathroom. So it is not surprising that aging brings with it a steady increase in the number of fractures.

Osteoporosis is the term used to describe bones that are so fragile they are at high risk of breaking. *Osteo* means bone and *porosis* means porous. So osteoporosis is a condition where the internal architecture of the bone starts looking like Swiss cheese and becomes structurally very weak. I was talking to my older sister about this recently. While she knew that osteoporosis could be in her future, she admitted she didn't know why this happens or if it could be prevented. To understand what occurs, it is helpful to begin with an overview of how our bones are structured and how the bone cells that comprise them are organized and regulated.

Our skeleton consists of 206 bones. If you've ever examined a beef bone while preparing a meal, you've likely noticed that there is an outer hard component and an inner softer core. The outer shell is called *cortical bone* and the inner center is composed of *cancellous* or *trabecular bone.* Cancellous bone consists of a fine network of boney filaments or spicules that act as a scaffold inside the harder casing of the bone. Within this matrix resides the bone marrow which basically is an incubator for our red and white blood cells and platelets. These elements are formed and stored in the marrow and released into the bloodstream as needed. Bones that have large amounts of marrow, such as the spinal vertebra and the top of our femur, are the ones that are most susceptible to being broken as women age.

We tend to think of bones as solid and inert, like the ones our dogs love to chew on. But in the living body, bones are in a dynamic state of activity. Specialized bone cells called *osteoclasts* are constantly tearing down tiny areas of bone, while builder cells called *osteoblasts* march behind and lay down new layers of bone filling up the voids. This process of bone removal and replacement is known as *bone remodeling.*

Visualize one of our bones, such as the femur which is the long bone inside the thigh. Imagine it as a rigid tube with a network of delicate struts crisscrossing back and forth inside it. This honeycomb-like interior is lined by rows of osteoclasts and osteoblasts that are constantly carving away bits of bone and then rebuilding it. The end result of this activity is that the interior architecture of the bone can be modified and redesigned as needed in response to the direction and degree of force being applied to it. Many fish, such as sharks, that float and swim in water their entire lives have hardly any boney structure at all. Whereas we humans, living on the surface of the earth, have developed skeletons strong enough to keep us from crumbling to the ground under the force of gravity.

The remodeling process can bolster specific areas of the skeleton in response to changes in activity. If you start jogging, your body responds by strengthening your leg bones. A right-handed professional female tennis player, who hits hundreds of balls a day, has stronger bones in her right arm and shoulder than on her left side (or her *non-dominant wing* as they say on the Tennis Channel). The fact that our skeleton is constantly adapting itself to changes in our activities is fascinating, and scientists are studying how this is accomplished. It is thought that specialized cells within the bone sense where stress is coming from, then instruct the remodeling cells to shore up the bone in that area.

This is why you hear your doctor encouraging weight-bearing exercise. Walking and jumping strengthen the bones but swimming doesn't have the same benefit since gravity isn't much of a factor. A big concern for NASA is that an astronaut spending prolonged periods in outer space will literally lose bone mass. An important piece of equipment in the International Space Station is a special exercise machine. Each astronaut must spend two hours a day working out on it. This is effective because research shows that doing weights in the gym adds to bone strength. When a muscle contracts and pulls against a bone, the stress transmits signals to the osteoclasts and osteoblasts to stimulate bone strengthening.

Now that you have an understanding of the bone remodeling process, you can see that there are two major ways the bones could get thinner. Either the breakdown process (osteoclast activity) proceeds too vigorously, or the buildup process (osteoblast activity) is too slow. For most of our adult life, this process is perfectly balanced and our bones remain strong. This is ensured because a number of hormones and other chemical messengers are involved in regulating this process. Estrogen, in particular, suppresses osteoclast activity and plays a major role in keeping a check on the bone breakdown process.

As we age: the difference between men and women

With normal aging, it is primarily the osteoblasts that slow down – so the bone buildup process starts to lag behind the bone breakdown activity. This results in a gradual net loss of bone mass. The width of the outer boney cortex decreases in thickness and the internal rungs and struts become thinner. So it is inevitable that all men and women will develop some degree of bone weakening as they age.

When a woman reaches menopause, however, there is a dramatic acceleration of bone deterioration. Without estrogen's suppressive effect on the osteoclasts, they go into overdrive chewing up bone at a rate far faster than the aging osteoblasts can keep up with. This causes a rapid loss in bone mass. To put things in perspective, after about the age of 50 men lose about 0.4% of their bone mass per year. Women going through menopause at age 50 start losing bone up to three times as fast.[4] Some women can lose up to five percent of their bone mass per year.[5] The most rapid period of bone loss begins just before menopause and tapers off about seven years post menopause.

The loss of estrogen particularly affects the integrity of the architecture inside the bone. On average women lose about 25% of their cancellous, or inner, bone within the first ten years past menopause. The revved-up osteoclasts enlarge the spaces within the honeycomb structure and without this extra internal support the bones become exceedingly weak and more susceptible to breaking.

I don't think many women think about what is happening to their bones as their menstrual cycles wind down. While hot flashes and mood swings are inescapably obvious, the rapid decline in our bone mass doesn't cause any noticeable symptoms. I think doctors should make more of an effort to discuss this matter when counseling women about HRT because in most cases, without immediate intervention, it is essentially impossible to recover much of what is lost. I will emphasize this point later because the existing guidelines do not recommend HRT, nor any other drug for that matter, for women with normal bone densities. It is not until the bones are nearly on the verge of fracturing that the guidelines advise some form of medical treatment.

Let's talk more about fractures

Having an outer hard shell with a honeycomb interior allows the bones to be very strong, but lightweight. (Can you imagine how much we would weigh if our bones were solid?) This construction also allows bones to have some flexibility. Have you noticed that while pulling apart the wishbone from your Thanksgiving turkey that there is quite a bit of bend before it breaks? This flexibility prevents many fractures from occurring. Of course, bones do break as any busy emergency room can attest to. Traumatic events like a car crash or a skiing accident can exert enough force to make anyone's bones snap. These types of fractures frequently involve the ribs as well as the bones in our extremities.

The major type of fracture that occurs with osteoporosis is called a *compression fracture*. Picture this type of fracture as a bone collapsing within itself. This can occur when a vertical force is applied to the bone, such as falling from a tree or landing on your butt while ice skating. In someone with severe osteoporosis, it can happen because of a severe sneeze! Bones that have a relatively high proportion of cancellous bone are the most vulnerable to compression and this most often occurs in one of the vertebrae of the spine.

Have you ever noticed an elderly woman walking on the street or in the mall clutching her walker – her upper back bent over like a half moon? Why does this happen? It is the end result of multiple compression fractures which invariably are due to severe osteoporosis. Think of the spine as a tower of spools – the spools being the vertebrae. If some of the spools compress (like squeezing a marshmallow) the vertebrae become thinner and the length of the spine shortens. This can cause a woman to lose over six inches in height! In addition, a vertebra doesn't always compress uniformly. Frequently just one side is affected so it winds up shaped like a wedge with the inner side shorter than the outer side. When several of these are lined up in a row, the spine starts to curve in a fan-shaped configuration forming a dowager's hump. We call this *kyphosis*.

As more vertebrae compress in this fashion, the spine becomes precariously bent. I have fond memories of one of my favorite patients, Elsie, who was so stooped over that in order to talk to her I had to lean way over onto my lap and turn my head up to see her face. She was remarkably resilient and didn't complain much, but her deformity severely impaired her quality of life. I knew that I would never want to end up in her condition, and it was patients like Elsie who motivated me to want to do everything I could to prevent any of my other patients from going down that path.

You may find it amazing that two out of three women who have a compression fracture are not aware of having one. The deformed vertebra usually shows up incidentally on a chest x-ray taken for some unrelated reason – such as for a bad cough. Even for those of us who are not trained radiologists, these abnormal-looking vertebrae are pretty obvious on the images. I have had the task of informing many a patient that her x-ray showed one of these fractures. Understandably it usually came as a big surprise.

It is unclear why these go unnoticed by so many women. How do you have a fracture and no clue when or how it happened? Most likely what occurs is that over a period of years, multiple tiny cracks develop in the vertebra. Each time one happens it may not cause much discomfort and perhaps is passed off as a slight strain. Over time the weakened vertebra eventually compresses and shrinks in size.

A compression fracture can also come on abruptly – frequently following a relatively minor event such as a misstep, a bumpy ride on an airplane, or while bending over to tuck in a grandchild. In these instances, a woman experiences

136

a sudden jolt of intense pain followed by severe back spasms brought on by movement.

Compression fractures of the spine can occur at any level – but generally in the middle part of the back, which is the thoracic spine, or in the lower back involving the lumbar vertebrae. Generally, there is not much that can be done for them, other than give them time to heal – which takes months. Sometimes a procedure known as *kyphoplasty* or *vertebroplasty* is performed. These are procedures where a radiologist inserts an epoxy-like substance through a large needle into the vertebra to bolster it up inside. These procedures have produced variable results – sometimes they can help immediately by relieving the pain; other times they can be totally ineffective or even cause a complication such as inadvertent damage to a nerve in the spinal canal. And the jury is out on how effective they are long-term and whether the adulterated vertebra can adversely affect the ones above and below it.

Spinal fractures can be a major cause of morbidity and mortality in older women. The pain leads to inactivity and in some cases prolonged bed rest. Frequently narcotic drugs are the only means to some relief – but prescribing these to older patients causes its own set of adverse effects such as nausea, constipation, confusion, or mental decline. Needless to say, managing the pain in these situations can be very difficult. Whether to withhold pain meds and let a patient suffer or administer them and deal with side effects is always a balancing act. One way or the other, the aftermath of a bad compression fracture usually leads to progressive weakness, an increased risk of another fall, and a susceptibility to other complications such as pneumonia.

The other fracture that is notorious for being osteoporosis-related is a "hip" fracture. It is commonly called a hip fracture but is technically a fracture of the upper part of the leg, or femur, where it joins the pelvic bone to form the hip joint. The femur is shaped like a hockey stick and it is the short segment that breaks. This part of the femur contains a great deal of cancellous bone making it vulnerable to a fracture. Even a simple fall can lead to one. Unlike putting a fractured arm or leg in a cast, a hip fracture requires surgery to hold the bone together to allow it to heal. This involves putting in large screws or doing a hip replacement.

Recovery from this can be very hard on elderly and frail patients. Hip fractures portend a poor prognosis for the future. The risk of death following a hip fracture can be up to ten percent following surgery; up to 35% of patients die within the first year after their fracture.[6,7] Overall, women who have suffered a hip fracture have considerably shorter life expectancies than women who have not.[8]

Diagnosing osteoporosis

The scary thing about osteoporosis is that in most cases a woman doesn't know if she has it because there are no symptoms. If she does happen to break her hip from a minor fall or if a compression fracture shows up on an x-ray – then, by definition, we diagnose her as having osteoporosis. This is because the formal definition is *a disease characterized by low bone mass and micro-architectural deterioration that leads to enhanced bone fragility and fractures.* However, the vast majority of women have no idea how weak or how strong their bones are without doing some type of test.

The gold standard diagnostic test is a *bone biopsy* where a tiny sample of bone is removed and analyzed. This is usually obtained by sticking a large needle into the iliac bone which is the boney prominence on one side of your back at the beltline. The specimen is examined under a microscope where the details of the internal bone architecture can be viewed. If I showed you two bone biopsy slides – one from a young woman and one from someone with osteoporosis, I bet it would be obvious to you which slide was which. The bone from the younger woman's sample would have a very dense honeycomb appearance, but the osteoporotic one would look like someone fired a shotgun through it!

Bone biopsies are invasive, uncomfortable, and expensive – so obviously they are not a very practical way to screen women for their bone densities. (It is hard enough to get all of our patients to come in for an annual flu shot, much less expect them to volunteer to have a very large needle jabbed into their backsides!) Bone biopsies primarily are used in research situations.

Fortunately, there are other more palatable tests to assess how the bones are doing. There are a number of urine and blood tests that measure bone activity – the common ones being the *NTX (N-terminal telopeptide)* and the *CTX (Carboxy-terminal collagen crosslinks)* tests. These are simple but informative tests. As discussed above, the bones are constantly remodeling. As the bones are being broken down, a number of leftover particles from the process are discarded into the bloodstream and cleared out of the body in the urine. Measuring these particles is the basis for these tests. If a woman's bones are being broken down at a fast rate, the number of NTX or CTX particles will be high. If the bone breakdown and buildup process is balanced, the numbers will be low.

These tests do not actually tell you if you have osteoporosis but indicate how fast you may be losing bone. If the numbers are quite high, you are probably on your way to a fracture. Almost all women past menopause will have elevated readings. If estrogen or another treatment is started, the levels go down gradually over a few months. These tests are particularly helpful in assessing response to treatment. If the levels do not go down, the drug is not working for some reason or, more commonly, the patient is not taking it correctly.

Although bones that are osteoporotic appear fainter than normal bones on a plain old x-ray, routine x-rays are not very useful as a way to diagnose osteoporosis because they don't give any quantifiable information. So, a more sophisticated x-ray test, a *DEXA* scan, is commonly used to assess bone density. This stands for *dual-energy X-ray absorptiometry*. In this test, X-rays are sent through the bone and then mathematical calculations are made to determine how dense (i.e., strong) the bones are. These machines use a tiny amount of radiation and pose very little risk to the woman being scanned or to the technician – so they can be done in a doctor's office without the need for special lead shielding to block the radiation.

The standard bones tested are those that are most prone to a fracture, i.e., the hip (upper femur) and the lumbar vertebrae. DEXA scanners can't accurately test the thoracic vertebrae because there is too much interference from the ribs and the breastbone. However, the density of the wrist, which is actually the radius bone just above the wrist joint where we wear our wristwatches, can be tested. A fall onto an outstretched arm commonly leads to a fracture of this bone.

When you have a DEXA scan performed, the machine reports two numbers – a *T-score* and a *Z-score*. The T-score compares your bone density to that of a typical 35-year-old woman. This value is used because it is assumed that the bones of a 35-year-old woman of your height and weight should be of normal strength and density. The normal value is 0.0. If your T-score is between -0.9 and +1.0 (which encompasses some wiggle room above and below normal) – you are considered to have normal bone density.

The lower the T-score is below 0.0, the thinner the bones. If the T-score is between -1.0 and -2.5 this indicates *osteopenia*. Osteopenia is the term used to describe bones that are thinner than normal but not to the point of being osteoporotic. Once the T-score is at or below -2.5, this is defined as osteoporosis. In technical terms, this number indicates a value that is 2.5 or more standard deviations below normal. This determination of osteoporosis is somewhat arbitrary. It's not a black and white condition (such as if you are pregnant or not pregnant!). Back in the 1990s the World Health Organization analyzed thousands of records and determined that women with T-scores less than -2.5 had the highest risk of fractures. So that is how this cut-off level was decided. It is much like the definition of high blood pressure. Many studies conducted over the years have shown that people whose systolic (upper number) exceeds 130 or whose diastolic (lower number) exceeds 80 have a higher risk of a stroke or heart attack than those with lower values. So we have defined high blood pressure as anything over 130/80.

So how does the T-score actually equate to the risk of a fracture? The lower the T-score, the greater the chance of a fracture. If the T-score is -2.5, a woman has roughly a six-fold higher risk of a hip fracture than if she has a T-score of 0.0, and an even greater risk of a spine fracture.[9] Another way of looking at this would be to imagine a woman and her grandmother out for a walk and they both tripped over a crack in the sidewalk. The older woman with a T-score of -2.5 would be six times more likely to break her hip than her 35-year-old granddaughter.

The other score reported by a DEXA scan is the Z-score. This score compares you to other women your age. It really isn't very useful to assess your risk of a fracture. Your Z-score may be normal for your age – but that doesn't mean your bones are normal density. It just means that you have the same amount of thinning as other women your age. A 90-year-old with a normal Z-score of 0.9 very well may have a T-score below -2.5.

The majority of women who live beyond age 90 will eventually develop osteoporosis.[9] This is because the total number of cells that make up our skeletons decrease with age causing a loss of bone mass – no matter how hard we try to prevent it. However, taking some form of osteoporosis-preventing treatment helps slow this decline and lessens the chance of a fracture.

The vast majority of women nearing menopause will have normal bone densities. There are of course exceptions. Women who were nutritionally deprived while growing up, particularly those with a history of anorexia, have low baseline densities as adults. Women with autoimmune diseases such as rheumatoid arthritis and lupus are at high risk for osteoporosis. Chronic or frequent treatment with prednisone or comparable types of steroids also causes low bone density.

Genetic factors play a major role in determining bone density. There are many genes that produce proteins necessary for normal bone remodeling. A minor genetic mutation in one of these genes can cause an increased risk of osteopenia or osteoporosis.[11] This may explain why a woman is at higher risk for osteoporosis if it runs in her family. Some ethnic groups tend to have thinner bones. This is in part due to lifestyle, but also due to certain inherited traits that affect the bone. Asian women tend to have lower bone densities than Caucasian women, whereas African American women have higher densities than most ethnic groups.

Conversely, genes that lead to a higher than normal bone density have been identified. Early in my practice one of my patients had an exceptionally high T-score, even at the age of 78. This puzzled me for years until I read about this research and now I realize she likely inherited a gene that affected her bone remodeling process, which led to a stronger than normal bone density. As genetic research is getting more sophisticated, analyzing how these genes affect bone remodeling is opening doors to discovering new treatments for osteoporosis.

It is important to understand several aspects of DEXA scans. While they measure overall bone density, they can't really tell us how the inside of the bone is structured. The characteristics of the interior of the bone can affect its intrinsic strength. One of the aspects of menopausal bone loss is that the lack of estrogen particularly weakens the matrix within the bone. Many of the tiny cross-links between the spicules disappear and this weakens the bone's strength. In this situation, the overall bone density score on a DEXA scan may be near normal, yet the loss of the internal structure decreases the bones' ability to withstand breaking. The analogy would be removing three or four rungs from a ladder. The overall weight of the ladder does not change too much, but it is much less sturdy.

Another factor not reflected by a DEXA scan is the stiffness of the bones. Bones that lack flexibility are more likely to fracture. One of the earlier drugs used to treat osteoporosis was fluoride. Although treatment with this mineral increased bone density, it caused the bones to be brittle and more prone to fracturing.

It should also be noted that there can be a moderate amount of variability in the results between one DEXA scan and the next. In other words, a woman can have a study done twice on the same day and the results may not be identical. The scores can vary as much as 0.2 to 0.5 units in difference. I have had many patients elated that their T-scores improved over the prior year, but then become disappointed when the scores went down the following year. I would counsel them that they should keep in mind that we are looking for a gradual trend up or down over a period of many years – not just year to year. So that is why it doesn't make much sense to do DEXA scans any more frequently than every one to two years.

Another issue to be aware of is there are several manufacturers of DEXA machines commonly used. The different machines may give a slightly different reading on the same individual. So it is important to try to have the same brand of machine do your bone density test each time. Otherwise, it is more difficult to know how your bone density is truly trending.

Before leaving the topic of bone tests I will mention a couple of other procedures used to assess the status of your bones. Ultrasound analysis of the heel is frequently done as a screening test, but it is not as accurate or definitive as the x-ray tests. It is a simple exam that many doctors' offices perform. If it is normal, it generally means you are in good shape, but if it is low, further testing, such as a DEXA, is needed. There are also more sophisticated CAT scans that measure bone density, but these involve more radiation and don't give that much more information than a DEXA scan in most situations.

Estrogen therapy and the bones

Let's now talk about estrogen replacement and our bones. It is well accepted that it is the loss of estrogen's effect on osteoclasts that causes accelerated bone loss at the time of menopause. So it seems logical that replacing estrogen should prevent this from happening. And indeed, there is really not much controversy about this. When started at the time of menopause, HRT retards this rapid bone loss and, more importantly, reduces the risk of future fractures. We have much data to support this. A plethora of older observational studies demonstrated that women on HRT have a lower risk of fractures. In addition, multiple major clinical trials have confirmed this. Even the WHI study showed a 33% reduction in fractures in women taking estrogen, either with or without a progestogen.

A 2016 meta-analysis reviewing 28 studies confirmed again that HRT treatment improves bone density.[12] In this review, just about any estrogen and progestogen formulation showed benefit, but estradiol appeared slightly more effective than Premarin. Even women starting HRT later in life demonstrated a benefit, albeit not as robust. This was demonstrated in another study, where estrogen treatment given to women over the age of 75 for nine months improved their bone densities compared to women on a placebo.[13]

This is an interesting point to call attention to. As you will see in other chapters of this book estrogen can confer significant health benefits in young postmenopausal women, but these same benefits are not always seen in older women who initiate hormones later in life. In some cases, HRT has been found to cause detrimental effects in this older population of women. This does not seem to be the case when it comes to the bones. This is probably due to the fact that estrogen improves bone health through several mechanisms – not all of which may be dependent on having functioning estrogen receptors. So even if there is a loss of receptors with age, which likely accounts for much of older women's loss of response to hormones, non–receptor functions may play a role.

Since estrogen treatment has been shown to prevent osteoporosis, and older women's bones appear to respond to it, what about treating women with established osteoporosis? It seems that it should help and there has been some data indicating it is effective. In one study, women with known osteoporosis and a history of vertebral fractures were treated with either transdermal estradiol or a placebo. The women receiving estrogen had an improvement in their DEXA scores, and a fifty percent decreased risk of a fracture.[14] Other studies have shown that HRT has even improved bone densities in osteoporotic women over the age of 75.[13]

Despite this, experts in the field are not ready to recommend estrogen as a treatment for established osteoporosis, and HRT is not approved for this purpose. The concern is that women are generally older when they develop osteoporosis and data from the WHI and other studies have led to warnings that the cardiac risks outweigh the benefits of initiating HRT in this age group.

HRT, however, is approved for *preventative* treatment of osteoporosis. Your initial thought may be that this opens the door for anyone going through menopause to be a candidate for treatment. As much as I would like this to be the case, it is far from how the guidelines are applied. The indication for prescribing HRT, or any drug for osteoporosis prevention for that matter, rests upon the qualifier that the woman should be at *high risk*. This means that a woman's bone mass must have declined substantially to the point where she has a high chance of getting a fracture. Relatively few women would be considered high-risk around age 50; the age when women go through menopause. So, just because we know a woman's bone mass is going to decline when her estrogen level goes down this is not considered a valid reason to start therapy with hormones or any of the drugs approved for osteoporosis prevention.

How do we determine *"high risk?"* Certainly, if a woman entering menopause has had an osteoporotic fracture or for some reason has a terribly low T-score, she would be a candidate for treatment. In both of these situations, there is a high likelihood that one or more fractures will occur in her lifetime. Other than under these circumstances, how do we determine who else would be considered high risk? The best way is to take a number of factors such as her age, weight, ethnicity, bone mineral content, family history, and other information and plug them into a program designed to determine fracture risk. The tool widely accepted for this purpose is called the *FRAX assessment* calculator. This is an online program where a woman's information is entered and the program churns out her risk of incurring a fracture over the next ten years. If the results indicate that a woman has a 3% chance of getting a hip fracture or a 20% chance of getting any type of fracture, then she is considered high-risk. If we were to run this analysis on every woman just as she enters menopause, the vast majority will not turn out to be high-risk candidates.

Even for those women determined to be at high risk, other drugs besides HRT have been approved for preventative treatment. And when one reads articles and guidelines about how best to manage these women, over and over again appear phrases like *"HRT is no longer considered first-line treatment."* So unless a woman in this situation wants to take HRT for her hot flashes, she will frequently be directed to one of these other options, which are discussed below.

If you sense that I am concerned about the current guidelines which don't explicitly address an opportunity to prevent osteoporosis, you are correct. It seems like we are really missing the boat by not encouraging the early and widespread use of HRT as a bone-preserving measure. Calcium and vitamin D and exercise are all helpful but don't prevent the bulk of the bone loss that occurs within the first five years of menopause. Why must we wait until we have lost a considerable amount of bone before we intervene? And then, even with treatment, we rarely see much in the way of bone-building. Generally, we are happy just to see that we can stop further deterioration. To me, it makes much more sense to replace our estrogen right away and prevent bone loss in the first place.

Even if you stretch the current guidelines and feel justified in putting a patient on HRT to prevent bone loss, recall that in the guidelines hormones should be prescribed *only at the lowest doses for the shortest period of time*. This really isn't going to be optimal treatment because, while low-dose therapy may help limit some bone loss, these regimens are not as effective as the standard doses of HRT and do not appear very effective for preventing fractures.[15] And certainly, just taking them for a few years is not going to have much long-term benefit for the bones. While the bone preserving effects of estrogen can persist for several years after discontinuation, bone density will decline if estrogen therapy is withdrawn.

The reason doctors are cautious about promoting HRT is because the presumed cardiac risks outweigh the bone benefits. However, the basis for this concern stems heavily from the WHI study, which primarily included women who were older and many had cardiac risk factors. Therefore, it is not appropriate to apply the WHI findings to all menopausal women. Most 50-year-old women are low in cardiac risk but essentially all will start losing bone when they reach menopause. The irony in this situation is that by the time these women may become high-risk there is an increasing likelihood that they will have developed cardiac disease – which further precludes consideration of HRT. So, at that point, non-hormone drugs are the only option for osteoporosis prevention. This is why I will address these alternatives. Knowledge of the benefits and risks of alternative therapies should be considered in the decision-making process regarding the choice to take HRT.

But first, what about progesterone?

It is known that there are progesterone receptors in our bones and that progesterone appears to stimulate osteoblast formation. Thus, progesterone should contribute to bone health. While there is not a plethora of studies looking at this, it appears that estrogen plus progestogen therapy is a little more effective than estrogen alone.[16,17] This has been shown to be true with both the synthetic progestins and natural progesterone. Unlike some other situations where a progestogen negates estrogen's effects, in the bones, it appears to augment its effects.

Now on to other drugs to prevent osteoporosis

There are several other drugs that have been developed that are effective in preventing bone loss, and these are all relatively new – or at least came out well after I left medical school! But like HRT, they are not indicated until a woman is at high risk for osteoporosis. The first non-hormone drugs to come out were the *bisphosphonate* drugs. The one familiar to many women is alendronate (Fosamax) which appeared in the late 1990s. The other oral bisphosphonates that followed were risedronate (Actonel), and ibandronate (Boniva – remember the F*lying Nun*, Sally Fields, who was the spokesperson for this drug?) There are also stronger bisphosphonates which must be given by an injection at a health facility every six to twelve months. These drugs, such as Reclast, have primarily been reserved for women with certain types of cancers known to cause severe bone thinning.

Bisphosphonates have been shown to improve bone density and decrease fractures on a magnitude comparable with estrogen. The phosphate part of these drugs hooks onto the calcium in the bone and the drug gets incorporated into the bone cells and kills the osteoclasts. By disabling some of the osteoclasts, the bone-building osteoblasts are able to stay ahead of the bone breakdown process. So these drugs work very much like estrogen. It is unclear, however, if they are as effective as estrogen in preserving the normal architecture inside the bones.[18]

When bisphosphonates became widely available in the late 1990s, they were heavily promoted. They seemed very promising. The pharmaceutical drug reps who regularly visited my office described them as a win-win intervention. Unlike estrogen, they did not seem to have any serious downsides. We were advised that there were only some minor issues we had to warn patients about. For one, they were poorly absorbed – so patients had to be very diligent in taking them on a completely empty stomach. They also could be very irritating to the esophagus – so it was imperative that they be taken with a full glass of water and that patients be instructed not to lay down immediately afterward (where the pill could float back up into the esophagus and cause damage).

Prescriptions for bisphosphonates greatly increased in the early 2000s following the WHI study when HRT lost its popularity. And while at first blush they appeared very safe, as time went on and with more widespread use, more serious adverse consequences of the bisphosphonates became apparent. Dentists noticed an increase in cases of *osteonecrosis of the jaw* (ONJ) following dental extractions. This is a condition where the tooth socket fails to heal leaving exposed, non-viable, boney tissue. ONJ is difficult to treat and may require multiple surgeries to remove all the dead tissue and it frequently persists as a chronic non-healing wound. It is unclear exactly how bisphosphonates predispose patients to this but may be related to its effects on the blood vessels in the bone around the tooth. The risk of ONJ is extremely rare, and certain women appear to be more prone to this than others. Women receiving intravenous bisphosphonates and those with poor dental health and other immune disorders are at the highest risk.[19]

Not too long after the ONJ problem presented itself, another complication attributable to prolonged use of bisphosphonates surfaced. Women on these drugs were appearing in emergency rooms with fractures of the femur (upper leg) but having no history of trauma. Normally these fractures are caused by a major accident such as a tumble down a ski slope. Since the typical fracture associated with osteoporosis is a compression fracture of the spine or hip, these fractures have been referred to as *atypical fractures.* Why these breaks occur is unclear, but somehow may be related to how the bisphosphonates affect bone remodeling. And it may have something to do with women who have a specific genetic susceptibility (although we can't predict at this point who is at risk). As more women are being treated with these drugs, we are seeing these fractures more often. The incidence appears to be about six to ten atypical fractures per 10,000 women treated.[20]

So, despite the initial impression that these drugs were without risk, it has become clear that they have some adverse effects on bones as well as the potential to cause other rare events (such as triggering a heart rhythm disorder, atrial fibrillation, and promoting esophageal cancer). While the specter of these complications has frightened many women, experts in menopause emphasize that the risks are extremely low and need to be taken in the context that treatment prevents many osteoporotic fractures. It is estimated that for every eleven atypical fractures that occur, 800 other osteoporosis-related fractures are prevented with bisphosphonate therapy.[21]

The recommendations for bisphosphonate therapy are evolving. Since long-term therapy appears to increase the risk for adverse bone events, current guidelines advise treatment for only five years and then discontinuation for a so-called *drug holiday.* The idea is to give the bone remodeling process some time to get back in sync. After discontinuing a bisphosphonate drug, its bone preserving effects persist for many months, but as with estrogens, bone density starts to decline after two to five years. There are ongoing discussions and research about how best to use these drugs to balance risks versus benefits. For most women, there is a reluctance to treat for extended periods of time. But for an extremely high-risk patient, a longer duration of therapy may be appropriate.

More drugs are being developed. In 2010 the FDA approved the use of the twice-yearly shot denosumab (Prolia). Like other osteoporosis-preventing drugs, Prolia is indicated only for high-risk patients. Prolia is in a class of drugs you will be seeing more and more of – drugs called *biologicals* – that are based on *monoclonal antibodies*. Antibodies are proteins that our white cells make to fight such things as bacteria and viruses. Scientists have learned to produce antibodies in laboratories and can create ones that can seek out specific targets in the body to cause specific actions. This can be anywhere from fighting bacteria like anthrax, killing cancer cells, or blocking proteins that cause inflammation. Whenever you see a drug's generic name ending in '*mab*' – this indicates a drug consisting of these man-made antibodies.

Prolia works by blocking a factor that stimulates osteoclast congregation thus slows down the bone removal process. Studies show that Prolia has been linked to ONJ, but may not cause the atypical bone fractures seen with bisphosphonates – so Prolia may be safer long-term. However it is a relatively new form of treatment and, with more widespread use, we may see some other adverse effects. One recent concern that Prolia is presenting is that if women stop treatment, their risk of a fracture can suddenly increase.[22,23] To avoid this spike, it is recommended that a bisphosphonate drug be prescribed upon discontinuation of treatment with Prolia. This may not be something some women are able or willing to do.

The other non-estrogen and non-bisphosphonate class of drugs for osteoporosis prevention and treatment are the SERMs, or selective estrogen receptor modulators. These drugs are designed to have positive estrogen-like effects on the bones but don't have some of the adverse effects associated with estrogen on other organs. The primary drug used for bone protection is raloxifene (Evista). It is approved for osteoporosis prevention in high-risk patients and also for osteoporosis treatment, but isn't as effective as estrogen in preventing fractures. A positive aspect of raloxifene is that it can help prevent breast cancer. The downside of this and all SERMs is that they can increase the risk of blood clots and don't help hot flashes and can even make them worse.

A very new estrogen-SERM combination, Duavee, which is bazedoxifene combined with medium-dose conjugated estrogens, has been approved for osteoporosis prevention in the U.S. When this drug first came out I was a little puzzled. We are discouraging estrogen use for osteoporosis prevention – but here is a new drug containing essentially the same estrogen used in the WHI. Although it is a slightly lower dose, one could not help but ask why using it wouldn't carry the same concerns as using estrogen. The answer is that, in theory, the SERM would block any negative estrogen effects. This drug has not been in use for very long, and we don't have extensive data on its long-term safety profile and its effects on the breasts and other organs.[24]

For women with severe osteoporosis, there is a daily injectable drug called teriparatide (*Forteo*). It is very expensive and reserved for the most advanced cases of osteoporosis. Unlike estrogen and the drugs described previously, it works on the bone-building segment of bone remodeling and activates the osteoblasts. It is limited to therapy for a maximum duration of two years because of concerns that it increased cancer in animal studies with long-term administration.

The final drug to mention is a brand new product, romosozumab, which was approved by the FDA in the spring of 2019. This biologic works to increase bone formation through a unique mechanism. Studies have shown that it is very effective in decreasing vertebral fractures. However, one study showed that one patient suffered an atypical femoral fracture and two women developed ONJ in a two year period[25] – raising some concern about whether these complications may occur more frequently with romosozumab than with bisphosphonates. There may be some other safety issues regarding this drug. There is a boxed warning that states this drug may increase the risk of a heart attack, stroke, or cardiovascular death, and should not be used in patients who have had a heart attack or stroke within the previous year. Likely its use will be limited to a very select group of high-risk patients.

A scheme to consider

A number of drugs have been developed to prevent osteoporosis – which is truly amazing since we had no options other than hormones until around 1980. However, none of these medications are prescribed until women have fairly advanced osteopenia. From my perspective, this doesn't make sense and it seems we should reevaluate the way we approach women's bone health. Shouldn't we think in terms of how we can preserve our bone strength over the continuum of our lives, rather than waiting until we are on the verge of a fracture? How about the following scheme?

Prior to menopause (and of course on an ongoing basis), it is important to do everything we can that is good for our bones. This means getting regular weight-bearing exercise and taking adequate calcium and vitamin D. The optimal doses recommended for these supplements have fluctuated over time and every provider has his or her own preferences. Generally, about 1,200 mg calcium (ideally through dietary sources) and about 800 to 1,000 units of vitamin D daily are adequate.

I believe that HRT has a special place in this scheme. In this approach, women entering menopause should start taking adequate doses of estrogen known to be effective in suppressing the osteoclasts (assuming there is no medical contraindication). This would prevent the inevitable rapid bone loss that occurs after the first few years post menopause. Since most experts in the field believe that the benefits of HRT outweigh the risks for the majority of women for the first five to ten years past menopause, why not continue estrogen for at least this duration? This has been shown to keep our DEXA scores from declining and estrogen is uniquely capable of helping preserve the internal structure of our bones – an effect which appears to persist for some time after it is stopped.[26]

After five to ten years, or when it is considered prudent to discontinue hormones, the need for ongoing bone-protective therapy should be regularly assessed. Although a gradual loss of bone will occur, it may be many years before another intervention is indicated. The need to take the next step in pharmacologic therapy may not happen until a woman is well into her 70s or older. At that point, a bisphosphonate or Prolia would be a reasonable option. And because taking HRT delayed the need for this type of drug, therapy may only be needed for a limited time.

This approach makes sense to me, and many of my colleagues agree. A long-term plan like this is particularly important in this day and age when women are living 30 or more years past menopause. Approaching bone health in this way would limit the need for long-term, non-estrogen therapy, which carries more adverse effects if taken for extended periods of time.

It is unfortunate that when the WHI study findings were announced there wasn't greater emphasis on the effectiveness of estrogen therapy in preventing bone loss and fractures. Following the study, not only have fewer women initiated HRT, many high-risk women were not switched to other osteoporosis-preventing drugs. Furthermore, if they were, they may not have continued taking them. Studies have shown discontinuation rates for this class of drugs are as high as 70%.[27,28] What concerns me is an entire generation of women have not been treated with any type of drug to prevent early bone loss. Possibly thousands of women have unknowingly become severely osteopenic. The fact that the incidence of bone fractures has risen since 2005 attests to this.[1]

This is not inconsequential. The growing number of women ending up with osteoporosis is going to have a substantial impact on public health. The downstream cost of caring for them, including hospitalizations, surgeries, and long-term rehabilitation will be astronomical – especially when you consider that three million of us baby boomers are reaching Medicare age every year!

In conclusion

Estrogen plays a vital role in maintaining healthy bones and the loss of estrogen at the time of menopause has serious consequences. Physicians should advise women that a decision not to take HRT at the time of menopause will result in an accelerated rate of bone loss – a loss they may not recover. Women who take HRT to deal with their hot flashes will get the added, and likely unrecognized, bonus of a decreased risk of osteoporosis. Since women not having hot flashes are not considered candidates for HRT, they will miss out on this bone-preserving opportunity.

In addition, women should be advised that by not taking HRT, there is a high probability a non-hormone drug may be advisable at some point in the future. An awareness of the benefits and risks of these alternatives should be considered in deciding whether or not to take HRT.

Decision Making Helper

Key considerations

All women will start losing bone mass rapidly the minute their estrogen levels fall, and they will lose a considerable amount of bone over the ensuing five to seven years if they do not take estrogen. Once this bone has been lost, taking any of the drugs approved for osteoporosis prevention will hopefully halt the loss, but will not build it up to premenopausal levels.

The thinner the bones become, the higher the risk of a fracture. Fractures place women at a high risk of long-term disability and premature death.

All of the standard dose estrogen preparations prevent bone loss and decrease the risk of future fractures. The addition of a progestogen does not negate the benefit and appears to add to the efficacy of HRT for bone preservation. Low-dose estrogen treatment has less benefit than standard-dose estrogen treatment.

Bone density is assessed with a DEXA scan. Many guidelines do not recommend obtaining one of these until age 65 in normal risk women, but many providers suggest that younger women have one sometime after menopause as a baseline. The blood or urine NTX or CTX tests measure how fast bones are breaking down, but they cannot be used to diagnose whether a woman has osteoporosis.

The FRAX calculator is an online tool to help predict a woman's risk of a fracture. Various factors that increase the risk of osteoporosis are tabulated to give an overall score – these include a woman's bone mineral content, her weight, her ethnicity, her smoking history, treatment with steroids, and whether she has a diagnosis of certain diseases such as rheumatoid arthritis.

A woman has generally lost a significant amount of bone mass by the time she is considered *high-risk* or a candidate for any of the drugs that prevent osteoporosis, including HRT.

A woman is considered to have osteoporosis if she incurs a vertebral or hip fracture not associated with a traumatic injury such as a car accident or skiing accident. Otherwise, having a bone density test with a T-score of -2.5 or lower is considered diagnostic of osteoporosis.

Initiating HRT at the time of menopause works most effectively to prevent osteoporosis, but studies show that starting them later (even up to 20 years later) has beneficial effects on bone loss.

Estrogen was the first drug found to be effective in preventing osteoporosis and reducing the risk of fractures. Several non-hormone drugs have been developed that are beneficial but not superior to estrogen therapy. Despite this, since the WHI study was published, estrogen therapy has not been considered first-line therapy for osteoporosis prevention because of concern of potential risks. First-line drugs include:

- Bisphosphonates, which may cause rare adverse bone effects such as ONJ. These should be avoided in women who may require dental extractions and are contraindicated in women who have had weight loss surgery.

- Denosumab, which can also rarely have adverse bone effects. After treatment with this drug is ended, the patient should continue on a bisphosphonate to avoid a sudden increase in fractures.

- SERMs, such as raloxifene. These can help prevent breast cancer but increase the risk of blood clots. They do not decrease hot flashes and may make them worse.

If any of the medications approved for preventing osteoporosis are discontinued, the bone-preserving effects will wane, and the bones will gradually weaken over the next three to five years.

At this time HRT is not recommended to be combined with other drugs used to prevent osteoporosis, such as Fosamax.

Current HRT guidelines with respect to the bones

The current guidelines specify that estrogen replacement is approved for the *prevention* of osteoporosis – but as discussed above, treatment is not recommended until a woman is determined to be at high risk for a fracture. The vast majority of women entering menopause would not be considered high-risk and thus not candidates for HRT for this indication alone.

HRT is not recommended for treatment of established osteoporosis.

What the guidelines don't acknowledge

HRT is not considered first-line treatment for preventing osteoporosis because of risk concerns. However, it is becoming increasingly clear that for most women entering menopause the benefits outweigh the risks. By not encouraging the early use of HRT, women will lose bone mass, putting them at an increased risk for osteoporosis.

Estrogen therapy likely benefits women with established osteoporosis.

Chapter 12
Estrogen and Your Heart

As a woman, are you more likely to die from breast cancer or a heart attack? Whenever I ask a patient this question, she usually gives me the wrong answer and is surprised to learn she is much more likely to die from heart disease than breast cancer. Over 250,000 women die of heart attacks every year.[1] This is in contrast to 41,000 deaths per year due to breast cancer. Even a woman who has been diagnosed with breast cancer is more likely to die from a heart attack than from her breast cancer! In fact, more women die from heart disease than *all* types of cancer combined.

While you may think men are more likely than women to have heart attacks, this is only the case up until the time a woman reaches menopause. At that point in her life, her risk of heart disease rises dramatically such that her risk of a heart attack is comparable to a man of her age.[2,3] In fact, the rate of new diagnoses of heart disease is rising faster in women than in men.[4] There is a great deal of speculation about why this is occurring. Is it because more women are smoking or in higher stress jobs? Do the increasing rates of obesity and diabetes play a role? All of these are risk factors for heart disease and much attention is being devoted to addressing and modifying these lifestyle issues.

However, something not discussed is that since 2002 far fewer women are taking hormones than were taking them prior to the publication of the WHI. *Is it possible that we are seeing more heart disease because fewer women are being treated with estrogen when they go through menopause?* This question may seem far-fetched, but as you read this chapter you will understand why I believe it could be a major factor and why, rather than running away from HRT fearful of breast cancer, women should be demanding that their doctors prescribe it.

Does HRT increase heart disease? The controversy in a nutshell

When I discuss HRT with my patients, I have found that most of them don't know whether hormones are "good" for their hearts or "bad" for them. This is because there has been a great deal of controversy regarding this aspect of hormone treatment. Prior to the year 2000, most of us in the medical field believed that hormones helped prevent heart disease. A large meta-analysis summarizing the results of a number of studies done prior to 1990 concluded that women taking HRT experienced lower rates of heart disease than those who went without them.[5] This was followed by the publication of the Nurses Study, which was the major observational study that followed 40,000 nurses over two decades after they had gone through menopause. This study found that women who took HRT experienced a 50% decrease in major cardiovascular events such as heart attacks.[6]

However in 2002, when the WHI results came out, opinions changed abruptly. The findings of this landmark study showed that rather than preventing heart disease, HRT increased the risk of heart attacks and strokes. As I have discussed in previous chapters, when those shocking results were released, thousands of women stopped their hormones and thousands more were discouraged from starting them. The guidelines generated from the WHI's conclusions emphasized that HRT should not be prescribed as a preventative treatment for heart disease; these same guidelines have persisted for almost two decades.

Why did the WHI study find that HRT was bad for the heart when earlier studies showed the opposite effect? This perplexing contradiction has been studied extensively. This chapter delves into the research and the theories that attempt to explain this discrepancy. I will describe how estrogen affects our cardiovascular system to help you understand why I believe that estrogen is "good" for our hearts.

The cardiovascular system – the basics

To begin, it is helpful for those who don't have a medical background to review some basic anatomy. The major components of the cardiovascular system are the heart, the arteries, and the veins. Visualize one of those anatomic diagrams of the human circulation you may recall seeing on a doctor's wall or in a biology book. Emanating from the heart, and colored red, are the arteries. These spread out in every direction – branching out to the top of the head and the tip of the toes – delivering oxygenated blood to every inch of the body. The arteries get progressively smaller in caliber and then terminate in capillaries – the tiniest of vessels. This nearly translucent network of capillaries surrounds essentially every cell in the body and is where all the blood and cellular interchanges take place. To complete the circuit, the capillaries connect to tiny veins that get progressively bigger as they carry blood back to the heart.

The vascular system holds about five liters, or a little over five quarts, of blood. Floating within the bloodstream are red blood cells – the vehicles that carry oxygen – and countless other elements including a variety of white blood cells (such as lymphocytes and neutrophils), disease-fighting antibodies and other proteins, glucose and other nutrients, electrolytes, clotting factors, hormones, and any other drug or supplement one has ingested. The bloodstream is the Amazon delivery system of our bodies.

If our heart stops beating, our body can't survive much more than five to ten minutes without oxygen and other life-sustaining elements. Similarly, if a blood vessel going to any of our limbs or organs is blocked, the tissues downstream will become damaged. If circulation isn't promptly restored, all or a portion of that body part will die.

Plaque formation and its consequences

The major disease process that affects our arteries is *atherosclerosis*, the technical term for "hardening of the arteries." Atherosclerotic plaques are cholesterol-laden deposits that can develop in any artery in the body. However, the areas where they cause the most medical complications are the arteries supplying the heart, which is known as *coronary artery disease*, and arteries traveling to and within the brain, which is known as *cerebrovascular disease*.

An artery is a flexible tube surrounded by a coating of muscle cells. The muscles around the arteries can contract and relax, causing the diameter of the artery to constrict or dilate. This is an important concept to appreciate because diseased and hardened arteries don't dilate well and this can limit adequate blood flow.

The inside of an artery is lined by a thin sheet of cells, somewhat like a layer of skin, called the *endothelium*. Our external skin is a pretty amazing organ. It is waterproof, protects us from harmful agents in our environment, and repairs itself quickly when damaged. Likewise, the internal skin lining the arteries, the endothelium, is equally proficient. It allows nutrients to be transported from the bloodstream into the cells, protects the artery from harmful substances, and plays a major role in directing the blood flow where it is needed most.

We are learning more and more about the vital role the endothelium plays in plaque formation. We use the terms *endothelial function* and *endothelial dysfunction* to refer to the general health status of the endothelium. When it gets damaged, its ability to protect the artery from further harm becomes compromised. Later in this chapter, you will read more about the critical role that estrogen plays in this process.

Up until young adulthood, the endothelial lining of the arteries is smooth and unblemished. As we age, areas along the endothelium can become irritated or damaged. This triggers formation of plaque which deposits on the walls of the arteries. Plaque is actually a complex conglomeration containing not only cholesterol and calcium, but protein, cellular elements, and even tiny blood vessels.

Everyone develops some degree of plaque. It starts as a little rough spot that can grow and thicken over time, eventually covering large stretches of an artery. Although you commonly think of plaque building up in the arteries on the heart, it can be found in arteries in the brain, kidneys, legs, intestines, and just about everywhere else. Generally, if plaque is present in one area, odds are it is fairly widespread. As the plaque deposits get larger, they can cause some turbulence in the flow, which sometimes can be heard with a stethoscope as a swishing sound, called a *bruit.*

If the buildup of plaque in any given area gets severe enough to compromise the flow of blood, the cells downstream don't get enough oxygen or nutrients. The tissue in these areas becomes damaged and inflamed, causing symptoms, such as pain. If there is a complete blockage large groups of cells can die. This is basically what leads to a *heart attack* – part of the heart dies due to a blockage in one of the arteries that supply it with blood. Similarly, a complete blockage of a blood vessel going to the brain causes a *stroke.* Depending on how much tissue is damaged, the heart attack or stroke can be a minor one or a massive and fatal one.

Many factors contribute to the build-up of plaque. It is believed that certain chemical and physical agents irritate the endothelium and this initiates the process. Then other factors come into play and add to the problem. The hydrocarbons and other nasty constituents of cigarette smoke that enter the bloodstream from the lungs are particularly damaging. Certain types of cholesterol molecules, particularly the low-density form (or LDL particles), cause oxidative damage to the endothelium. High blood pressure, diabetes, inflammation, and certain genetic abnormalities also promote plaque. All of these factors that lead to arterial damage are referred to as *cardiovascular risk factors.* Addressing these risk factors – such as lowering the LDL cholesterol or quitting cigarettes – helps retard plaque development. In addition, measures that increase the HDL, which is the "good" cholesterol, can help prevent plaque formation.

Once plaque forms, it does not dissolve and is not likely to diminish without some type of surgical treatment. That is why patients end up having their heart arteries opened up with stents, or bypassed with grafts. These are invasive procedures and can be risky. Ideally, the goal should be to prevent plaque formation in the first place. This is why those of us in health care devote so much energy encouraging people to eliminate or modify the risk factors that they can control.

It was originally thought that a heart attack was caused by plaque building up to the point where it completely blocked the artery, but now we know that this is usually not the case. Scientists have studied the makeup of plaque and we have learned that it is not as inert as we once believed. While most of the plaque gets calcified and becomes hardened, there generally is a squishy center inside, known as *soft plaque.* This is covered by a tougher outer covering or cap of varying degrees of thickness.

At some point, this covering can be abraded exposing the inner area to the bloodstream. This can trigger a series of events that can literally cause the plaque to explode – forming a large clot that suddenly completely plugs the artery and blocks all downstream flow. This is what technically causes a heart attack. There is much research exploring why some plaque deposits are more vulnerable to rupturing than others and what sorts of agents promote erosion of the surface of the plaque. There is a suspicion that hormones may actually be detrimental to established plaque. I will be going into more detail on this theory shortly, but to pique your curiosity this may explain why older women who start hormones late in life face a higher risk of cardiac complications than younger women who start them at the time of menopause.

Most of the time, the presence of plaque does not lead to an acute heart attack or other sudden catastrophic event. If it does get to the size where it impairs blood flow, it will cause some symptoms. This usually doesn't occur until the blockage occupies over 70 to 80% of the diameter of the artery. If the arteries supplying blood to the heart are involved, this can cause chest pain, or *angina.* Angina is usually brought on by exertion because with exercise the heart needs more blood and the blocked areas restrict the flow. Typically angina is described as a deep ache over the chest that can radiate toward the neck or left arm. However, angina can cause other symptoms. This frequently happens in women and can come in the form of nausea, heartburn, or shortness of breath. Sometimes there is only a sense of unexplained fatigue or dizziness. One explanation for why women present with atypical symptoms is because they are more prone to blockages of very small arteries on the heart. This has been referred to as *microvascular angina*.

You may have heard the term *sudden death*. This usually is a consequence of a heart attack where the injured heart cells trigger a fatal irregularity called *ventricular fibrillation*. This essentially causes the heart to stop beating and, without CPR or other intervention, death can ensue within minutes. An electrical shock from a defibrillator can jar the heart rhythm back to normal and can be a life-saving measure.

If a person has multiple heart attacks, more and more of the heart muscle can become permanently damaged. This weakening can lead to *congestive heart failure* (CHF). When this occurs the heart becomes enlarged and inefficient at circulating blood through the lungs and body. The hallmark symptoms of CHF are weakness, shortness of breath, and leg swelling. Heart failure can also be due to other causes such as severe hypertension, heart valve problems, viral infections, or other diseases.

I have spent time describing the consequences of atherosclerosis because when you read studies that contend taking HRT increases or decreases the risk of cardiovascular disease, the authors are referring to these conditions. Understanding what they are and knowing the role our hormones play in heart health should be considered when it comes to making your HRT decision.

Ways to detect plaque

Short of having any symptoms, such as angina, how do you know if you have plaque in the arteries around your heart? Many patients think that when we listen to their hearts with a stethoscope we are able to detect cardiac plaque. I wish that were so, but that is not the case. We can hear heart rhythm irregularities, such as skipped or missing beats, or swishing sounds called *murmurs* that indicate heart valve problems – but we can't hear anything that may be a sign of a blocked coronary artery. Even a resting *electrocardiogram* (ECG or EKG), the test where electrodes are taped to the chest to measure the electrical activity of the heart, can't detect plaque. Plaque can only be determined by doing more sophisticated tests.

Fortunately, with the advent of technology over the last 50 years, ways to detect and measure plaque buildup have been developed. In the 1970s *angiograms* came into routine use in cardiology. An angiogram is performed by injecting a dye into the bloodstream. Then using x-ray machines called *fluoroscopes*, we are able to observe the arteries which are outlined by the dye. This innovation revolutionized our ability to diagnose and treat coronary disease. Today, most patients having an acute heart attack or suspected of having severe plaque formation undergo an angiogram. The blockages can usually be successfully opened by inflating tiny balloons at the site of the obstruction and then can be kept open by inserting small stents (which look much like the spring in your ballpoint pen).

Angiograms are considered invasive procedures because cardiologists need to insert long catheters into arteries in the arms or legs and thread them through delicate structures to reach the heart. Complications can occur such as puncturing a vessel or causing heart rhythm disturbances. Other downsides are that these tests involve considerable radiation exposure and that the injected dye can damage the kidneys. So, while angiograms can be invaluable procedures, they are used as diagnostic tests only if necessary.

Fortunately, other non-invasive ways to detect plaque have been developed. One such test is an *EBCT* (*electron beam computed tomography*) or *CT/CAT* (*computerized axial tomography*) of the heart. These scans deliver small doses of radiation and utilize computer technology to make 3-dimensional pictures of the heart and blood vessels. The radiologist then scrutinizes the scans looking for any evidence of calcium deposits on the heart – which only should appear if there are plaque deposits present in the heart arteries. The location and amount of calcium deposits give an indication of which arteries are involved and how extensive the plaque may be. Serial scans done over time can show if the plaque is growing.

Another technique to assess plaque utilizes ultrasound technology. The carotid arteries, which are the two main arteries that travel from the heart up on either side of the neck, can be easily imaged using sophisticated ultrasound machines. A hand-held device is placed on the neck and sends sound waves that are used to measure the thickness of the arterial wall, providing a reading called the *carotid intima-media thickness* or *CIMT*. The test is based on the premise that any thickening noted represents an early sign of plaque because the presence of plaque would make the lining of the artery slightly wider. Many health care providers are using this technique to assess if their patients have atherosclerosis. If plaque is present in a carotid artery it likely is present

161

in other areas, especially the heart. CIMT measurements have been very useful in research, but because large-scale studies have not confirmed how reliable a CIMT is to accurately predict one's future risk of a heart attack or stroke, it is not currently recommended as a routine screening test.[7]

However, these tests are frequently used in clinical studies. Since it takes years for plaque to form and progress, it would take many years and many patients in a study to show if an intervention increased or decreased the risk of a heart attack. So, many studies use these non-invasive tests to assess if a treatment is beneficial. If the treatment prevents plaque from developing as measured by these tests, it is presumed that the treatment would be effective in preventing a heart attack down the line. These tests, used in this manner, are referred to as *surrogate markers*.

As an example – let's say a new cholesterol-lowering drug is developed. It may take ten or more years to gather enough data to see if this drug prevents heart attacks. However, if the researchers could show that patients on this drug form less plaque on a CIMT test over a three-to-five year period, this would be an indication that the drug would be effective in preventing a heart attack or stroke in the future.

I feel it is important to discuss these tests and their implications because when you read studies about a drug or treatment preventing an outcome it is important to know what was actually measured or recorded to arrive at the results. Did the study assess actual events, such as the number of heart attacks, or did it rely on results of a substitute test such as a CIMT? A surrogate endpoint does not always equate to a true endpoint.

Assessing the risk for plaque – cardiovascular risk factors

It is well established that there are a number of factors that increase one's chance of developing heart disease. These are known as cardiovascular risk factors and include high cholesterol, smoking, diabetes, high blood pressure, inflammation, and genetics. The more risk factors a person has, the higher the risk of having a heart attack or stroke.

Being a male has consistently been considered a risk factor for heart disease despite the fact that the mechanism for this is not well understood. This does not appear to be due exclusively to lifestyle issues such as stress or smoking – or to the fact men have more testosterone. Women have two **X** chromosomes and men have an **X** and a **Y** chromosome. There has been some speculation that there may be other factors derived from the **Y** chromosome that are responsible.[8]

Once a woman goes past menopause, her risk of a heart attack increases dramatically. Does this mean that the loss of estrogen is a risk factor? I find it interesting that in all my years of going to lectures and looking at lists of cardiac risk factors there is rarely any mention of this probability. I think many health care providers simply assume that older women start having more heart disease because they tend to have more diabetes, hypertension, inactivity, and other factors that would increase their risk. But this doesn't explain why women who had their ovaries removed at a very young age who did not take HRT have almost a two-fold increase in the rate of cardiovascular disease![9] Or studies that consistently show the younger a woman is when she goes through menopause, the more she is at risk for developing heart disease.[10-13]

So while information such as this suggests that estrogen therapy would appear to be a preventative treatment for heart disease, the results of the WHI closed the door on any further debate about whether women should be advised to take HRT for this purpose. Even though we have accumulated considerable data from various clinical trials and observational studies that taking estrogen is good for the heart, none of them trump the credentials of the WHI. Because it is considered to be the gold standard of studies, it remains the cornerstone for the justification of the guidelines.

However, I believe it is important for women to be aware of the large body of evidence that contradicts the findings from the WHI and shows that estrogen has many beneficial effects on our cardiovascular system. To better appreciate all the areas where estrogen affects our risk factors, let's discuss each in more detail. Awareness of the following information should play a role in a woman's decision about whether or not HRT is right for her.

Estrogen effects on cholesterol

Cholesterol is a molecule found in almost every plant and animal and plays many roles in the human body. It is present in the lining of all of our cells and is converted into many hormones, including all of our sex hormones. Cholesterol circulates in the bloodstream in little packets called *lipoproteins*. These consist of fatty (lipid) balls with various proteins called *apoproteins* stuck on the surface. Each type of lipoprotein has different ingredients and exerts different effects in the body. Some promote atherosclerosis formation while others actually decrease its formation.

The LDL or *low-density lipoprotein* is a "bad" type and increases the tendency for plaque formation. It causes oxidative damage to the endothelium and promotes cholesterol buildup inside the plaque. I have described this to patients by saying the LDL is like a "dump truck" – dumping cholesterol onto the lining of the artery. On the opposite side of the spectrum is HDL, or *high-density lipoprotein*. It is more like the "garbage collection truck", acting in ways to "pick up" cholesterol from the plaque. So we refer to HDL as the "good" cholesterol as high levels of HDL correlate with a low risk of heart disease.

As their names imply, these lipoprotein compounds vary in density as well as in size. There are sophisticated blood tests that further classify each of these cholesterol types based on particle size. You may have heard that the worst types are the small dense ones, and the best ones are the large "fluffy ones." Some doctors order an extensive analysis of these various lipoproteins in your blood to further characterize cardiac risk – as there are some particles that are considered worse than others. One in particular is the Lp(a) particle. A high level of this leads to a high risk of plaque formation.

The total amount of cholesterol in each of these lipoproteins can be measured. Traditionally, we measure *total cholesterol* as a screening test and the ideal value is below 200. This number is the sum of the LDL and HDL (plus other less prevalent forms of cholesterol).

It is a well-established fact that women tend to have better cholesterol profiles than men – primarily in that we generally have higher HDL levels. The average HDL for women is in the 50 to 60 range and for men, 40 to 50. Studies have shown that for every point increase in HDL, there is a substantial decrease in cardiovascular risk. So, this is one reason that may explain why women, before the age of fifty, have a lower risk of a heart attack than men of comparable ages.

However, within two years after menopause, a woman's lipid pattern changes markedly, with an increase in the unfavorable LDL levels.[14] The HDL level is not significantly affected by menopause.[15] Studies have shown that *oral* estrogens, including estradiol and Premarin, lower LDL and can raise HDL. They also lower the very bad Lp(a) levels. These effects on lipids are related to the first-pass phenomenon described previously. Transdermal estrogens don't have these beneficial effects.

It should also be pointed out that the addition of a synthetic progestin appears to counteract some of the LDL-lowering benefits. Natural progesterone appears to have a neutral effect on cholesterol.

Estrogen effects on blood pressure

High blood pressure, or hypertension, is another major risk factor for plaque development. Think of an artery as a garden hose. When you turn up the pressure, more force is exerted on the inside of the hose. In the arteries, the increase in force caused by high blood pressure puts stress on the endothelium which leads to injury and inflammation. This causes chemical messengers to be released, which triggers a cascade of reactions that initiate plaque.

It has been shown that keeping the blood pressure below 140/90 tends to prevent damage to the arteries. When the pressure runs higher than this, we recommend treatment with drug therapy if other measures, such as weight loss, exercise, and salt restriction, are not effective. There are a variety of medications that act to lower the pressure through different mechanisms. The most effective ones are agents that make the arteries relax and dilate which, in turn, lowers the pressure inside the artery. Interestingly, the natural estrogen produced in a woman's body tends to have this effect on the arteries.

High blood pressure is very common and becomes increasingly likely as people age. Men below the age of 50 tend to have hypertension more frequently than women, but after menopause, the incidence of hypertension in women increases sharply.[16] It is postulated that this has something to do with our loss of estrogen, and it would seem logical that hormone replacement would have a beneficial effect. Evidence for this has come from animal studies. Removing the ovaries from mice forces them into a menopausal state. Mice can be subjected to agents that cause hypertension. If these mice are treated with estradiol, they are more resistant to developing high blood pressure than those not given estrogen.[17]

However, the results of studies where estrogen is given to humans are mixed, and experts are hesitant to conclusively say that HRT lowers blood pressure after menopause. Below is a summary of a number of studies that demonstrate why there is uncertainty about the relationship between HRT and hypertension.

- In the WHI study combined hormone treatment did not have a blood pressure-lowering effect, and, in fact, tended to increase it.[18]

Recall that the hormones used in this study were Premarin and Provera, and the average age of the women was older.

- The KEEPS study did not show that estradiol (oral or transdermal) with or without natural progesterone had any effect on blood pressure.[19]

- In a study that recruited women with known hypertension, estradiol lowered blood pressure in younger women close to menopause, but not in older women who were further beyond menopause.[20]

- Adding estradiol to blood pressure pills helped control blood pressure more effectively than blood pressure pills alone in a study assessing 24-hour blood pressure control.[21]

- A review of a large number of articles published between 2000 and 2013 showed that oral estrogen therapy neither raised nor lowered the blood pressure in women with or without a diagnosis of hypertension. However, transdermal estrogen tended to lower blood pressure in women who did not have known hypertension but didn't seem to benefit women with known hypertension.[16]

It should be noted that most of these studies were not designed with the principal goal of testing the outcome of taking hormones on blood pressure. So, we really don't have enough data to make definitive conclusions. In addition, not all the studies distinguished whether women were taking some form of progestogen. Studies have shown that synthetic progestogens, such as Provera, can cause blood vessel constriction, which can raise blood pressure, whereas other progestogens can have a diuretic effect – which would have a tendency to lower blood pressure.[22] Natural progesterone appears to have either a neutral or slightly beneficial effect on blood pressure.[16]

The bottom line is that we can't say HRT will have a beneficial effect on blood pressure, but it likely does not have a negative effect. The progestogen component may be a factor in why there are variations in the outcomes between studies. And finally, the timing issue may come into play – where HRT given early in menopause may be beneficial but not so if given at a later time.

Estrogen and diabetes

Another major risk factor to discuss is diabetes. Patients who have diabetes have a markedly increased risk of developing a heart attack or stroke. Diabetes prevalence is on the rise. The risk of diabetes increases as women age.[24]   One out of four women will be diagnosed with diabetes by age 65.[23] Whether the loss of hormones plays a central role in increasing this risk is controversial, but several lines of evidence suggest this. For one, there is a clear association of an increased risk of diabetes in women who go through menopause early, or who have had their ovaries removed.[25,26] It has also been shown in both human and animal studies that estrogen deficiency is associated with an increased deposition of central fat (belly fat).[27] This pattern of fat accumulation greatly increases the chance of developing *insulin resistance*, which is the major mechanism behind adult-onset diabetes.

If it is the loss of estrogen that leads to diabetes, then HRT should help prevent it. And indeed, this has been demonstrated in many studies. Two well-respected studies, the PEPI and HERS studies found that women on HRT had up to a 30% lower chance of developing diabetes than women on a placebo.[28,29] And, believe it or not, the WHI study even confirmed this.[30] Women taking estrogen/progestogen had a 19% decrease in new cases of diabetes and women on estrogen alone had a 14% reduction.[31]   A meta-analysis published in 2014 found that HRT reduced the risk of diabetes by almost 40% and improved women's overall blood sugar levels.[32]

How menopause and HRT affect diabetes is discussed in more detail in Chapter 15, but the bottom line for this discussion is that HRT clearly plays a role in decreasing this major risk factor for heart disease.

Estrogen and inflammation

Over the last ten years or so you may have read a lot about the CRP test or *C-reactive protein*. This is a blood test that has traditionally been used by rheumatologists to measure the level of inflammation going on in the body from such diseases as lupus and rheumatoid arthritis. Cardiologists recently have discovered that even minor increases in the CRP, which are detected by running a *highly sensitive* assay for CRP (known as the *hs-CRP*), correlate with an increased risk of having a heart attack. The simple explanation for this is that if there is an inflammatory process going on anywhere in the body, the body's immune system is activated and some of these factors are harmful to the lining of the arteries. Indeed, patients with autoimmune diseases have a higher risk of heart attacks. So inflammation is now recognized as a risk factor for developing cardiovascular disease. Unlike some of the other modifiable risk factors such as high cholesterol, the vexing problem is what to do about this. Taking ibuprofen or some other anti-inflammatory drug hasn't been shown to counteract this risk.

While it is believed that the natural estrogen in our bodies has strong anti-inflammatory effects, whether hormone replacement retards or promotes inflammation has been difficult to sort out. Some immune diseases seem to get worse with estrogen therapy and some better. It has frequently been cited that HRT raises CRP levels – this was a finding in the WHI study as well. This has led to the assumption that estrogen therapy increases inflammation. However, the rise in CRP may be primarily related to the first-pass effect (described earlier) which only occurs with oral estrogens. Transdermal estradiol does not appear to affect the CRP level.[33]

In addition, CRP is only one of countless components involved in the inflammatory process. We have identified a number of blood "markers" that are associated with immune activity in the body. Some are "good guys" playing a beneficial role; others are "bad guys." Estrogen administration has been shown to decrease many of the deleterious inflammatory markers.[34] A number of studies in the lab have demonstrated that at the cellular level estrogen can exert potent anti-inflammatory activity.[35,36] A recent review of this subject concluded that, overall, HRT appears to improve the immune response in postmenopausal women.[37] So while more research is needed, there is a strong suspicion that estrogen's effect on inflammation is another reason why HRT may decrease the risk of plaque formation.

Other risk factors

Before leaving this discussion I want to comment on some of the other risk factors that aren't affected by HRT. Smoking is one harmful habit that women can easily avoid. Many of my patients assume that the biggest risk from smoking is lung cancer – but the truth is that cigarettes cause way more heart attacks than cancer. The toxic hydrocarbons and carbon monoxide inhaled with every puff travel throughout the bloodstream wreaking havoc on the endothelium. A woman increases her risk of getting a heart attack six-fold if she smokes one pack per day and the risk increases the more she smokes.[38,39] I like to point this out because I think it is important for women to realize that smoking is exponentially more likely to lead to heart disease than taking HRT. I overheard a conversation between two women smoking at a bus stop about how they would *never* take estrogen because of all the risks, and it was all I could do to not walk over and set the record straight about their uninformed choices to choose cigarettes over hormones!

Even second-hand smoke is likely more harmful to the heart than HRT. According to a study published in the *New England Journal of Medicine*, being exposed to second-hand smoke can increase the risk of developing heart disease by 25% to 30%![40] This is roughly the same degree of risk that the researchers in the WHI attributed to taking combined Premarin and Provera, which increased the risk of a heart attack by 26%. This interesting comparison may help put some perspective on the relative risks of taking HRT – especially if you happen to be living with a smoker.

Genetics also play a role in determining cardiac risk. Patients who have a first-degree relative who suffered a heart attack prematurely (defined as men younger than age 50 and women younger than age 65) are at higher risk for heart disease. That is why doctors ask about family history. There are many genes that play a role in one's predisposition to a heart attack – such as genes that dictate an unhealthy cholesterol pattern, or ones that predispose one to hypertension. However, there are also other, yet to be identified, genetic defects that appear to promote early and severe plaque development. That is why we occasionally come across a young patient who presents with a heart attack out of the blue despite having none of the known risk factors.

Other conditions that increase cardiovascular risk are HIV infections, chronic kidney disease, and a history of chest radiation treatment. Many women may not realize that radiation therapy for breast cancer can harm their hearts.[41] Although great pains are taken to specifically target the cancer and shield other parts of the body, some of the ionizing rays cause damage to the deeper structures inside the chest, especially the sensitive endothelium of the heart arteries. I recall one patient in particular – a 64-year-old woman who ran three marathons a year and had excellent blood pressure and cholesterol, who suddenly developed chest pain requiring an emergency cardiac procedure to put a stent in a nearly completely blocked artery on her heart. We were both very surprised because, in addition to having no risk factors, she had had a heart CAT scan about ten years earlier that showed no evidence of plaque. However, she did have a history of breast cancer and had received radiation treatment that year. Her cardiologist agreed that this played a role. Radiation damage to the coronary arteries happens more frequently than many women realize, especially if their breast cancers occur in the left breast.

Assessing cardiac risk

A person who has multiple risk factors will develop hardening of the arteries at a much earlier age than someone with no risk factors. Formulas have been developed to assess one's degree of risk by plugging in information such as age, weight, cholesterol levels, blood pressure, smoking history, and other factors to come up with an estimate of the likelihood of experiencing a major cardiac event within a ten-year window. A classic early version of one of these calculating tools is the *Framingham Risk Score.* More recently the American Cardiology Association and the American Heart Association have promoted their version, known as the *ACA/AHA CVD risk calculator.* This can be found online. You or your doctor can put your information into this program to get an assessment. If the risk is over a certain level, experts in the field advise doctors to more aggressively treat the patient's risk factors – such as prescribing high-dose statin drugs.

In looking at these risk assessment tools and reviewing the internal medicine and cardiology websites that discuss cardiac risk factors, I find it interesting that there is essentially no mention of the use or non-use of menopausal hormone therapy in most of these discussions. (Whereas in a popular and respected medical practice database, called *UpToDate*, I noted an entire paragraph discussing the effects of testosterone deficiency in increasing a man's cardiac risk!)[42] The reason this bothers me is that it is clear that taking estrogen has a beneficial effect on several cardiac risk factors, yet there continues to be a huge reluctance to formally acknowledge this information, much less disseminate it to women. This undoubtedly is due, in large part, to the findings from the WHI that have raised a red flag on the safety of HRT and the heart. However, there are many reasons why women should question whether relying on the WHI as the final word on HRT and cardiac risk makes sense. Hopefully, you can come to an informed opinion as you read the rest of this chapter.

A review of the studies on HRT and the heart

Now that I've described how estrogen impacts specific cardiovascular risk factors, let's look more closely at some of the key studies that have helped us understand how hormones affect the heart. Over the last 50 years, a tremendous amount of information has been generated. This has come from research in the lab at the cellular level, as well as studies examining the effects of various hormones on both animals and humans. Some of the studies that I will be discussing in the rest of this chapter have been introduced in earlier chapters, but I feel it is important to refresh your memory and provide further details about them.

Prior to 2000, the Nurses Study and the Leisure World Study showed that HRT substantially decreased a woman's risk of having a heart attack, and textbooks published at the time acknowledged that estrogen was beneficial for the heart. So up until 2002, the preponderance of evidence indicated that HRT was an effective cardioprotective agent.

It had also been assumed HRT would be beneficial for women with established heart disease. However, this assumption was shaken by the Heart and Estrogen/Progestin Replacement Study (HERS).[43] The goal of this study was to enroll women with known heart disease and assess how hormone treatment impacted their status. The investigators recruited 2,763 women who had a history of a heart attack, coronary artery surgery, or angiogram evidence of coronary disease. The average age of the enrollees was 66.6 plus or minus 6.7 years, and they were 10 to 26 years past menopause. Premarin and Provera were the hormones given for treatment. After four years there was no difference in heart outcomes between the placebo and treatment groups – indicating that HRT did not appear to improve the status of women with known heart disease.

Then on the heels of HERS came the WHI. Unlike the HERS, the intent of the WHI was to enroll *generally healthy* women without known heart disease. The results of the WHI showed an increase in heart attacks and strokes in women taking Premarin and Provera, and an increase in strokes in women on Premarin alone.[44,45] So the upshot of this was that we had two highly reputable clinical studies that showed that HRT not only did not benefit women with known heart disease but increased the risk of heart attacks and strokes in healthy women! These two studies shattered the presumption that HRT was good for the heart and tipped the scales regarding the safety of hormones. Doctors and patients were warned that the risks of HRT outweighed the benefits, and this was primarily because of cardiovascular issues.

The discrepancy between the earlier studies and the WHI and HERS results spurred much consternation and further inquiry. Why were the outcomes so disparate? To explore this, it is helpful to review some significant points regarding these studies.

- The earlier observational studies primarily included younger women who were placed on HRT around the time of their natural menopause.

Conversely, in both the WHI and the HERS studies the women were older and many were at least ten years beyond the time of natural menopause.

- Because most of the women in the earlier studies were younger, it would be unlikely they would have developed heart disease. This is in contrast to the women in the HERS study all of whom had established heart disease and, while the WHI study recruited *generally healthy* women, the majority had at least two cardiovascular risk factors.

- The only hormones used in both the HERS and WHI were oral Premarin and the synthetic progestogen, medroxyprogesterone. In many of the observational studies, the exact type of hormones taken by the women being assessed wasn't always differentiated, and in many early studies estrogen alone was being used for HRT.

- And finally, a relatively small number of women in the HERS and WHI studies were having hot flashes. (The WHI study specifically excluded women having significant hot flashes.) It can be assumed that most of the women in the earlier studies were having hot flashes, as most women experience them when they initially enter menopause. The reason to mention this is that women with hot flashes may be at a higher risk for heart disease – and they may be the ones to most benefit from HRT.

The significance of these points will become increasingly clear as you read on in this chapter. The important issue to note is that neither the WHI nor the HERS study really represented the typical 50-year-old symptomatic woman going through menopause, which was the case in the bulk of the earlier studies. But because the WHI has been the only truly gold-standard study assessing hormone use and the heart, its conclusions have been the foundation for the guidelines since 2002, and have been applied to all menopausal women without regard to their age or health status.

To overcome the shortcomings of the WHI, the ideal solution would be to design a study comparing hormone therapy in younger premenopausal women versus older women. It wasn't until 2016 that such a study was published, the Vascular Effects of Early vs. Late Postmenopausal Treatment with Estradiol (ELITE study). As described in Chapter 7, the investigators recruited two groups of women – newly menopausal women (the early group) and women at least ten years past menopause (the late group). The aim of this study was to assess the difference in outcomes of HRT between these two groups. The 650 women in the study were placed on oral estradiol and natural progesterone. A CIMT (carotid thickness test) and a sophisticated heart CAT scan were done at the beginning and end of the study. As discussed earlier in this chapter, these are tests used to detect plaque.

At the end of five years the investigators found the following:

- At the start of the study, the older women generally had more plaque in their arteries than the younger women – which you would expect due to their age. At the end of the study, treatment with hormones neither worsened nor improved the degree of arterial thickening in these late menopausal women.

- In younger women, treatment with hormones *decreased* the rate of progression of hardening of their arteries compared to women on a placebo.

The significance of this study is that it formally addressed the Timing Hypothesis, thus supporting the theory that hormones have different effects depending on the age they are initiated. This study showed that HRT prevented the progression of plaque in younger women, but not in those who were ten or more years away from menopause. I recall the morning when I opened up my copy of the prestigious *New England Journal of Medicine* and read this article for the first time. I was excited about these results as it reinforced what many of us believed – that taking HRT early at the time of menopause carries many cardiac benefits. It further suggested that it was something about being well past menopause that prevented HRT from having the same effect. However, my bubble of elation burst when I read a subsequent editorial that stated,

> *"Despite a favorable effect of estrogen in the ELITE trial, the relevance of these results to clinical coronary heart disease remains questionable."*[47]

The author of the editorial noted that while the CIMT tests used in the study can correlate with plaque development, they do not necessarily predict who is going to have a heart attack or stroke. To me, he was saying that while this study appears to support the Timing Hypothesis, further research is needed and there is no reason to consider any changes to the guidelines.

Quite frankly with all of the paranoia about HRT safety in older women and the lack of money for research in this area, I was amazed (but pleased) to see that the ELITE study had been undertaken. I am not sure if we will be seeing any more studies of this nature which directly compare younger women to older women. No doubt this reticence is due to the continued stronghold the WHI has placed on the advisability of prescribing HRT for older women, or for extended periods of time.

So how else can we gather data to build support for the case that hormones are good for the heart and challenge the findings of the WHI study? Several approaches can be followed. These include:

- Proceeding with clinical studies that recruit only younger menopausal women to further solidify the belief that HRT carries more benefits than risks in this age group.

- Reanalyzing data from older studies to compare the effects of HRT in younger vs. older women.

- Continuing to gather and analyze data from large observational studies and from basic research.

An example of the first approach noted above was the KEEPS study, introduced in Chapter 7. The study's goal was to determine whether hormone therapy prevented plaque progression in younger women. This study enrolled 727 women between the ages of 42 and 58 and placed them on Premarin, transdermal estradiol, or placebo. If a progestogen was needed, natural progesterone was prescribed. While I was hopeful that the results of this study would be a breakthrough moment attesting to the benefits of HRT in young women, the final conclusion was that hormone administration had no effect.

However, we can't say that it "disproved" the premise that estrogen prevents heart disease. The five-year length of the study was likely not long enough to see significant plaque development in these younger women. In addition, as noted above, the changes measured by using CIMT testing cannot definitely predict whether or not a patient will eventually have a heart attack. And finally, other data from the KEEPs study supported the potential cardioprotective benefits of HRT. Women in the study on hormones demonstrated improvement in their cholesterol readings and those on transdermal estrogen showed a decrease in insulin resistance which is a precursor of diabetes. Both of these are measures that correlate with a decreased future risk of heart disease.

Studies using the second approach have also appeared. Although most of the women in the WHI study were older, researchers have teased out data on the approximately one thousand women who were younger than age 59 when they entered the study. Some of these women had serial cardiac CAT scans. Recall this is the test that shows calcium deposits on the heart – which correlate with the amount of plaque in the coronary arteries. After five years, women taking HRT demonstrated lower levels of calcium in their heart arteries compared to those women taking a placebo.[48] This supports the premise that taking HRT soon after menopause decreases the development of hardening of the arteries that can go on to cause a heart attack.

Back in 2007 when this information came out, I found it to be very reassuring (especially since I was taking HRT!). Of course, there were those who reminded us that CAT scans are substitute tests for the presence of an actual disease (i.e., surrogate markers) and we can't assume that these findings prove these women will be less likely to have a heart attack. But I am happy to report that a subsequent paper came out in 2013 that reported further on the status of this group of women who started hormone replacement therapy before turning 59. In this 13-year follow-up analysis of data from the WHI study, women in the HRT group demonstrated 40% fewer heart attacks than women on a placebo.[49] This impressive beneficial effect of estrogen was not seen in women who started HRT later than age 60.

Other studies have continued to build the case that taking HRT at the time of menopause correlates with a lower risk of developing heart disease.[50,51] In 2012 we learned of the results of the Danish Osteoporosis Prevention Study (DOPS).[52] This study involved 1,006 recently menopausal women, average age 50, who were treated with HRT. The investigators found that women who had taken HRT had a significant decrease in cardiac events after ten years of treatment compared to women who did not go on HRT.

Subsequently, in 2015, a major review of 19 clinical trials found that oral hormone therapy initiated less than ten years after menopause lowered the risk of cardiovascular disease as well as all causes of death, and did not increase the risk of a stroke.[53] In women who started treatment more than ten years after menopause, HRT did not have any significant effect on death or coronary heart disease.

New observational studies continue to appear showing the cardiac benefits of HRT. A study published in 2017 looking at HRT use and heart CAT scan findings was done in Iceland.[54] A large group of women over the age of 70 who had had CAT scans of their hearts were sent questionnaires regarding their hormone use history. The authors found that women who had used hormones had 30% less calcium buildup (which correlates with the amount of plaque) than women who had never used them. The longer a woman had taken HRT (many for greater than 15 years) the lower were their calcium scores. They also found that women who had started HRT within five years of menopause had the lowest accumulation of calcium deposition.

Animal studies have been helpful in assessing how timing of initiation of HRT affects cardiac outcomes. Estrogen therapy has been shown to prevent plaque development and progression in younger menopausal mice but had no effect in older mice that already had established plaque.[55] Similar findings were found when monkeys underwent this type of experiment. Estrogen given to younger menopausal monkeys decreased the onset of atherosclerosis by almost 70% but did not benefit the older ones.[56]

Collectively these studies help build the case that HRT is beneficial for the heart, at least in younger, newly menopausal women. Why this may not hold true for older women, who are 10 or more years beyond menopause, is the next major subject to address.

The difference between young arteries and old arteries

The million-dollar question is why does the timing of hormone therapy make a difference when it comes to plaque? What is it about hormones that are beneficial for younger arteries and not older ones? Much of our understanding comes from research focusing on the role the endothelium plays in preventing atherosclerosis. Recall that the endothelium is the lining inside an artery. It plays a very active role in preventing plaque from forming, progressing, and even rupturing.[57]

As described above, when the endothelium is not functioning optimally we call this *endothelial dysfunction.* A number of articles have demonstrated that estrogen plays a vital role in preventing endothelial dysfunction.[58] It has been shown that the endothelium is rich in estrogen receptors and when estrogen interacts with them many positive actions are induced. In summary, these include:

- ***Stimulation of nitric oxide production.*** Arteries are not fixed diameter tubes. They constrict and relax. A primary factor that promotes dilation is nitric oxide, a chemical produced by the endothelial cells. It has been shown in the lab that estrogen rapidly stimulates the release of this substance. When nitric oxide is released, the pressure in the artery decreases and there is improved blood flow to the cells which increases the delivery of oxygen and nutrients.

- ***Anti-inflammatory action.*** Inflammation is a major contributor to the build-up of plaque. Estrogen blocks some of the chemical changes that cause inflammation within the endothelium.

- ***Anti-oxidant effects.*** The bad cholesterol particles, primarily the small, dense LDL particles, get oxidized and burrow into the endothelium. Estrogen works to limit the damage from oxidation.

All of these artery-protective effects conferred from estrogen occur even before menopause and contribute to women's lower risks of heart disease. The loss of estrogen and thus the loss of these functions ostensibly would allow plaque to develop at an accelerated rate. This would also explain why women who go through menopause earlier than expected get more cardiovascular disease than women who go through menopause later.[59,60,61]

If women are given estrogen as they transition through menopause and beyond, these positive effects on the endothelium should continue uninterrupted. However, if some period of time goes by – presumably around ten years – the endothelium can't respond to estrogen as it did prior to menopause. This is the underlying premise of the Timing Hypothesis.

One approach to study how timing of HRT affects endothelial function is to examine in more detail how estrogen affects nitric oxide production. Both in animal and human experiments, it has been shown that higher levels of estrogen correlate with higher levels of nitric oxide production.[58] Scientists have come up with ways to test how well our endothelium is able to generate nitric oxide by measuring how much blood flow goes through a particular artery. Since nitric oxide makes the artery dilate, the more nitric oxide that is made and released, the greater the flow. This can be measured in patients in the lab with monitoring equipment and the technique is called *flow-mediated dilation.*

Studies have been conducted testing the differences between how estrogen administration affects nitric oxide production in younger versus older women.[62,63] In younger women, pretreatment with a course of estrogen improved their flow-mediated dilatation. In older women, there was no improvement. This implies that in the older women estrogen was not able to effectively trigger the release of nitric oxide. It appears that after prolonged estrogen deprivation, administering estrogen is unable to restore endothelial function.[64]

Why would this occur? Does something happen to the arteries if they are not exposed to estrogen after a number of years? As discussed in Chapter 7, the answer is likely related to the loss of estrogen receptors. Without receptors, estrogen is unable to interact with the arteries to promote beneficial effects.[65,66,67] With aging, there is a general loss of receptors in many tissues and studies have documented that the number of receptors on women's arteries declines the further she is beyond menopause.[68]

Without a receptor, estrogen cannot cause good things to happen. So, if estrogen therapy is withheld and then given some period of time beyond menopause, it would simply float around in the circulatory system. There would be plenty of estrogen detectable in the bloodstream, but since it can't find any receptors it can't exert any effects. Credibility for this theory comes from animal studies. "Menopause" can be induced in mice by removing their ovaries causing them to develop atherosclerosis prematurely. If they are given estrogen, this is prevented. However, in mice that been genetically altered to lack estrogen receptors treatment with estrogen is ineffective at preventing atherosclerosis.[69,70]

Why would HRT be harmful in older women?

While the loss of receptor function is a very plausible explanation why delaying HRT may not be effective in preventing plaque formation, a very important question to address is why would giving HRT to older women actually be detrimental, as was shown in the WHI? This is a major issue that has yet to be fully clarified, but we are coming closer to an understanding.

A likely explanation stems from the theory that hormones may cause some adverse effects in certain types of plaque. It is speculated that in some women, especially those with large amounts of plaque, hormones may interact with the plaque in some detrimental way, which sets off a cascade of events that cause the plaque to rupture and form a blood clot.[71] The end result can be a complete blockage of the artery causing a heart attack or a stroke. The fact that oral estrogens cause the blood to coagulate more readily can exacerbate the situation.

This theory would explain an interesting finding noted in the WHI, HERS, and some other studies – that most of the heart attacks that occurred happened within the first year of treatment. The likely scenario was that a substantial amount of plaque was already present in these older women and the hormones destabilized the plaque shortly after treatment was initiated. In other words, these were the women most likely to develop cardiac complications. Women without major plaque on their arteries would not run into problems and HRT would either have beneficial or neutral effects going forward.

I haven't come across a universally accepted explanation why hormones would irritate plaque and look forward to future research in this area. One current theory is that it has something to with hormone-induced stimulation of certain enzymes that normally play a role in creating a woman's menstrual cycle. Each month these enzymes help "dissolve" part of the lining of the uterus to allow it to shed leading to the monthly blood flow. These same enzymes may also weaken the cap that covers arterial plaque.[72] Older women with large amounts of plaque could theoretically be harmed by this. Younger women, who by virtue of their age have less plaque, would not be affected in this manner from hormone administration.

Currently, the guidelines discourage initiating HRT after the age of 60 because of a presumption that these women have plaque. However, this is not always the case. There are many extremely healthy women this age and older who likely have very little plaque. Older women who have negligible cardiac risk factors and no evidence of calcium on their heart scans potentially could even benefit from HRT. How to predict who may be at risk from taking HRT, other than being of advanced age, is an area in which we need more research and more direction.

The role of progestogens

In the WHI study it was the women taking combined estrogen and the progestogen Provera who were found to have an increased risk of cardiac events (whereas the women taking Premarin alone did not). This has raised the question whether it was the progestogen that made the difference in the WHI outcomes. But, other studies have not consistently shown that the addition of a progestogen increases cardiac harm.[73]

As noted, most of the studies prior to the WHI concluded that women on HRT had less cardiac disease. However, most of them did not differentiate the exact HRT regimen taken by the women in the studies. This clouds our understanding of how progestogens affect the cardiovascular system. It likely depends on the particular type taken. Some synthetic progestogens may attenuate the beneficial effects of estrogen on lipids as well as on endothelial function.[74,75] Other synthetic progestins may have positive effects, such as blood pressure-lowering effects.[76] Natural progesterone probably has a neutral effect on all these parameters, including its effect on the clotting system.[77]

In conclusion

It will be interesting to see how things evolve with respect to the guidelines as we learn more and more about the Timing Hypothesis. Many experts agree that starting HRT at the time of menopause presents very little risk and appears to protect against heart disease in younger women.[76] However, current guidelines emphasize that HRT should not be used for preventing cardiovascular problems no matter a woman's age. The good news is that hormone therapy is appropriate for treatment of hot flashes, so women taking them for this reason will reap some cardioprotection. Unfortunately, women without hot flashes may miss out on these potential benefits. The wisdom of using them only for the *"shortest period of time necessary"* is also possibly shortsighted as once HRT is discontinued, the beneficial effects on the endothelium will be lost.

Decision Making Helper

Key Considerations

Much research and many studies, including the WHI, have shown that initiating HRT at the time of menopause carries very little cardiac risk and may be cardioprotective. Starting hormones ten years after menopause appears to increase cardiac risk. However, this may be confined to women who already have pre-existing cardiac disease.

Heart CAT scans are useful to assess if there is any plaque in the arteries on the heart. If the scan does not show any signs of calcium, there is a low probability of significant plaque.

Women with severe hot flashes may be at a higher risk for cardiac disease and may be the ones to benefit the most from taking HRT early in menopause.

Women tend to have better cholesterol profiles than men, but after menopause, their LDL increases. Taking oral estrogen has been shown to lessen the rise in LDL, but transdermal estrogen does not appear to do so. Oral estrogens can raise triglycerides but transdermal estrogen does not. These effects on lipids may be related to the first-pass phenomenon.

Estrogen does not appear to increase blood pressure. Some synthetic progestogens may have a negative impact on blood pressure. Natural progesterone appears to have a neutral effect on blood pressure and may be slightly beneficial.

HRT appears to decrease the risk of metabolic syndrome and diabetes, which are risk factors for cardiovascular disease.

Oral estrogen appears to raise the inflammatory marker CRP, whereas transdermal estrogen does not appear to do so. The elevation of CRP is of questionable significance, however, because research indicates that estrogen has a major anti-inflammatory effect on the endothelium.

Both oral and transdermal estrogen improve endothelial function by promoting nitric oxide production and by their anti-inflammatory and antioxidant effects. These properties of estrogen retard plaque development.

Natural progesterone may be preferable to synthetic progestogens with respect to cardiac risk because it appears to have a neutral effect on the endothelium, blood pressure, cholesterol, and the clotting system. Synthetic progestogens may attenuate some of the beneficial effects of estrogen.

Current guidelines regarding HRT and the heart

HRT is not recommended as a preventative therapy for heart disease or for treatment of high cholesterol or hypertension.

What the guidelines don't acknowledge

Most experts in menopause agree that initiating estrogen at the time of menopause decreases a woman's risk of future heart disease. Initiating HRT in older women, ten or more years beyond menopause, may increase cardiac risk but the risk is very small and likely depends on whether the woman already has established plaque.

Chapter 13
Estrogen and Your Clotting System

It's always heart-rending to hear about a person dying from a blood clot. Suddenly, without any warning, a person loses consciousness, collapses, and cannot be resuscitated. In many cases this happens to someone on a plane returning from a dream vacation or shortly after a patient has had an otherwise successful surgery.

Frequently, the sequence of events preceding these tragedies is the development of a clot, known as a *deep vein thrombosis* (DVT), which formed inside a vein, subsequently dislodged, and traveled to the lungs – causing a pulmonary embolism. These clots originate in one of the deep veins inside our bodies – generally in the thigh or calf. Three out of every 2,000 people will experience one of these in their lifetime. Blood clots conjure up scary thoughts, and they should. They can cause sudden death even in a young, healthy person.

How blood clots occur and why they are dangerous

When we are injured, veins lying within the skin, muscles or deeper organs can become damaged and disrupted. This causes a leakage of blood into the surrounding tissue. Depending on the severity of the injury this will result either in a small bruise or a larger collection of blood called a *hematoma*. Fortunately, in almost all cases the body is able to contain the bleeding because a complex cascade of chemical reactions immediately begins to make the blood congeal and clot. This is obviously a life-saving process – preventing someone from bleeding to death. However, overzealous clotting can also be hazardous as this could cause massive blockages throughout the circulatory system. So our bodies have developed an intricate system to finely regulate this process to keep blood flowing through our body, as well as being able to plug holes as they occur. Our clotting system has multiple components that work in concert. These include platelets which are tiny particles made in the bone marrow, clotting factors made primarily in the liver (*Factors I through XII*), and a number of other proteins and enzymes.

Clots formed outside of vessels, such as hematomas, are contained within the skin or other tissue layers and don't travel anywhere. The body slowly resorbs the blood over time and the bruise disappears. It is the clots that form inside the vessels of our circulation that are the troublemakers. They can cause a blockage of blood flow where they first form or can dislodge and travel to another area.

In the last chapter I discussed how plaque develops and causes problems in the arteries. Veins are structurally different than arteries and don't develop plaque. Veins are much thinner, and rather than supply blood to the tissue, they are the conduits for returning blood back to the heart. In the legs, they have to work against gravity and facilitate blood flow all the way up from the toes. This is accomplished by the presence of delicate valves positioned every six to twelve inches inside the veins that act like little fish ladders. Each beat of the heart pumps the blood up to the next level and, eventually, it flows into the heart.

Over time these valves can become damaged and blood will pool in the veins below them causing them to swell. Dilation of the superficial veins just below the skin causes varicose veins – those ugly, swollen blue vessels that bulge on the surface of our legs. Chronic dilation of the deeper veins inside the legs distends them to the point where the pressure causes fluid to seep through the vessel walls and out into the surrounding tissue. This leads to swelling of the legs. This condition is referred to as *venous insufficiency.* Wearing compression (support) stockings helps prevent the legs from swelling. In some cases, vein surgery may be needed.

The more serious vein problem occurs when blood clots form along the *inside* wall of the vein. This can occur anywhere in the venous system – in the arms or in the vessels that supply our internal organs – but most commonly occurs in the legs. An injury can cause one of these deep vein clots, but they can also develop when the blood flow in the veins is constricted or becomes sluggish. These conditions occur with prolonged inactivity such as bed rest, immobilization from a cast, or sitting for extended periods of time with flexed hips and knees such as on an overseas plane ride.

In the legs, the extensive system of small, superficial veins under the skin drain into several large, deep internal veins. Small clots can form in the surface veins and cause tender, swollen, inflamed lumps, and this condition is called *superficial phlebitis.* Because these superficial veins form a tight, lattice-like network, clots in these areas usually are contained where they form.

Most of the time, superficial phlebitis is not a serious condition and is treated with heat and anti-inflammatory drugs such as aspirin. Superficial phlebitis usually resolves over several weeks.

The dangerous clots are the DVTs, the ones present in the deep internal veins of the legs. When a clot such as this forms it may progressively enlarge and at some point potentially dislodge and travel up into the heart and then out into the arteries supplying the lungs. Because these arteries get progressively smaller as they branch out into the lungs, the clot eventually becomes wedged within one, blocking blood flow to a section of the lung, causing a *pulmonary embolism* (PE) – damaging the lung tissue downstream. If a large amount of the circulation to the lung is blocked, this can be fatal.

Generally, a DVT in the leg causes symptoms – primarily leg swelling and pain. While other medical conditions can cause both legs to swell, when only one leg becomes swollen, we are more suspicious of a clot. The swelling can be fairly subtle, just some puffiness around the ankle, or the patient may have an impressively fat leg. The pain caused by a DVT can be variable in intensity and is usually felt in the thigh, calf, or behind the knee. However, up to one-third of patients with a DVT don't present with any of the typical symptoms. So, diagnosing a DVT can be difficult. Doctors frequently need to rely on clues that may raise suspicion of a clot such as a history of prolonged sitting or other extended time of immobility.

If a DVT is suspected, the next step is to perform an imaging test to confirm the diagnosis. Ultrasound tests are very effective in detecting clots. If it is a small clot below the knee, generally no specific treatment is required other than to monitor it to make certain that it doesn't progress. If it is a large clot or one that occurs above the knee, strong blood thinners are prescribed for three to six months or longer to treat it. For years the mainstay of treatment has been heparin, given by injection, or warfarin (Coumadin) pills – the infamous *rat poison*. Now, there are multiple other oral blood thinner drugs available. Although aspirin thins the blood, it is not sufficient to treat a DVT. Aspirin has also not been recommended as a measure to prevent blood clots, although recent studies are showing that it may be more effective than we realized.[1]

Prompt and aggressive treatment is important to keep a DVT from enlarging or breaking loose and traveling to the lungs and causing a pulmonary embolism. The typical symptoms of a pulmonary embolism are shortness of breath and a type of chest pain called *pleurisy*. Pleurisy is pain that is aggravated by breathing. CAT scans or other imaging tests of the lungs are needed to confirm the presence of a pulmonary embolus. Fortunately, most DVTs do not dislodge and cause pulmonary emboli.

Conditions that affect our clotting system

It is quite remarkable that our body has perfected the ability to keep our blood flowing smoothly, yet rapidly create clots to stop excessive bleeding when we are injured. Because the clotting system has so many intricate components, a minor defect in any of them can interfere with this delicate balance. When evaluating a patient with a clot, physicians attempt to discover if there is an underlying reason that predisposed the patient to form the clot. This can impact decisions on the initial and long-term treatment.

When someone is abnormally prone to blood clots we refer to this as having a *hypercoagulable condition.* There are a number of reasons why this occurs. Sometimes a leukemia-like process causes the bone marrow to make too many platelets. Some other cancers, particularly lung cancer and cancers of the gastrointestinal tract, cause the production of abnormal clot-producing factors.

There are also common genetic defects that affect the clotting proteins and make the blood clot too quickly – such as the *Factor V Leiden mutation* or the *prothrombin mutation.* Approximately 5% of the population harbors one of these abnormal genes. But fortunately, since we get one gene from our mother and another from our father, it is fairly unusual to get the same defective gene from both – which is generally necessary for someone to get into significant trouble with excessive clotting. People who have only one abnormal gene may be at a slightly increased risk for developing a clot under some conditions, but most never have any resulting complications.

Drugs can also affect the clotting process. Many drugs tend to "thin" the blood or make it less prone to clotting. Aspirin, most anti-inflammatory drugs, and prescription products such as heparin and warfarin fall into this category. However, there are a few agents that work the other way, making the blood more prone to clots. This is where hormone treatment comes in.

Hormones and blood clots

Birth control pills, which generally contain both an estrogen and a progestogen, have been used by millions of women since they first became available in the 1960s (although it wasn't until the 1970s that unmarried women were legally allowed to use them!). It has long been known that a risk of taking birth control pills, albeit fairly low, is the chance of a blood clot. So it is not surprising that hormones prescribed for menopause treatment also were found to increase the risk of blood clots – even though they are much less potent than the hormones used in birth control pills. A large study published in 1997 analyzing the medical histories of over 300,000 women in England found that women on HRT had a two to three times increase in the risk of developing a clot.[2] Shortly after that, researchers reviewed the results of 12 other studies and discovered similar findings.[3] Interestingly, both of these reviews noted that the highest risk of getting a clot was during the first year of treatment.

One of the findings from the WHI that was widely reported by the press was that taking HRT *doubled* a woman's risk of getting a blood clot. This announcement was alarming. However, although blood clots are serious, it is important to keep things in perspective and look at the *absolute risk* of getting a clot. In the WHI study, for every 10,000 women treated for one year with estrogen and progestogen, there were 18 more cases of blood clots compared to women taking a placebo. In the estrogen-only group, there were six more cases per 10,000 women per year. While these numbers are not insignificant, in counseling patients on the risks and benefits of HRT, I frequently point out how the risk of getting blood clots from HRT compares to other choices a woman may make in her lifetime. Hormone replacement therapy, in general, is thought to increase the risk of DVT by *two to four times*. Taking birth control pills increases the risk by *three to six times*. And finally, something many women may not be aware of – pregnancy increases the risk of getting a blood clot by *six to ten times*![4] In my opinion, it seems we unduly frighten menopausal women about the risk of HRT causing blood clots but seem to minimize this risk when counseling younger women when it comes to their choices of using birth control or contemplating pregnancy.

It is interesting to reflect on why pregnancy increases the risk of a blood clot. Pregnancy induces a mild hypercoagulable state – presumably as a defense against women bleeding to death if they have a miscarriage or during delivery.[5] However, the exact mechanisms accounting for this are unclear. Since estrogen and progesterone levels are extremely high during pregnancy, it has been assumed that they are the culprits, but it has never made sense to me why our natural hormones would cause detrimental effects. It very well may be that other factors, and not hormones, are the guilty parties. Substances made by the placenta have been shown to affect the coagulation system. In addition, other factors unique to pregnancy increase the risk of clots – such as pressure from the enlarged uterus on the veins in the lower abdomen, which constricts blood flow and causes leg swelling.

Does the specific type of estrogen make a difference?

Evidence is emerging that the mode of estrogen administration may be an important factor affecting the clotting system. Oral estrogens have been the mainstay for HRT regimens and so the vast majority of studies utilized this mode of administration. However, as discussed in previous chapters, we are learning that oral estrogens behave differently in the body than those applied onto the skin or into the vagina. A number of studies have been published that compared the effects of orally administered estrogen to those topically applied to the skin. In 2008 a review of eight observational studies and nine randomized controlled studies on HRT concluded that oral estrogen increases the risk of deep venous disease whereas transdermal estrogen does not.[6] A subsequent meta-analysis, updated in 2010 to include observational studies conducted since 2008, confirmed the findings that oral, but not transdermal, estrogen was associated with a higher risk of DVT.[7] Since that time, even more studies have found that transdermal estrogen is very unlikely to cause blood clots.[8]

While we don't have a large, randomized clinical trial to give us a definitive answer, enough evidence has surfaced to make most experts agree that it is the oral route of taking estrogen that contributes to clot formation, and that we can advise our patients that the risk of developing a clot will be exceedingly low if estrogen is applied to the skin.[9-13]

The question you may be asking is why would estradiol, taken as a pill, have different effects than estradiol applied to the skin? The answer lies in the fact that, as described in Chapter 3, all orally administered hormones undergo the first-pass effect – where drugs make their first stop in the liver after being ingested. It is speculated that the chemical changes that are triggered by going through this pathway cause the abnormalities in the clotting system that predispose women to blood clots.[14] And because there are so many steps involved in the coagulation cascade, it just takes one or two minor perturbations to significantly affect how easily a clot can form.

Is pure oral estradiol less risky than the conjugated equine estrogen, Premarin? There is scant data available to answer this question, so there is not a clear answer. Because both of these trigger the first-pass effects, there likely is little difference. As noted, oral contraceptives are more likely than HRT preparations to cause clots. One reason accounting for this is that all contraceptives contain the extremely potent synthetic estrogen, ethinyl estradiol, and the risk of blood clots appears to be correlated with the strength of the estrogen dose.

We also have little data on the effects of vaginally administered estrogen, but it would appear that the risks for blood clots are very low when using these preparations – probably comparable to transdermally-applied estrogen. Furthermore, women using very low-dose vaginal estrogen preparations, designed specifically to treat postmenopausal vaginal dryness, have a negligible risk of blood clots.[15]

Does the progestogen make a difference?

The next issue to address is how progestogens affect the coagulation process. There is evidence that some of the synthetic progestogens increase the risk of blood clots. This has become apparent in studies of women on birth control pills which contain various synthetic progestins. It has been found that some contraceptive formulations are more prone to cause blood clots than others – despite the fact they contain an identical form of estrogen.

With respect to HRT, it is believed that adding a progestogen may further increase the risk of a clot when an oral estrogen is taken. This was demonstrated in the WHI as well as in a number of other large studies.[10,11,16] The difference in risk can be as much as two to three times.[10] Whether there are differences in risks between the types of synthetic progestins used in HRT regimens is unclear. Most of the earlier studies on HRT in the U.S. used medroxyprogesterone (Provera), whereas other progestogens have been used more commonly in Europe. There is little data on how natural progesterone affects the clotting system, but research is indicating that it may not add any additional risk of blood clots.[17,18,19]

Risks of HRT in women who have had a blood clot

Blood clots are treated with blood thinners for at least three months and sometimes longer depending on the circumstances. Sometimes indefinite treatment is indicated. So, the question comes up whether it would be wise for someone with a prior history of a clot to take hormones. At the present time, most doctors would say absolutely not, and this is based on studies that have shown that oral estrogen therapy (especially combined with a synthetic progestin) can increase the risk of a recurrent DVT by as much as six times in these patients.[20] It appears that transdermal estrogen therapy does not carry this degree of risk, but there is not enough data to know for sure, and women in this position need to have an extensive discussion with their providers before considering HRT.[21]

If a woman is known to have a genetic defect that increases her risks of a clot, most providers do not recommend HRT. However, as the safety profile of transdermal estradiol and natural progesterone becomes clearer, this combination may be an option in cases where a woman clearly understands the benefits and risks of her choices.

SERMs and blood clots

As discussed in previous chapters, SERMs are being used for many conditions associated with menopause. All of the SERMs on the market increase the risk of blood clots, on a scale similar to the oral estrogens. This should be taken into account as women weigh their options for alternative treatments to hormones. It is generally not advisable for women who have a history of blood clots, or who are at increased risk for them, to take a SERM.

Decision Making Helper

Key considerations

Oral estrogens can increase the risk of clots; however considerable evidence has accumulated that indicates that transdermal estrogen causes a negligible risk.

A synthetic progestin taken along with an oral estrogen may increase the risk of clots more than treatment with estrogen alone.

Natural progesterone appears to have a low risk of promoting clots.

Certain situations that cause prolonged immobility increase the risk of blood clots. This includes prolonged sitting (such as a long airplane ride), extended bed rest, recuperating from surgery, or wearing a cast. Since HRT may further increase the risk of a clot, it may be advisable to temporarily interrupt HRT treatment or take extra measures known to prevent blood clots in these situations.

Women with a history of blood clots and women with an inherited or other increased risk for blood clots are generally advised not to consider HRT.

However, recent evidence suggests that transdermal estrogen poses considerably less risk in these circumstances.

Current guidelines for HRT with respect to blood clots

Prescription inserts for estrogen and any progestogen warn that estrogen can increase the risk of blood clots and are contraindicated in women with a current or past history of DVT.

What the guidelines don't acknowledge

It is becoming clearer that estrogens applied transdermally and intravaginally have a significantly decreased risk of causing blood clots compared to oral estrogen. In addition, it is probable that natural progesterone also has a significantly decreased risk compared to synthetic progestogens.

Chapter 14
Estrogen and Your Brain

My college roommate's mother, Norma, was a delightful lady with a Kansas accent who appeared regularly at our dorm room with care packages – like some Twinkies, toothpaste, and four or five pairs of socks or some other great bargain she picked up at Sears. While we were in college, Norma was having a rough time with menopause. She finally saw her doctor and he placed her on hormones. She rushed over to tell us that she felt so good on them that she thought she'd *"died and gone to heaven."* Norma loved her estrogen.

After I started my own practice some years later, I inherited her as a patient (when her beloved Dr. Jones passed on). I felt comfortable renewing her estrogen prescription every month. She was remarkably spry and independent, although perhaps a little more forgetful than expected for a 72-year-old.

One day a malignant tumor showed up on her mammogram. As was the standard of care, once breast cancer develops, it was prudent to stop the hormones. She was not for this at all but quit them at her oncologist's insistence. Within a year of being off estrogen, the family noticed a rapid decline in her memory and level of functioning.

Norma's daughter came in one day to discuss her Mom's condition. She was no longer a safe driver and they had a difficult showdown taking away her car keys. The family reported Norma was demonstrating more and more bizarre behavior – hiding money throughout the house and not remembering where she put it (her son reported finding a $20 bill in the flowerpot outside the front door). The family was convinced her decline was from going off hormones and requested that I resume prescribing them. However, her oncologist vehemently objected to this and I wasn't about to go against her specialist's advice. Unfortunately, her condition rapidly worsened and within several years she died – Alzheimer's disease stripping away every last bit of her Midwest dignity. I felt sad that her life ended this way and wondered if the outcome would have been different if we had continued her estrogen.

How our hormones affect our brains is a fascinating subject. Estrogen is necessary for the maintenance of normal brain function and health – in both women and men. Receptors for estrogen have been identified throughout the brain particularly in the hypothalamus, an area that plays an integral role in memory and cognition. This is also where much of the control of temperature regulation, food intake, and energy expenditure takes place. So it is easy to imagine that a lack of estrogen could have a major impact on all these functions.

In this chapter I describe the effects our sex hormones have in the brain and address these important questions:

- Is HRT good for the brain, or can it cause harm?
- Do different types of hormones and duration of use make a difference in brain function?
- Does the timing of initiating hormone replacement matter in the brain?

Brain basics

To begin, let's review the basic anatomy of the brain and nervous system and how it functions. The brain is made up of millions of cells called neurons that compose our grey and white matter. A nerve is a bundle of neurons (some as long as three feet!) strung together to transmit information back and forth from our skin and other organs to our brain. All of our senses – our eyes, ears, nose, mouth, and touch – have specialized nerve endings whose job is to collect information about our environment. They detect and transform the fragrance of a rose or the prick of a pin into electrical impulses that race along cellular pathways that enter and branch out into the brain where this input is processed. Specialized centers in the brain control every bodily process ranging from regulating our heartbeat and coordinating our movements, to creating our emotions.

A neuron looks like a miniscule octopus with multiple tentacles, which are called *dendrites*. The dendrites from neighboring neurons interconnect with each other in tangled masses, separated by tiny spaces called *synapses*. Each cell has one long dendrite called the *axon* which contains packets of chemical *neurotransmitters*. When an electrical signal moves through the cell it triggers the release of one of these agents – which floats across a synapse and then is snapped up by a neighboring neuron. These chemical messengers include *serotonin, dopamine, acetylcholine, norepinephrine,* and others. Each of these neurotransmitters has unique properties that can trigger various reactions within a given neuron and initiate new waves of electrical activity that miraculously dictate what we do, how we feel, and ultimately, who we are. A deficiency of any of these neurotransmitters can have major effects on how our brain functions.

Intertwined throughout the brain cells, a network of tiny blood vessels are the lifeline for taking care of the neurons. They deliver a constant supply of oxygen, glucose, and other nutrients, and transport out waste products left over from cellular functions. We tend to focus on how critical it is to nourish our cells, but we are now learning that the efficient functioning of the brain's waste management system is equally important. If leftover cellular debris is not bound up and transported out of the cells, it accumulates and causes damage and eventually cell death. The buildup of this toxic material appears to be the basic problem that leads to the devastating consequences of Alzheimer's disease.

Estrogen effects on the brain

Any disorder that impairs the integrity of the brain's circulatory system will cause problems. As I described in Chapter 12, the lining of the arteries, the endothelium, is rich in estrogen receptors. When estrogen connects with a receptor it triggers the release of nitric oxide – the powerful chemical that dilates blood vessels and increases blood flow to the cells. This allows oxygen and nutrients to be delivered to all of our cells, including the neurons, to enable them to function efficiently. Estrogen deficiency impairs the release of nitric oxide, so it follows that this is one mechanism where menopause can lead to detrimental effects on brain function.

Estrogen is also important in maintaining our neurotransmitters. Optimal supplies of our neurotransmitters are necessary for the brain to communicate within itself. Research in the lab has shown that estrogen administration increases the synthesis of several of these important brain chemicals, specifically acetylcholine, and serotonin.[1,2,3] Acetylcholine plays a major role in memory and cognition. The drugs commonly prescribed for Alzheimer's disease, such as Aricept, act to increase the availability of acetylcholine in the brain. Similarly, SSRI (*Selective Serotonin Reuptake Inhibitors*) drugs such as Prozac and Zoloft, which are used in treating depression, increase serotonin levels in the brain. (Isn't it interesting that a natural product, estrogen, can have similar effects as these multi-million dollar pharmaceuticals?)

195

In addition to improving blood flow and increasing neurotransmitter production, estrogen plays a major role in protecting neurons from damage.[4] Part of the aging process is caused by an accumulation of oxidized molecules – the infamous *free radicals* – that lead to cell injury. Neurons are particularly susceptible to these agents and estrogen has been shown to exert powerful anti-oxidant properties.[5] Estrogen also promotes the production of other anti-inflammatory chemicals that help fight brain damage.[6]

After menopause, there are very low levels of circulating estrogen. So it is logical to assume that with less estrogen bathing our neurons, the brain will function less efficiently, become more vulnerable to aging and be less able to withstand injury from other insults, such as damage from a stroke. The fact that more women than men are diagnosed with Alzheimer's disease raises speculation that the loss of estrogen may be a factor. Roughly 16% of women over age 65 have this diagnosis compared to 11% of men, and these percentages increase as people age.[7]

You may be surprised to learn that men over the age of 60 actually have higher circulating levels of estrogen than women of the same age who aren't taking estrogen replacement![8,9] This occurs because men don't go through menopause and they continue to make considerable amounts of testosterone – much of which is converted to estrogen. I find it ironic that women are discouraged from taking estrogen as they age, and yet men appear to benefit from estrogen because their bodies produce it naturally!

Ways we can study the brain

Much of our knowledge about estrogen's effects on the brain comes from radiology studies. Advanced imaging techniques are opening up many doors. For years we just had plain old x-rays. These virtually don't show anything about the brain – since the skull obscures the brain on these images. To obtain more detail on the structure of the brain, the next refinement developed was *angiograms*. These involve injecting an iodine dye into a blood vessel in the arm or leg and then taking x-ray images (like filming a video). As the dye travels through the circulatory system, the interior of the blood vessels are outlined – identifying areas of plaque and whether there are any blockages in the arteries. The dye quickly fills up the massive network of blood vessels within the brain creating an image that displays its anatomy. The downside of angiograms is that they are invasive, involve a considerable amount of radiation exposure, and iodine can cause allergic reactions and kidney damage.

When CAT (*computerized axial tomography*) scans were developed, this was a major advancement. The CAT (also referred to as CT) scan renders 3-D images of the inside of the body. It does this by taking x-rays in different planes and then uses computer manipulation to render images that show ¼ inch thick or less cross-sections anywhere in the body. These are then displayed on a screen, laying each image side by side, much like slicing a sausage and arranging each piece next to each other. This technique shows the size and shape of any abnormality deep in the brain such as a tumor. An iodine dye is frequently injected in the vein to help outline the vascular structures.

MRI (*magnetic resonance imaging*) was the next major advancement. This technique provides images similar to a CAT scan but in considerably more detail. Rather than using x-rays to obtain the pictures, these machines utilize strong magnetic impulses that minutely change the molecular pattern inside our tissues. Since each tissue has a unique composition, it utilizes these differences to outline our internal structures. A dye called *gadolinium* is usually used, which is not iodine-based and is not so toxic to the kidneys.

I remember when MRI scans first came out. I marveled at how amazingly clear the images were. Those of you who are baby boomers may appreciate the analogy when I say they are like the difference between viewing an old black and white TV and the new ultra high definition LED screens that greet you when you walk into Best Buy. The exquisite detail of MRI images allows radiologists to see previously undetectable problems not visible on CAT scans, such as sub-BB sized tumors, infectious processes, and small strokes.

These basic CAT and MRI studies are the electronic versions of an anatomy book in that they create static pictures of our organs. With advances in technology, refinements have been developed where not only can we see the brain's structure but gather information on how it works such as the specific locations where our various hormones interact with the brain. Scientists have created compounds with tracers attached to them that can hone in on specific receptors in the brain and light up these areas on an image. For instance, a marker can be attached to an estrogen molecule and this is injected into the circulatory system where it seeks an estrogen receptor and hooks onto it. The location of the marker can be identified allowing researchers to map where the estrogen receptors reside. This is the sort of technology that has shown us that estrogen receptors appear not only in the brain but just about everywhere else in our bodies.

None of these tests tell us anything about the dynamic functioning of the brain. This brings us to some of the latest imaging tests, which to me are truly amazing. Since our neurons require oxygen and blood sugar as sources of energy, scans have been developed that can map areas of the brain where these nutrients are being actively consumed. These are called *functional MRI* scans and *positron emission tomography* (PET) scans. In studies, these scans are performed while volunteers perform some sort of task. The areas that "light up" indicate which parts of the brain control this function. For instance, the area of the brain that is responsible for doing math can be pinpointed while someone is solving a math problem. These studies are being used to assess how HRT affects memory and other brain activities.

Many of the studies examining how HRT affects the brain utilize the types of tests that I've described. Having some knowledge of what these tests are will better help you understand the information to be presented in this chapter. With this background, let's move on and address the many areas where hormones are known to play a role in the brain and how we have come to learn this information.

Cognition

Let's start with the area of cognition. Cognition refers to your brain's ability to understand and interact with the world around you and determines your ability to learn, perform tasks, and communicate. Cognition encompasses multiple mental processes including memory, attention, spatial ability, language, learning, and living skills. It refers to a current level of functioning in time and can change over time. One can have temporary and reversible changes in one's level of cognition – such as being under the influence of drugs or alcohol or being delirious with a high fever. Once these external factors are removed, your mind returns to its normal level of functioning.

Some degree of impaired cognition generally occurs gradually with aging. We see these changes frequently in our older patients. This is manifested by having mild memory loss, slowness in processing things, and difficulty learning new tasks – but otherwise being able to be independent and functional. Doctors refer to this condition as *mild cognitive impairment*. It is important to note that these brain-aging changes do not necessarily lead to dementia – a more serious condition to be discussed next. This is an important point because many people assume these changes signal the start of Alzheimer's disease, which is not necessarily the case.

As I was working on this book, I happened to review a recent article that caught my attention. It was an analysis of studies that followed patients who had been diagnosed with mild cognitive impairment. Patients were given a series of cognitive tests. Of those who performed poorly, approximately 20% of these patients "reverted" to normal cognitive function after several years.[10] The reason this study is important is that it highlights the point that mild cognitive impairment is not necessarily a forerunner of dementia. It also raises awareness that when cognitive testing is used to study an intervention and finds a worsening or improvement over time, there should be some doubt as to whether the intervention tested was responsible for the difference.

There are many cognitive tests that have been studied that are felt to be highly predictive of brain function. However, many factors can interfere with one's ability to perform on these tests. For example, how many times have you been in a situation where you are nervous and under stress and don't perform as well as you know you can? Medicare requires that primary care doctors annually screen patients for cognitive impairment. One test we use is the clock-drawing test. We ask the patient to draw a clock depicting a time, such as ten minutes to five. One of my patients was so flustered that she initially failed the test and felt absolutely humiliated. This was a lady I then followed for another 15 years who remained mentally sharp and independent until age 95!

There are a number of other more sophisticated tests used to measure cognition that are typically administered by psychologists who have training in this area. These are used to assess a person's competency and to monitor for any deterioration in one's brain function. They are also used extensively in research. In this setting some tests are done, then repeated at a later time after some treatment is given. Then the studies are compared to see if the patient performed better or worse. But as pointed out, one's ability to perform will likely vary from one day to the next and can be influenced by all sorts of things, including the person's state of mind, where the test is done, and even the personality of the person administering the test. In the situation where a menopausal woman is being tested, one factor that can influence performance is whether she was having a hot flash, which many of us know can be very distracting.

The reason that I have spent so much time discussing the potential pitfalls in studies that assess cognition is to emphasize how difficult it is to interpret the significance of some of the findings. As opposed to studies that measure hard values, such as your cholesterol level, these studies are based on more subjective tests. So I tend to be less confident accepting the conclusions of some of the studies that measure how hormones affect cognition. I always look to see what type of testing was done. Was it a full battery of specialized tests, or a twice-a-year phone call with only a short questionnaire?

This brings us to the question: does menopause bring on a worsening of our cognitive function? Many women going through the menopausal transition would tend to say it does. At some point we occasionally find ourselves going into a room and not remembering why we went there or forgetting where we parked our car at the mall. It probably is not a coincidence that this starts happening around the time our ovaries are winding down. Sometimes these mental slips can be downright scary. I remember one moment when I went to the gym for a quick workout before preparing Thanksgiving dinner and accidentally left a pot of turkey giblets on the stove. I came back to billows of putrid grey smoke throughout the house and was lucky to get there before the kitchen caught fire. I think it was at that point that I had to acknowledge that I wasn't going to escape the inevitable decline in memory that greets you at midlife. Since I was in the throes of having hot flashes, I questioned whether estrogen loss was a factor.

There is good reason to believe the declining and fluctuating levels of our hormones during perimenopause may cause problems like this.[11,12] A number of observations suggest that menopause affects cognition. These include:

- Women who have higher estrogen levels perform better in memory performance tests.[13]

- Prior to menopause, women tend to perform better than men of the same age in memory testing, but after menopause, their performance becomes more comparable.[14]

- Women younger than age 50 who had both ovaries removed show a significant decrease in performance in cognitive tests compared to age-matched women who still had their ovaries.[15] This observation supports the presumption that it is not just getting older that affects memory, but also the loss of hormones.

If one accepts the results of studies that indicate that loss of estrogen affects memory and cognition, then replacing the missing hormones should be beneficial. Various avenues of research support this. Animal studies have shown that estrogen administration plays a major role in maintaining the pathways for neuronal communication and preventing inflammatory damage in rats.[17,18] Other studies in humans have utilized functional MRI exams obtained while women perform cognitive tests. It was found that there was more brain activity in women taking estrogen compared to women on a placebo.[16] This suggests that estrogen appears to facilitate the electrical communications going in the brain. In a similar study, researchers followed a group of women for nine years and did annual cognitive testing and PET scans. They found that women on estrogen showed enhanced brain activity while doing memory tests and performed better on these tests compared to women given a placebo.[17]

All of this information derived from research in the lab suggests that HRT should improve cognition and you would expect that the large clinical studies would corroborate this. However, these studies have not been definitive.[18] In the HERS and WHI studies it was concluded that HRT *worsened* cognitive function.[20,21] However, as you recall, these studies involved predominantly older women. While this may suggest that HRT negatively affects cognition in these situations, several other studies around that time, predominantly involving older women, did not show that HRT worsened cognition.[22-25]

What about studies looking specifically at younger women going through menopause? Does HRT benefit their cognitive abilities? A review of a number of studies performed between 1995 and 2000 concluded that symptomatic women (such as those having hot flashes) treated with estrogen demonstrated some improvement in verbal memory and other areas, but the conclusion was that hormone treatment did not lead to an overall enhancement of cognitive function.[19]

Following this, other studies examined the effect of HRT in younger women. The investigators of the WHI evaluated the small fraction of younger women enrolled in the study to assess the effects of HRT on cognition. About seven years after the study ended, researchers contacted approximately one thousand of these women.[26] Assessment of their cognitive function was obtained via telephone interviews. The authors reported that there was no difference in global cognitive function between the women who had taken hormones during the study versus those who had been on a placebo. In 2015 the KEEPS study of 643 younger menopausal women followed for four years did not find any overall effect of hormones on cognition.[27] The ELITE study published in 2016 included younger (as well as older) menopausal women placed on hormones. The investigators concluded that estradiol therapy neither harmed nor benefited cognitive abilities in either age group.[28]

Collectively these studies don't support the contention that HRT improves cognitive function. Based on the research discussed earlier in this chapter indicating estrogen has many positive effects on our brain cells, it is disappointing that clinical studies have not confirmed this. However, I am not too surprised because these studies are difficult to do. There is a great deal of subjectivity in the testing process. There are also a number of variables that haven't been clearly addressed that could have confounded the results. For instance, it is unclear if the type of hormone matters. There are some studies that suggested that women on estradiol performed better on cognitive tests than women on Premarin.[29] In addition, although progesterone has been shown to play many important roles in the brain, it is conceivable that the synthetic progestogen used in some of the studies may have negatively affected cognition. Hopefully, studies in the future will address how different hormone regimens compare to each other. But for now women who are experiencing "brain fog" as they go through the menopausal transition should not be worried that they will be harmed by taking estrogen for their hot flashes.

Dementia

Dementia is a term reserved for a permanent level of brain dysfunction. As emphasized above, mild cognitive impairment does not necessarily imply the person has or will go on to get dementia. But in cases where one's cognitive function clearly shows a progressive decline, the end result is likely going to be a permanent case of dementia – a condition where so many brain cells have died that the brain shrinks and loses many critical functions.

Dementia is a frightening diagnosis we all dread. It eventually affects about one in ten people.[30] Dementia can progress slowly or alarmingly quickly. It leads to a progressive decline in functioning to the point where patients become completely unaware of their surroundings and completely dependent on others for their survival.

Alzheimer's disease accounts for over half of the cases of dementia. The second major cause is due to cumulative brain damage occurring from a series of strokes. We call this *vascular dementia* or *multi-infarct dementia*. People who have risk factors for hardening of the arteries (such as smoking, high cholesterol, and high blood pressure) are the most at risk for this type of dementia. The rest of the cases of dementia are due to a variety of causes. Lewy body dementia, which is associated with Parkinson's disease, accounts for many cases. Repetitive brain injury – like that which is the result of one too many head-on tackles in football players – has recently been recognized as a cause of dementia. Other conditions such as tumors, excessive brain pressure, drugs, viruses, and inflammation account for the rest of the cases.

More about Alzheimer's

Alzheimer's disease causes permanent brain damage due to an accumulation of protein-like deposits (called *amyloid and tau*) that build up within and around the brain cells and this ultimately leads to progressive nerve cell death. Genetic defects appear to play a major role in this disease. Scientists have discovered that there are a number of genes that make products that are important in providing a "housekeeping" function for the brain cells. They facilitate the removal of amyloid and tau and other molecular debris that needs to be cleared out of the neurons. If a person has a defective gene that renders one of these "housekeepers" ineffective at its job, waste products build up and choke out the healthy cells. As more brain cells die the communication pathways in the brain are disrupted. The brain's ability to efficiently run all the processes in our bodies falters − leading to problems not only with cognition and speech, but personality, balance and, eventually, motor function.

One of the genes that plays a role in this housekeeping system is the *APOE* (*apolipoprotein E*) gene. Three types of APOE genes have been identified, named epsilon 2, 3, and 4. We inherit one version from each parent. The APOE epsilon 4 gene (APOEe4) confers an increased risk of developing Alzheimer's − two to three times the risk if you have one e4 gene and up to a twelve-fold increase risk if you inherited two of these defective genes (one from each parent).[31,32] It is important to realize, however, that a person doesn't necessarily go on to get Alzheimer's even if unfortunate enough to inherit two of these unfavorable genes. Also, 40% of people with Alzheimer's do not have this gene abnormality because other defective genes and processes can contribute to this disease.[32]

Some of the more recent studies on HRT included this type of genetic testing. The KEEPS study, which was discussed earlier, was designed to test how HRT affected a number of health-related outcomes in younger women who were within a few years of menopause. Specialized brain PET scans (called *Pittsburg compound B* or *piB scans*) that detect the toxic Alzheimer's proteins were performed in the women at the beginning and the end of the study. Women taking transdermal estradiol showed less accumulation of these deposits compared to women on a placebo over a four-year period. This was most pronounced in women who carried an APOEe4 gene.[33] Other lines of evidence suggesting that estrogen treatment may help defray Alzheimer's come from lab studies where it has been demonstrated that exposing brain cells to estrogen facilitates removal of some of the harmful products that make up amyloid and tau protein.[34,35] It is not yet known for sure why estrogen helps, but there is speculation that it is related to its anti-inflammatory properties and beneficial effects on blood flow.

Does HRT prevent dementia?

Despite the evidence that estrogen plays an important role in limiting neuron damage, clinical studies are needed to make substantive conclusions about how hormone replacement affects the risk of dementia. A number of early observational studies addressed this and found very favorable results. The Leisure World study, which has been mentioned previously, was a long-term study where 8,877 female residents of this retirement community were closely followed for many years. This study, published in 1994, found that the risk of dementia was less in women who had been taking estrogen, and the risk decreased significantly with a higher estrogen dose and longer duration of use.[36] Other early studies came up with similar findings.[37] A meta-analysis published in 2001, which reviewed studies from 1996 through 2000, found there to be an overall decrease in the risk of dementia in HRT users.[19] Those of us in practice at that time found the studies very convincing and I felt comfortable advising my patients that one of the benefits of taking HRT would be that it would likely help protect them from developing dementia.

However, things changed in 2002 when the results of the WHI study were released. Recall that the WHI was the largest randomized clinical trial done to date on HRT and carried tremendous impact. Its findings once again blindsided us as we read disparaging headlines announcing that estrogen therapy causes dementia. The basis for this conclusion came from an ancillary study of the WHI, called the WHIMS (Women's Health Initiative Memory Study) which assessed global cognitive function in 4,532 postmenopausal women who were *over* age 65 and presumed not to have dementia when they entered the study. The investigators found that hormone therapy increased the risk of dementia.[38]

This is why your package insert for estrogen carries a disclaimer in bold print that reads estrogen therapy *"should not be used for prevention of dementia."* In looking at the conclusions of the WHIMS study, however, a couple of points need to be noted. The absolute number of affected women was very small. Of the 2,229 women taking HRT, there were 40 cases of dementia diagnosed by the end of the study period. Of the women on a placebo, there were 21 cases out of 2,303. This equates to 19 more cases of dementia occurring that may be attributable to taking hormones. It also must be emphasized that these women were over the age of 65 when they entered the study and started taking hormones. This is in contrast to many of the earlier observational studies which generally involved women placed on HRT around age 50.

This brings up the question of whether we are once again dealing with a timing issue. As discussed in Chapter 12, starting hormones around the time of menopause has different effects on the heart than when starting them a number of years beyond menopause. Is this also an issue when it comes to dementia? To investigate this possibility, the next step would be to examine studies specifically involving younger women. Fortunately, we have some data. In 2005, two papers were published that concluded that women who initiated HRT treatment early in the menopausal transition had a *decreased* risk of developing Alzheimer's.[39,40] Another large study, known as the Cache County Follow-Up Study, was published in 2012. The investigators found a reduced Alzheimer's risk if hormone therapy was started within five years of menopause and continued for more than ten years.[41]

I read these studies with great interest as they appeared to validate our previous belief that starting HRT early in menopause would protect against dementia. However, a subsequent review analyzing 15 observational studies was published in 2014.[42] The authors concluded there was not enough evidence to definitively show that administering HRT early in menopause prevented dementia, but at least it did not appear to bring it on any sooner than women not taking hormones.

Three years after this review, the results of a large study from Finland that followed 8,195 women over a 20-year time span were published.[43] It's findings revealed that while women treated with short-term therapy did not show a benefit in cognition, women treated for over ten years showed a 50% reduction in the onset of Alzheimer's disease. The estrogen used in this study was estradiol, and the principal progestogens used were norethisterone and levonorgestrel – formulations commonly used in that country.

This study once again fired up the debate on the merits of HRT for the brain and added support for the claim that hormones may help prevent dementia. However, experts in menopause caution that this study was an observational one and doesn't "prove" that taking HRT will boost brain health. More research is needed and many questions remain, such as:

- Does the type of estrogen matter?
- Does the addition of a progestogen help or hinder?
- Does the type of progestogen make a difference?

It has only been relatively recently that women have had the option of using transdermal rather than oral estrogens, so most of the large studies on HRT predominantly involved women taking estrogen pills. As we have seen in previous chapters, estrogen applied to skin escapes some of the negative metabolic processes that occur with oral estrogen. So, while it may be speculated that transdermal estrogen may be less likely to cause adverse effects in the brain, we don't have much data to go on.

The next issue is whether the addition of a progestogen increases the risk of dementia. In the WHI study it was only the women taking estrogen and progestogen who developed a higher rate of dementia compared to women on a placebo. Women prescribed estrogen alone did not show a significant increase in the risk of dementia.[44] Similarly, in the Finnish study, women taking long-term estrogen alone were at lower risk for dementia than the women on combined therapy.

In both the WHI and the Finnish study, synthetic progestogens were used. The question that comes up is whether natural progesterone may be less likely than synthetic progestogens to cause any negative effects on the brain. As in other areas of our body, it is very probable it would be neutral in its action. Some evidence comes from studies where researchers performed functional MRI scans on women taking either natural progesterone or a synthetic progestin along with estradiol for several months.[46] Recall that these are studies that show how the brain is functioning while performing a mental task. Women taking natural progesterone demonstrated much greater brain activity than women on a synthetic progestogen, implying that there were differences between these two agents in their effects on the brain.

Although the information I have presented demonstrates that hormones support brain health in a number of ways, physicians can't advise patients that HRT will protect them from dementia without future large-scale clinical studies. However, it is probable that starting HRT at the time of menopause is not harmful. Starting hormones later – ten or more years beyond menopause – may not be advisable. This is similar to the situation that we are seeing with respect to HRT and the cardiovascular system. Hormones may help preserve healthy arteries but be detrimental to diseased ones. In the brain, they may protect healthy neurons but may not be so good for neurons that have been damaged from age or other insults.

Whether or not discontinuing hormones after long-term use may accelerate dementia in susceptible women, like my dear patient Norma, is unknown. There is evidence that hormone treatment, particularly with higher doses of transdermal estrogens and natural progesterone, may improve functioning of women with Alzheimer's[47,48] but at this point using HRT as a treatment for dementia is not advised by the experts.

Does HRT affect mood and depression?

How often have you watched a movie or TV show where a menopausal woman appears? Besides desperately fanning herself, she is often portrayed as depressed or cranky. While it is true that most women get hot flashes, is there evidence that menopause is also associated with mood changes? As it turns out, the data is quite convincing that it does – depending on where in the premenopausal to postmenopausal journey a woman happens to be.

It has been estimated that anywhere from 15% to 50% of women experience mood issues during the perimenopausal period. Studies show that the risk of depression increases as women approach and go through menopause. Women with a prior history of postpartum depression appear to be particularly vulnerable.[49] Since these are both situations where there is a fall in estrogen levels, this suggests that a decline in circulating estrogen is a factor. Furthermore, women who have had their ovaries removed prior to natural menopause, which causes an abrupt drop in hormone levels, have a higher risk of depression than their age-matched controls.[50]

Menopause is associated with fluctuating and decreasing levels of serotonin.[1,51] This is the neurotransmitter that plays a major role in mood control. Its chemical name is *5-hydroxytryptamine (5-HT)*. Lack of serotonin in the brain leads to depression and anxiety. To treat depression, more serotonin must be delivered to the neurons. We can't simply buy a bottle of serotonin – since it is not something that can get into the brain directly by ingesting a pill – so the pharmaceutical industry developed drugs such as the SSRIs (selective serotonin reuptake inhibitors). These agents work by increasing the concentration of serotonin in the synapses to make it more available to more neurons. The first SSRI drug on the market was Prozac, but now we have Zoloft, Paxil, Lexapro, and a dozen others. Another class of drugs, called SNRIs (serotonin-norepinephrine reuptake inhibitors) is also commonly prescribed for depression. Because this type of drug is designed to raise not only the level of serotonin but also the level of an adrenaline-type neurotransmitter, it may be less sedating and more energizing. All of the SSRI drugs can be helpful for treating depression associated with menopause; one SNRI, Pristiq, has also been found to be helpful in perimenopausal women with depression.[52]

Although antidepressant drugs are recommended as the first-line treatment for women with perimenopausal depression, there has been considerable research showing that adding estrogen to one of these drugs works much better than treatment with an SSRI alone.[53] It also has been shown that in women on HRT, their depression symptoms worsen if their hormones are discontinued.[54] These observations raise the question of whether simply taking HRT would be effective as a primary treatment for perimenopausal depression. Theoretically, this should be helpful because estrogen treatment can increase serotonin levels.[55] In addition, estrogen also raises *endorphin* levels. Endorphins are our natural opioids and play a major role in mood and pain modulation.

A number of clinical studies have shown that HRT can improve mood problems in perimenopausal women. One study assigned 50 women between ages 40 and 55 to treatment with either transdermal estrogen patches or a placebo.[56] The women treated with estrogen showed substantial improvement in their level of depression compared to women on no treatment. Another study of 286 women treated with estrogen showed significant improvement on mood scores after 12 months.[57] In an ancillary part of the KEEPs study, younger menopausal women treated with Premarin showed greater improvement in mood compared to women on a placebo.[58] Interestingly, the women on transdermal estradiol did not witness this benefit.

Certainly alleviating hot flashes, night sweats, and sleep disturbance with estrogen should help improve mood – so the question arises whether hormone replacement is effective simply because it relieves these distressing symptoms. An interesting study that addressed this found estrogen prevented depressive symptoms in women going through menopause regardless of the degree of initial vasomotor symptoms.[59]

Current guidelines, however, recommend hormone treatment only for women having bothersome hot flashes. Women without such symptoms are not considered candidates for treatment. This is unfortunate because, in my opinion, it seems reasonable to try treating depressed perimenopausal and early menopausal women with estrogen before resorting to an SSRI. These antidepressant drugs can have their own set of side effects (decreased libido for one!). I have also had patients complain that after starting SSRI drugs, they had a worsening of their night sweats. This is actually not an uncommon side effect of these drugs. Another area that concerns me is that SSRI drugs have been shown to increase bone loss[61] – not something we should be exacerbating during the time a woman's bone mass is rapidly declining.

So far I have been discussing using HRT for mood issues for women as they approach and go through menopause – the phase where there is a fairly high incidence of depression and other mood disorders. In contrast to this period, women further down the menopausal road tend to have less depression, rather than more.[62,63] Studies have shown that using hormones to treat depressed women who are more than five to ten years beyond menopause is not very effective. In addition, many experts do not advise initiating HRT for these women because of the uncertainty of other potential adverse effects of HRT in older women. It is not clear why hormones would not be helpful under these circumstances, but there is speculation that the estrogen receptors in the brains of older postmenopausal women may no longer respond to estrogen in the same manner as they did when younger.[64]

HRT and Parkinson's disease

Another neurologic condition affecting midlife adults is Parkinson's disease. The hallmark of this disorder is a deficiency of *dopamine* in the brain. Dopamine is one of the neurotransmitters that play a major role in how our motor system works – thus the symptoms of Parkinson's are tremors, slow movement, muscle stiffness, and rigidity. There is diminished fine muscle movement of the face, so patients appear to have no facial expression, and get the "mask-face" appearance that is a feature of this syndrome. Another interesting observation is that these patients write with very small characters. During my years of practice when I suspected early Parkinson's, I would check the patient's intake form, and more often than not my suspicion was corroborated when I saw a tiny little cursive signature.

Parkinson's disease affects more men than women and usually appears after the age of 60. I feel terrible for my patients who shoulder the burden of caring for a spouse with this disease. As Parkinson's progresses, it robs people of their strength, balance, and eventually cognitive function. Those affected require an extraordinary level of caregiving and invariably long-awaited retirement dreams never become a reality.

After menopause, the risk of Parkinson's disease increases in women. It has been shown in animal and other studies that estrogen appears to be beneficial in maintaining dopamine activity in the brain.[9,65] So it is logical to suspect that the loss of estrogen at the time of menopause would predispose women to develop Parkinson's disease. One of my absolute favorite patients, Bernice, developed breast cancer at age 62, so she was advised to discontinue her estrogen. She subsequently was placed on Arimidex – the powerful anti-estrogen drug that is now commonly used for breast cancer treatment. This therapy essentially bottomed out any remaining estrogen in her body. About two years later we both noticed a mild tremor. As it progressed we had to face the possibility that her symptoms were from Parkinson's, and this was later confirmed by a neurologist. I still wonder if there was a connection between her developing this disease and depleting her estrogen.

Whether taking HRT can prevent Parkinson's is an area of research. Studies have shown that removing one or both ovaries prior to menopause puts a woman at a significantly higher risk of developing Parkinson's, [66,67] and taking estrogen reduces this risk.[68] Studies on women going through natural menopause have been mixed, but evidence suggests that hormone replacement, especially if taken early, may help prevent this disease.[69,70,71] It is also thought that there may only be a finite window for the initiation of estrogen to be preventative, and delaying HRT some period after menopause may not provide any benefit.[72]

HRT and migraines

Twice as many women as men suffer from migraine headaches, and almost every woman who gets them will agree that their female hormones must be a factor. This is because these women have had to plan their lives around their monthly menstrual cycles – knowing that the surest way to sabotage a great evening or vacation is to schedule a special event at certain times of the month. For years migraine sufferers have known that the peak time for a headache is right before or during their menstrual flows. This is the time when both estrogen and progesterone levels drop precipitously. Migraines are unequivocally affected by fluctuations in these hormones.

A migraine is a severe headache that lasts about 24 hours. It is usually felt only on one side of the head and typically is accompanied by nausea. It's the kind of headache that makes you want to shut out the world and seek refuge in a dark and quiet bedroom. A unique feature of migraines is a distinctive warning sign that alerts some patients that one is coming on. We call this an *aura*, or a *prodrome event*. It usually consists of a visual disturbance such as glittery wavy lines or a blank spot in the visual field. Or, more alarmingly, an aura can present as transient numbness or weakness of an extremity (which would cause one to worry, appropriately, is this a stroke?). Sometimes the symptoms of an aura can be very strange, such as a bad odor or a déjà vu feeling. Auras typically last 15 to 30 minutes before resolving and then, boom, the headache comes on. While an aura is clearly a characteristic of a migraine headache, only about 25% of migraine patients have them, and we describe these patients as having *classical migraines with aura*. There are multiple other variations of migraines that are not so straightforward and sometimes it takes an astute primary care doctor or neurologist to come up with the diagnosis. Many times migraines are confused with sinus headaches.

A migraine is caused by a series of complex changes in the brain. Initially, an artery constricts – temporarily restricting blood flow to a small region in the brain. This leads to the aura. Then the artery suddenly dilates (that's when patients feel like their heads are exploding). Other brain chemistry changes occur which contribute to the headache and associated symptoms.

There are specific anti-migraine medications (such as Imitrex) that act on the arteries to prevent them from dilating and can sometimes abort an attack. Other drugs, taken on a daily basis (or other schedule), are also prescribed to prevent migraines from occurring. Once a migraine is in full force, the only option for relief is medication to treat the pain and nausea.

During perimenopause, which is characterized by major fluctuations in hormone levels, migraines become much more frequent. To even out these hormonal ups and downs, many physicians will place patients on low-dose birth control pills or estrogen supplements. Keeping estrogen levels at a steady state helps prevent a migraine from starting. Many women have found this type of approach very effective. However, women who have clear-cut aura symptoms are not candidates for this type of treatment because of concerns that taking hormones may cause a stroke. This became apparent over 50 years ago when an increase in strokes was observed in young women on birth control pills. However, the potency of the pills used back then was much higher than the pills used today and were considerably stronger than the hormones used in HRT.

After menopause, when hormones have fallen to low levels, migraine headaches tend to diminish and sometimes completely go away.[73] So the question to address is whether a woman with a history of migraines should ever consider HRT – or is she just asking for a return of those dreaded headaches? Interestingly, most women placed on HRT do not experience a reappearance of their migraines. It is believed this is because when estrogen is administered in fixed doses, the hormone levels don't fluctuate the way they did during the reproductive years. This explanation is further supported by the observation that the transdermal estradiol patches, which have been shown to supply a more steady level of estrogen than pills, are less likely to trigger migraines.[74] Occasionally, however, HRT therapy may increase migraine headaches. This may be related to the fact that some women are extremely sensitive to very slight fluctuations in hormone levels.[75]

In summary, it is generally considered safe for most women with histories of migraine headaches to be candidates for hormone therapy.[76,77] The exception is that women whose migraines were associated with auras are generally advised to avoid any type of hormone treatment.

HRT and strokes – "brain attacks"

One of the most frightening events that can happen to a loved one is a stroke. The family is gathered around the dining room table and suddenly grandma starts talking gibberish, her eyelid and face droop on one side, and then she slumps over – awake but unable to move her right arm and leg. This is how many strokes manifest themselves. They require urgent recognition and treatment if there is any chance of preventing permanent disability.

A stroke is frequently referred to as a "brain attack" since the most common cause is similar to what causes a heart attack – an interruption of blood flow to a part of the brain due to a blocked artery. Within minutes the lack of oxygen causes damage to the brain cells and they soon die if circulation isn't promptly restored through emergency treatment. The stroke symptoms a patient experiences depends on where in the brain the blockage occurs. If the area responsible for vision is affected, partial or total blindness can result. If it involves the part of the brain that controls motor function, paralysis of the arms and/or legs can occur. A stroke to the part of the brain that controls balance can cause a lack of coordination, vertigo, nausea, and vomiting. A massive stroke causes so much damage that the end result can be sudden collapse and death.

Blood flow travels to the brain via two major arteries along the front part of the neck (the *carotid arteries*) and two smaller arteries in the back of the neck (the *vertebral arteries*). The carotids supply the *cerebrum* – the large part of the brain that controls our speech, muscles, sensations, memory, emotions, and essentially all of our other "cerebral" functions. The vertebral arteries supply blood to the *cerebellum* which is responsible for our coordination and balance.

The most common cause of a stroke is from a *thromboembolic event.* A thrombus can either be a clump of plaque that was jettisoned off from an artery, usually the carotid, or a blood clot, which usually arises from coagulated blood within the heart itself. The thrombus gets propelled through the circulation until it gets stuck in a narrow artery and cuts off the downstream flow.

Although the symptoms may be the same, there are other things that can cause a stroke. A blood vessel in the brain can burst and create a blood clot which expands and damages cells around it. This is usually caused by an *aneurysm,* which is a ballooned-out area from a weakened section of an artery. This type of stroke is called a *hemorrhagic stroke.* A tumor that either arises in the brain or that has traveled from another part of the body can slowly grow and compress normal brain tissue and cause symptoms of a stroke. All of these entities can cause irreversible brain cell damage that results in some level of permanent functional disability. The cause of a stroke can generally be determined by performing diagnostic tests such as an angiogram or MRI of the brain.

A warning sign of a stroke can be an event called a *TIA* or *transient ischemic attack.* This is usually caused by a spasm or blockage of an artery, which temporarily interrupts blood flow to a part of the brain. Frequently it is due to a bit of plaque that has broken off from a larger blood vessel, usually the carotid artery. When this occurs a patient may experience frightening neurologic symptoms that last for about 15 minutes. This could be anywhere from difficulty speaking, being unable to move a limb, or feeling dizzy and off-balance. The symptoms then disappear – either because the material clogging the artery dissipated or other arteries in the brain were able to quickly take over and supply blood to the cells in jeopardy. If the symptoms persist over 24 hours, however, it is inevitable that permanent damage has occurred – which then indicates that a stroke, rather than a TIA, has occurred.

When doctors suspect a patient has experienced a TIA, further tests such as an ultrasound of the carotid arteries are done. This can detect the presence and amount of plaque. Generally, blood thinners are prescribed, but if the blockage is severe, surgical intervention may be recommended.

Sometimes a patient may not even be aware that she or he has had a stroke. This is usually because the blocked vessel supplied a part of the brain that was not in a critical area and the deficit was so subtle that it didn't cause obvious symptoms. However, with repetitive small strokes, symptoms will start appearing as more grey matter is lost. These can include disturbances in memory and thinking or coordination problems. This leads to the syndrome of *multi-infarct dementia* mentioned above. Over time, the loss of cognitive and motor function can develop slowly and gradually or take sudden jumps where the level of cognition or motor function appears to drop in a stepwise fashion.

The risk of having a stroke increases with age; a person has a one in four chance of suffering one before she or he dies.[78] Women have lower rates of strokes than men until after menopause. Then the risk increases. Does this indicate that the loss of our female hormones plays a role? Evidence that supports this comes from data showing that the earlier a woman goes through natural menopause, the higher her risk of a stroke.[79,80] One study found that women who went through menopause before the age of 42 had a 103% increase in their stroke risk.[79] Similarly, women who have had their ovaries removed prior to their natural menopause have a significantly higher risk of stroke.[81] Conversely, the later a woman goes through menopause the less her risk of a stroke.[79]

The mechanism by which estrogen helps prevent strokes is not completely clear, but likely is related to the positive effects that estrogen has on preventing plaque formation – which is the underlying factor leading to the majority of strokes. As discussed in Chapter 12, the presence of estrogen throughout a woman's life is believed to have a powerful protective effect on the lining of the arteries – arteries that supply blood to the heart, to the brain and everywhere else.

Although it would seem logical that taking estrogen after menopause would decrease a woman's chance of a stroke, this hasn't been clearly demonstrated. Much of the controversy regarding this came from the results of the WHI study. It was frightening to read headlines that proclaimed that a woman's risk of a stroke *increased* by 41% if she took HRT. Certainly this was distressing news and was another reason many women threw their pills into the trash. However, the actual number of women who suffered a stroke during this study was quite small. In terms of absolute risk, these results would equate to eight more cases of stroke per year for each 10,000 women treated with combined estrogen and progesterone, and twelve more cases in women treated with estrogen alone.

Furthermore, the WHI findings were in contrast to previous studies that did not implicate hormones as a cause of stroke. A study that came out shortly before the WHI found no increased rate of stroke in women treated with estrogen.[82] In the Leisure World Study – where a large group of retired women was followed over many years – twice as many women died from a stroke if they *didn't take* HRT compared to women who were taking HRT.[83] Similarly a large study from Finland noted that women on HRT had an 18% decreased risk of stroke.[84] A number of other studies both before and after the WHI were reviewed in an article published in 2015. The authors found that women who, for whatever reason, discontinued hormone therapy had a higher rate of strokes than women who continued HRT.[85] To compare this with the WHI numbers, which showed that women on combined HRT had eight *more strokes* per 10,000 women years, this study concluded that women who continued HRT had *five fewer strokes* per 10,000 women years than those who had stopped them.

Once again the disparities between the outcomes of the WHI study and other studies led to an inspection of whether the Timing Hypothesis was a factor. It was suspected that women who were older and started HRT later in life would likely have a higher risk of a stroke. So it was not surprising to discover that women in the WHI who were below the age of 59 when they entered the study did not demonstrate an increased risk in stroke.[86] Several large reviews and a meta-analysis have confirmed this observation: women initiating HRT within ten years of menopause are not at any higher risk of having a stroke than women not on hormones.[87,88]

Why then would older women not benefit from HRT or possibly even be harmed by it? The explanation would be similar to what we have learned about heart attacks. Younger women, who likely have clean arteries as they enter menopause, would benefit from estrogen's tendency to prevent plaque. Older women likely have some degree of plaque on their carotid arteries as well as in the smaller arteries in the brain. Initiating estrogen therapy under these conditions may make the plaque less stable and more vulnerable to breaking apart and causing problems. In addition, as has been seen in other organs, women lose estrogen receptors as they age. Without estrogen receptors in the brain, estrogen may not be able to exert its beneficial neuroprotective actions.

Another reason that older women are at higher risk for strokes is that one out of ten women will eventually develop atrial fibrillation. Atrial fibrillation is an irregular heart beat that predisposes blood clots to form inside the heart.

They can dislodge and be propelled into the brain causing a stroke. Because oral forms of hormones can increase the risk of blood clots, women who unknowingly harbor atrial fibrillation and who take oral HRT may be at a higher risk of a stroke of this nature occurring. It should be noted however, that women with known atrial fibrillation who are on appropriate blood thinners are not at an increased risk for a stroke if they take HRT.[89]

More research is needed to know whether the type of hormone regimen makes a difference in stroke prevention or provocation. Oral estrogen has been the predominant form of estrogen used in most of the studies, including the WHI. There is reason to believe that transdermal estradiol would be much less likely to pose a stroke risk and studies are pointing to this.[90,91] Furthermore, the type of progestogen taken likely makes a major difference in the risk of strokes as it does in the risk of heart disease. In the large Finnish study, where HRT appeared to help prevent strokes, the progestogen predominantly prescribed was norethisterone, whereas medroxyprogesterone was the agent used in the WHI study.

Decision Making Helper

<u>Key considerations</u>

HRT and cognition and dementia

There is a debate about whether initiating HRT within five to ten years after menopause helps prevent cognitive decline and dementia. Many studies show a benefit. It does not appear that taking HRT is harmful to women experiencing the "brain fog" they may encounter as they go through their menopausal transition. There is data that indicates that HRT may confer some benefits in preventing Alzheimer's disease in women who go through early menopause and women who carry the APOEe4 gene.

Initiating HRT ten years after menopause will likely not help cognition or prevent dementia and possibly could be harmful.

Natural progesterone may have either a slight beneficial or neutral effect on cognition. Some synthetic progestogens may have a slightly negative impact.

We do not have enough data to know if there is any benefit in using HRT to treat established dementia and experts do not recommend this in view of the potential negative cardiovascular effects of HRT in older women.

HRT and depression

HRT is approved for the treatment of menopausal symptoms. This typically refers to hot flashes and vaginal symptoms. Mood changes such as depression are not typically considered an indication for HRT treatment, although studies show that mood changes are common during perimenopause. Hormone therapy has been shown to help depression during perimenopause, particularly in conjunction with anti-depressant drugs.

Taking HRT does not appear to be helpful for depression in women who are well past menopause.

HRT and Parkinson's disease

The risk of developing Parkinson's disease increases after menopause; taking HRT may help prevent this.

HRT and migraines

It is believed that fluctuating hormone levels that occur during perimenopause aggravate migraine headaches. Taking estrogen supplementation to even out these fluctuations can help prevent migraines.

For most women with a history of migraines, taking HRT has not been shown to be dangerous and generally does not bring on migraines. If women do experience continued or worsening migraines with HRT, switching to transdermal estrogen has been shown to be beneficial as this mode of administration produces a more steady level of estrogen in the bloodstream.

HRT is not advised for women with migraines associated with auras because hormone treatment in this situation could possibly increase the risk of a stroke.

HRT and strokes

Estrogen therapy initiated at the time of menopause appears to carry a very low risk of a stroke and may help prevent one.

Women more than ten years beyond menopause may be at a slightly increased risk of stroke if they take HRT.

Current guidelines for HRT with respect to the brain

HRT is not approved as a treatment for depression and other mood disorders, or as a preventative treatment for cognitive decline and dementia. The FDA package inserts for hormones warn that HRT can increase the risk of strokes, and should be used with caution in women with migraines.

What the guidelines don't acknowledge

Considerable evidence shows that estrogen is helpful in treating mood disorders and depression in perimenopausal women. While it is unclear if hormones prevent dementia, the bulk of evidence does not show that taking HRT at the time of menopause increases the risk of dementia. Taking HRT shortly after menopause may help prevent Parkinson's disease. There is also substantial data indicating that HRT, when taken within ten years of menopause, decreases the risk of a stroke. Hormone therapy may help prevent migraine headaches during the perimenopausal period and has not been shown to increase migraines post menopause; although they should not be used in women with a history of aura.

Chapter 15
Estrogen and Your Fat Cells and Diabetes

Do you think that many doctors talk to women about how hormone therapy may affect their figures? I seriously doubt that this subject comes up during a discussion of the benefits and risks of taking HRT. Yet research is showing that estrogen loss at the time of menopause greatly affects the location and type of fat that appears in our bodies as we age. As you will see, this is not just a cosmetic issue – this carries much more medical significance than meets the eye.

I have three sisters and we are all within two years apart in age. Over the last ten years all of my sisters, to their dismay, have gained weight around their middles while I have been fortunate enough to still fit into my old bell-bottoms from high school! One of my sisters was recently diagnosed with borderline diabetes, which came as a surprise – since it is not something that runs in our family.

This marked difference between my siblings and me has been puzzling. We all share similar genetics and we all have enjoyed fairly active lifestyles. What has occurred to me is that we all went through menopause around the time the WHI study came out – right when there was nationwide hysteria about the safety of HRT. So while I chose to take estrogen replacement therapy, my sisters' physicians did not recommend it.

Perhaps I should have been more vocal in voicing my opinion to them about the advisability of HRT. But, at the time, I didn't think it was appropriate to push them to discuss hormones with their physicians because my distrust of the WHI conclusions was more of a gut reaction than one founded on all that I know now. Besides, I generally followed the unwritten rule that doctors should not play the physician role to family members. So I didn't feel it was my place to tell my sisters to ignore the prevailing medical guidelines and encourage them to take HRT.

I can't help but wonder, however, if their not taking hormones affected their body changes, and possibly even their future health. The more I study

219

how HRT affects our metabolism, the more convinced I am that this was a factor. In this chapter, I will try to answer the following important questions:

- *Does menopause cause weight gain?*
- *Does menopause increase the risk of diabetes?*
- *Does hormone replacement therapy prevent any of this?*

The answers to these questions carry enormous significance. Obesity and diabetes cause severe medical complications and consume a tremendous amount of health care resources. Any measure that might deter weight gain or decrease the incidence of diabetes and its related health problems should be aggressively pursued.

Does menopause cause weight gain?

Both women and men tend to gain one pound a year (or more!) after the age of 50 and this is attributed to many factors.[1] However, more women than men become obese in later life.[2] Obesity occurs three to five times more in postmenopausal women than in premenopausal women.[3] These observations suggest that there is something about menopause that causes weight gain. Could it be due to the loss of estrogen?

Basic science in the lab supports this possibility (as well as my very non-scientific personal observation that my black Labrador retriever dramatically gained weight after having a complete hysterectomy!) Mice whose ovaries have been removed gain more weight compared to their cage mates who were spared this surgery.[4] In related experiments, it has been shown that mice genetically altered to eliminate their alpha estrogen receptors become obese.[5] In this situation, estrogen is present but unable to exert its biological effects.

It's not clear what causes these mice to gain weight. There is research that suggests that estrogen has an effect on parts of the brain that regulate food intake and energy expenditure.[6] But there is likely much more to it than that. We know that fat cells aren't simply inert storage lockers for extra calories. They are rich in estrogen receptors and it has been shown estrogen stimulates them to secrete hormones and other proteins and factors that are associated with weight maintenance.[7,8] One of these is leptin. Leptin plays a major role in regulating our metabolism. It is often referred to as the "satiety hormone" because it suppresses our appetite. A loss of leptin causes weight gain, so it is logical to assume that at the time of menopause our bodies will tend to put on fat in the absence of the weight-modifying effects of estrogen.

However, despite these findings, large-scale studies in humans have not been able to conclusively "prove" that menopause, per se, causes weight gain.[2,5,9] While it is generally observed that women gain weight at an increased rate after menopause, other factors that occur at this point in women's lives, such as changes in activity and lifestyle, cloud the picture so much that definitive conclusions have not been reached.

However, while there may be inadequate data to clearly assert that menopause causes weight gain, there is a strong consensus that menopause and the lack of estrogen dramatically affects *where* the fat goes as women go through this transition.[10,11] As many of you may have noticed, midlife weight gain seems to have a predilection to go around our middles. We call this *central*, or *abdominal, fat*. This fat is not just an extra roll around the waist; it also appears on the inside of us in and around our internal organs.

I vividly recall a moment in medical school when I saw a CAT scan of an obese person for the first time. As mentioned previously, a CAT scan uses x-rays to create a 3-dimensional picture of a person and displays the images in a series of slices – as if you sliced the body in narrow sections and laid out all the pieces in sequence. When the radiologist brought up the images on the screen, I recall being a little surprised. My first impression was that I was looking at a line of donuts. On each image there was a thick role of fat tissue wrapped around a normal size body. But what was equally impressive was seeing streaks and globs of fatty deposits within and surrounding the internal organs – like a well-marbled steak! For some reason, this experience has stuck with me as a visual memory that illustrates how fat can infiltrate every nook and cranny inside our bodies and not just on the outside. We tend to think that carrying extra weight puts a strain on our muscles and joints but the internal fat permeating within the abdomen and organs also can have serious medical consequences.

It is well established that it is menopause and not just aging that greatly accelerates the development of this extra belly fat. Women going through menopause have a much greater rate of central fat deposition than men of the same age.[12] Almost 75% of women over the age of 60 are considered to have abdominal obesity.[2] Even if a woman does not show a weight gain on the scales, her proportion of central fat increases when she goes through menopause.[6] Central fat accounts for about 5% to 8% of the total amount of fat in premenopausal women but up to 15% to 20% in postmenopausal women.[13]

Some interesting studies have provided further evidence that it is the loss of estrogen rather than aging that is responsible for this unwelcome change in our figures. There is a treatment that is given to women that temporarily shuts down ovarian hormone production, essentially creating a fake menopause. (This is used to treat certain conditions such as endometriosis.) Young women, well below the typical age of menopause, who have undergone this treatment develop an increase in central fat deposition.[14] Animal studies have also corroborated this. Animals deprived of estrogen develop more central fat than those with normal levels and this can be prevented by estrogen administration.[6]

The accumulation of central fat isn't just a matter of appearance. This type of fat behaves differently in the body than fat elsewhere. It plays a role in how our insulin and other hormones work and promotes inflammatory changes that have adverse effects in other areas of the body. This is why you may have heard that having an "apple" body shape (being round in the middle) is not as healthy as having a "pear" shaped figure (smaller waist and larger hips). This is the reason why many organizations include a waist circumference measurement in their health risk assessment screenings for their employees.

It was discovered many years ago that a large percentage of people with an "apple" shape also tend to have several other traits, which include high LDL (low-density lipoprotein) levels, high triglyceride levels, and *insulin resistance* – a condition that increases the risk of diabetes. This clustering of health factors has been described as the *metabolic syndrome*. This syndrome is something that receives a great deal of attention from cardiologists. People with this condition have a high risk of developing heart disease and other vascular complications.

Overall, about 20 to 25% of adults in the U.S. and Europe are believed to have the metabolic syndrome. However, 31% to 55% of postmenopausal women fit the criteria for having this diagnosis.[15,16,17] Furthermore, the earlier a woman goes through menopause the more at risk she is. Women who have their ovaries removed surgically before the age of natural menopause are more likely to develop the metabolic syndrome compared to women of comparable ages.[18,19]

If the loss of estrogen leads to the metabolic syndrome, and this syndrome is associated with diabetes, does this imply that menopause increases the risk of diabetes? It would be logical to presume that this is the case. Before embarking on examining this relationship, it's important to have an understanding of diabetes.

Diabetes 101

Diabetes is a condition where the blood sugar, or *glucose,* level in the blood is consistently above normal. In order for our bodies to function optimally, a set level of glucose needs to be maintained in the bloodstream at all times. If it gets too low our cells are deprived of fuel and the first organ to suffer is the brain. Low blood sugar, or *hypoglycemia*, can cause a person to have difficulty thinking or talking, or even lose consciousness. If the situation is not quickly corrected this can lead to death.

The term that denotes high blood sugar is *hyperglycemia*. Persistently high blood sugar levels, over time, can cause cellular damage – particularly in the eyes, nerves, kidneys, and circulatory system. Extremely high blood sugar can disrupt the chemical balance in the bloodstream and cause a severe life-threatening condition called *ketoacidosis.*

To regulate blood sugar, various hormones are produced in the body that either raise or lower it as needed. If the sugar level gets too low *glucagon* is secreted, and this stimulates the production and release of stored sugar. If the blood sugar level gets too high, *insulin* is released from the pancreas. Insulin lowers blood sugar in multiple ways. It drives sugar out of the bloodstream into the cells, it prevents the breakdown of glycogen (which is the storage form of sugar), and it inhibits the internal production of glucose. If someone takes too much insulin, their blood sugar can drop to dangerously low levels.

The blood sugar-regulating hormones are constantly working to keep the glucose level in a range from about 70 mg/dl to 140 mg/dl. (When you look at your lab report, mg/dl stands for milligrams per deciliter – this is the standard way of reporting blood sugar concentration). The level fluctuates up and down depending on when and how much a person eats. After a meal, the sugar level goes up, but then it comes down within a few hours as the body distributes the sugar into the cells.

We diagnose diabetes if the fasting blood sugar (meaning a sample taken first thing in the morning after having nothing to eat after midnight) is equal to or over 126 mg/dl. If the sugar level is over this value when you first get up, it will run much higher than this throughout the day because as food is consumed it will keep the blood sugar elevated. If the blood sugar goes above 200 mg/dl

223

it is eliminated from the circulation by the kidneys and spills out into the urine. Centuries ago diabetes was diagnosed by detecting sugar in the urine and in fact, the name, *diabetes mellitus,* comes from the Latin term meaning *"sweet like honey."*

One way to assess how well the body is regulating blood sugar is to perform a test called the *hemoglobin A1C.* This test gives us a value that reflects what the blood sugar has been averaging over the preceding three months. A normal A1C value is between 4.5 and 5.6. If the value is between 5.7 and 6.4 this is considered to be *prediabetes.* Values over this are diagnostic of diabetes. The higher the A1C level, the higher the average blood sugar. An A1C between 6.5 and 7.0 indicates a mild case of diabetes. Levels can go as high as 12 to 14 and a person with a number in this range has severe and poorly controlled diabetes with blood sugars frequently over 300 to 400 mg/dl.

You wouldn't think that something as innocuous as sugar would be bad for us, but persistently high glucose levels cause damage to our tissues. This adversely affects the lining of the arteries and promotes the buildup of plaque, which leads to blockages in the arteries. This is why diabetes greatly increases the risk of having a heart attack or stroke. High levels of glucose can also infiltrate the sheaths around nerves causing numbness and pain. These detrimental effects on the circulatory system and nerves lead to skin ulcers that heal poorly and are the reason diabetics can develop gangrene of the feet requiring amputation.

There are two basic types of diabetes, *Type 1* and *Type 2* diabetes. Although the hallmark of both types is elevated blood sugar levels, they are caused by different mechanisms. Type 1 diabetes accounts for only about 10% of the cases of diabetes and is due to a deficiency of insulin. In this situation, something destroys the insulin-producing pancreatic cells so that they can no longer make insulin. This is usually the result of an infectious or inflammatory process. This type of diabetes is called *insulin-dependent diabetes mellitus* (IDDM) since patients are dependent on insulin for the rest of their lives. Since it usually occurs in childhood, it is also referred to as *juvenile-onset diabetes.* Patients with this type of diabetes require insulin administration, which is typically given by injections multiple times per day.

The other form of diabetes, Type 2 diabetes, occurs because insulin has become ineffective in its ability to lower the blood sugar. Patients with this type of diabetes make insulin but their cells are resistant to its actions – so we describe this type of diabetes as being due to insulin resistance. The mechanism behind insulin resistance is extremely complicated. Rather than try to explain the complex chemical processes that are involved, I typically use the following simplistic description. A typical cell has insulin receptors attached to its surface. These are protein complexes that act like "catchers' mitts" for insulin. When people gain weight, excess fat gets deposited inside their fat cells. This affects the cell's receptors, making it difficult for insulin to attach to the cell and interferes with its job of lowering the blood sugar. The result is that the blood sugar stays in the blood vessels and glucose levels remain elevated.

The fascinating aspect of Type 2 diabetes is that with weight loss the fat in the cells diminishes and the receptors become functional – enabling the insulin to start working again. So the insulin resistance can reverse itself and for all intents and purposes the diabetes "goes away." This is why the most important aspect of treating Type 2 diabetes is weight loss. Achieving and maintaining an ideal weight literally can prevent and "cure" this type of diabetes.

Type 2 diabetes does not usually require insulin for treatment, although in some cases it is used. It is generally managed by taking pills or some of the newer injectable non-insulin drugs. This form of diabetes is also known as NIDDM or *non-insulin dependent diabetes mellitus*. At least one in four people have a genetic tendency to this type of diabetes but generally don't develop it until late in life, and so it is also referred to as *adult-onset diabetes*.

Aging and other factors bring on NIDDM in people with a genetic predisposition to it. The onset is particularly accelerated by weight gain. As more people are becoming obese, we are seeing Type 2 diabetes developing more frequently and much earlier in life – leading to alarming numbers of children and adolescents coming down with this form of diabetes.

With this background, let's now proceed with a discussion about the relationship between menopause, estrogen therapy, and diabetes. Surprisingly few women (and many of their health care providers) are even aware there is a link.

Does menopause increase the risk of diabetes?

There is quite a bit of literature attesting to the association of menopause, the metabolic syndrome, and insulin resistance. [20,21,22] This association strongly implies that menopause increases the risk of diabetes. In addition, there are other reasons to suspect there is something about the loss of estrogen that increases this risk. These reasons include:

- Men are at a higher risk for diabetes than women until about the age of 50. Thereafter women are more likely to be diagnosed with diabetes than age-matched men.[23,24]

- A number of studies, including a large meta-analysis published in 2019, have found that the younger a woman is when she goes through menopause, the higher her risk of diabetes.[25-28]

- Women who have their ovaries removed prior to natural menopause are at increased risk for developing diabetes.[29,30] In one study, women undergoing a bilateral oophorectomy demonstrated a 57% increased incidence of diabetes compared to age-matched women who did not have this surgery.[31]

- In animal studies it has been shown that mice that have their ovaries removed and mice without estrogen receptors develop diabetes at high rates.[32]

- Estrogen receptors are present on the insulin-producing cells in the pancreas and estrogen appears to play a role in insulin production.[33]

- Estrogen plays a role in facilitating the transport of glucose out of the bloodstream into muscle cells. A lack of estrogen would affect this important pathway which lowers blood sugar.[34]

Despite all of this, it is surprising that clinical studies have been mixed regarding whether natural menopause, per se, increases the risk of diabetes.[35-38] Although this seems perplexing, it is an understandably difficult condition to study. In order to make some determination about the effects of menopause on diabetes, women with underlying, predisposing conditions need to be excluded from studies. These include attributes such as obesity, an increased waist circumference, and even having the metabolic syndrome. However, we know that estrogen loss at the time of menopause contributes to these issues. So in my mind, by eliminating women with these conditions from the studies, the role that menopause plays in causing diabetes would be discounted. You can see why this gets murky.

Because of a lack of firm data, you will hear expert opinions, such as the 2017 statement from the American Association of Clinical Endocrinology that ". . . *menopause has not been associated with an increased risk of diabetes.*"[39]

While I can see why scrutiny of the studies to date may justify this opinion, the observations and research I have described strongly suggest that the loss of estrogen predisposes women to diabetes. If this is not the case, why would treating women with estrogen help prevent diabetes? This puzzling issue is explored in the next section.

What effect does HRT have on weight gain and diabetes?

Many women, as well as their providers, have the impression that taking estrogen causes weight gain. A lot of this perspective comes from their experience with oral contraceptives. Over the years, a number of my younger patients complained that their birth control pills made them gain weight. In some instances, this may have been the case because the hormones in these preparations are fairly potent and may stimulate appetite and cause some fluid retention. However, studies have not conclusively shown that contraceptive pills cause weight gain.[40]

Similarly, there is a large amount of evidence that indicates that the hormones used in HRT do not cause weight gain.[5] In fact, many studies show that women taking them gain *less* weight than women who do not take them. In the WHI study, women on estrogen and a progestogen showed small but significant *decreases* in body mass index and waist circumference during the first year.[41] Other studies have shown that HRT either has no effect on weight or is associated with less weight gain compared to women who are not on hormones.[42]

I came across an interesting study that was done to examine if estrogen prevented weight gain even in younger women.[14] Researchers gave a group of women who had not gone through menopause a medication that shut down their ovarian production of hormones, inducing a "fake" menopause. They then gave half of the women estradiol, and the other half a placebo. The women who took the placebo gained more weight than the women who were given estrogen.

Whether taking HRT prevents weight gain or not is probably not as relevant as whether it prevents central fat deposition. After all, it is the sinister abdominal fat that promotes the development of insulin resistance, which leads to diabetes and other heart complications. So the million-dollar question is – what impact does HRT have on central fat deposition? Does it prevent the dreaded belly bulging and protect us from becoming "apples?"

A number of studies have demonstrated that estrogen helps prevent the accumulation of abdominal fat.[43,44,45] I think most women would be surprised to learn this, as I doubt many doctors include this information when discussing the pros and cons of HRT with their patients. This is very unfortunate because we know that the widening of the waistline is not simply a cosmetic issue but portends an increased risk of future health problems – not the least being diabetes.

This brings us to the next important question. Does HRT prevent diabetes? I bet if you polled primary care doctors today, many would not be able to give the correct answer. Even if they knew the answer is *YES*, they may not be aware of the impressive amount of evidence that supports this. So let's review some of it.

Starting with studies in the lab:

- It has been shown that removing the ovaries from rodents and primates leads to an increase in blood sugar levels that are improved with the administration of estrogen.[32]

- Estrogen treatment can delay the onset of diabetes not only in female mice but even in male mice.[32]

- Estrogen receptors have been found in the insulin-producing cells in the pancreas. Estrogen treatment has a beneficial effect on insulin production.[46,47]

In addition to the information gained from this type of research, there have been numerous observational studies over the years, both in the U.S. and Europe, that have found that women taking HRT had lower rates of diabetes than women not taking hormones.[48-52] However, as we have learned, we need clinical trials to give us definitive answers. And guess what? Regarding this issue, the results actually agree with the observational studies!

In the WHI study, women who were treated with estrogen had a 21% decreased incidence of diabetes compared to women on a placebo.[41] Two other major clinical trials, the PEPI study and the HERS study, also showed that HRT decreased diabetes.[44,53] In the HERS data that was analyzed, treating 30 women with HRT prevented one case of diabetes.[53] (When you consider that 6,000 women in the U.S. become menopausal every day, this equates to a lot of women!). Other more recent studies support these findings.[54] A meta-analysis of studies between 1997 and 2011 reported similar findings – a 39% reduction in the incidence of diabetes in women treated with HRT.[55]

These studies strongly attest that HRT plays a role in preventing diabetes. This has led the North American Menopause Society to come out with the following conclusion in their 2017 position statement: *"Hormone therapy significantly reduces the diagnosis of new-onset Type 2 diabetes."*[56] This statement has huge significance and I find it strange that people are not paying more attention to this. Diabetes is a major health issue across the globe. I have managed hundreds of diabetic patients over the years and this diagnosis greatly impacts their lives. They frequently struggle to keep their diabetes under control. Managing their disease interferes with their daily activities, the medications are expensive, and complications from diabetes can be devastating. I would jump at a chance to be able to offer my patients any intervention that might prevent them from developing this disease.

However, because of the issues raised by the WHI that HRT may increase cardiac complications, the guidelines do not recommend HRT for diabetes prevention. To me this is very disappointing. Furthermore, I find it ironic that we have a treatment, i.e., estrogen therapy, which both improves cholesterol and lowers blood sugar – two major cardiac risk factors. Yet, because of a perceived increased cardiac risk, we are unwilling to recommend it!

Does timing and the type of HRT matter?

The question arises whether timing is an issue when it comes to the benefits of HRT for diabetes prevention. As discussed in earlier sections, the time at which postmenopausal women start HRT can impact how the hormones behave in the body. Is this the case with respect to diabetes? It appears so.

Studies have been done that can measure the degree of insulin resistance that occurs in the body. The more insulin resistant a person is the more likely they are to develop diabetes. It has been demonstrated that giving women HRT early in menopause decreases insulin resistance, but delaying it until after ten years may not be beneficial.[57]

Furthermore, as described previously, women lose hormone receptors as they age. There are several areas in the body where the loss of receptors, and thus the loss of estrogen effect, would promote diabetes. The loss of estrogen receptors in the pancreas would lead to lower insulin production; a loss of estrogen receptors in muscles would prevent blood sugar uptake into the cells.

229

Loss of both of these actions leads to elevated blood sugar levels and promotes diabetes. This suggests that hormones given to older women may not help prevent diabetes.

However, in both the WHI and HERS studies, which primarily consisted of older women, hormone treatment appeared to have a favorable impact on preventing diabetes. In the HERS study, where all the women were over age 65, fewer women entering the study who had mildly high blood sugar readings went on to develop diabetes if they were given estrogen compared to those who were given a placebo.[53] In the estrogen-only arm of the WHI, the most pronounced benefit of diabetes risk reduction occurred in women younger than age 70, but even those over this age showed a modestly decreased risk compared to women on a placebo.[58] These findings suggest that, although timing is important when it comes to HRT's effectiveness in preventing diabetes, estrogen may have some benefit even in older women.

One issue to point out, however, is that in the WHI, older women taking estrogen and medroxyprogesterone did not see a decreased rate of diabetes. [58] This suggests that progestins may attenuate estrogen's beneficial effect on diabetes. Whether natural progesterone would be less likely to have a negative impact is unclear, but generally, progesterone is considered to have neutral metabolic effects.

Whether the type and mode of administration of estrogen makes a difference is also unclear. We don't have much data to go on. One study that gave us a little information was the KEEPs study, discussed in Chapter 12. The women in this study were close to the age of natural menopause and were treated with either oral conjugated estrogens or transdermal estradiol along with natural progesterone.[59] The women on transdermal estrogen showed a slight benefit in their blood sugar readings suggesting this mode of administration may be preferable. However, a meta-analysis of clinical trials conducted between 1966 and 2004 concluded that oral estrogen was more effective than transdermal estrogen in reducing insulin resistance and new-onset diabetes by 30%.[48]

What about women with diabetes?

Do women who have diabetes go through menopause earlier than average? Some studies indicate this; others don't.[60] A very large study called the European Prospective Investigation into Cancer and Nutrition study (EPIC study) did not find an association of diabetes with the age at menopause.[61]

230

The next question that frequently comes up is whether women with diabetes can safely take HRT. With the increase of diabetes occurring nationwide, it is important to discuss menopausal treatment options for women who have diabetes.

One of my diabetic patients, Jill, who I had referred to a cardiologist for evaluation of a mild heart murmur, called me frantically after she had been to see him to report that he insisted she stop her estrogen. Needless to say, I was disturbed that he took the liberty of making this treatment recommendation to Jill without consulting me! Not only was her diabetes under excellent control, she was 53 years old and having hot flashes. She was in excellent health and had no hypertension or high cholesterol issues or other evidence of heart disease (other than the heart murmur, which turned out to be nothing of concern).

The cardiologist's presumptiveness perturbed me because I was aware that a number of studies had been published that included women with Type 2 diabetes that consistently showed HRT was not harmful to diabetic women and, in fact, taking oral hormones actually improved control of their diabetes.[62,63,64] In the HERS (the Heart and Estrogen/Progestin Replacement Study) one third of the patients had diabetes or pre-diabetes. The fasting blood sugars in the women on HRT remained stable, whereas it increased in the women in the placebo group.[51]

Despite this favorable data, there has been reluctance on the part of many medical providers to treat any woman diagnosed with diabetes with HRT. This is reflected in a number of guidelines such as the 2011 American Heart Association position statement that basically suggests that women with diabetes should avoid HRT.[65] I suspect that this is because of the ongoing concerns raised by the WHI conclusions that HRT increases the risk of heart disease and, since diabetics are at increased risk, caution is in order. Needless to say, however, this caution should only apply to older women initiating HRT a number of years beyond menopause. Younger women, like my patient Jill, represent an entirely different category of women. Unfortunately, there have not been many studies performed since the WHI assessing HRT treatment in younger women having Type 2 diabetes (and even fewer involving women with Type 1 diabetes).[66]

In summary

After reading this chapter, you probably are still trying to digest all of this information. To recap, it's not clear how much menopause contributes to the weight gain that typically occurs at midlife, but there is considerable evidence that indicates that the loss of estrogen predisposes women to an increase in abdominal fat. This, in turn, increases the risk of insulin resistance which increases the likelihood of diabetes. Yet studies don't consistently show that menopause increases diabetes even though quite a bit of data shows that the earlier a woman goes through menopause the more likely she will develop diabetes. And finally, data from both observational and clinical studies have shown that women who take HRT have lower chances of developing diabetes than women who don't.

While it appears that hormone replacement therapy potentially could save thousands of women from developing diabetes, HRT is not recommended or approved as a preventative treatment for diabetes. From my perspective this is unfortunate and I believe it is important for women to be aware of this very significant potential benefit of HRT.

Decision Making Helper

<u>Key Considerations</u>

HRT should not cause weight gain and may help avoid it.

Menopause leads to an increased deposition of belly fat. HRT likely will decrease the amount of central fat deposition and help prevent an increased waist circumference. This decreases the risk of developing insulin resistance and the metabolic syndrome.

HRT has been shown to prevent the development of diabetes when initiated at the time of menopause and may also have some preventative effect in women starting them ten or more years beyond menopause. Synthetic progestins may lessen this benefit. Natural progesterone does not appear to have a negative impact, but studies are limited.

In women who have diabetes, HRT does not appear to adversely affect blood sugar control and may improve it. However, experts in the field of cardiology and endocrinology are reluctant to recommend that diabetic patients take HRT.

Current guidelines for HRT pertaining to weight and diabetes

Current guidelines do not recommend HRT for prevention of weight gain or diabetes. Women with diabetes are discouraged from taking HRT.

What the guidelines don't acknowledge

HRT does not cause weight gain and appears to decrease the deposition of central fat and the risk of developing the metabolic syndrome. HRT may prevent diabetes, especially when initiated at the time of menopause. HRT has not been shown to adversely affect blood sugar control in women with diabetes.

Chapter 16
Estrogen and Your GU System (and Sex)

One of my fondest memories was the day when 75-year-old Ruthie Ann visited me, her face aglow and appearing very excited. She had been a patient for over 20 years and together we had struggled through her husband's long battle with pancreatic cancer until he had passed away some five years earlier. They had been childhood sweethearts and had spent over 60 years together. Losing her soul mate had been rough, but when I saw her recently, it appeared she had finally risen above her grief. She girlishly told me that an old high school friend had contacted her. They had been seeing each other and were going to get married!

Like so many women, Ruthie had stopped her HRT when the WHI study came out and had been off estrogen for over ten years. Until this visit, she hadn't mentioned that she had been putting up with quite a bit of vaginal dryness and discomfort. She just assumed it was aging and, until romance showed up at her doorstep, she hadn't really paid much attention to that part of her body. She and her fiancé were interested in a sexual relationship and she had promised him she would discuss this with me. Even as close as we were, she still found it embarrassing to bring up the subject. I helped ease her into it by teasing her and telling her I was noticing a little twinkle in her eye. She confided in me that it seemed like her vagina was very small and she couldn't imagine that any sort of intercourse was possible, much less enjoyable. But she was hopeful that perhaps there might be something that could be done.

Ruthie Ann was dealing with the condition known as *vaginal atrophy*, the thinning and shortening of the vaginal wall. Although this occurs gradually with aging, her lack of hormones for so many years was a major contributing factor. Studies show that over 50% of menopausal women have vaginal complaints[1] but this is likely a gross underestimation of the true number because both patients and their providers frequently do not initiate conversations about these delicate issues. Sadly, it has been estimated that only about 10% of women are being treated for these problems.[2]

This chapter deals with the *genitourinary (GU) system* and how menopause and HRT affect it. The GU system consists of the external genitalia (vulva and clitoris), vagina, urethra (the opening where the urine comes out), and the bladder. The tissues in these areas are sensitive to the effect of hormones and the loss of estrogen after menopause leads to not only dryness, burning, itching, and pain with intercourse, but problems with urinary control and an increased risk of infections – all of which greatly impact a woman's quality of life. The general term for the problems caused by estrogen loss in these areas is the *genitourinary syndrome of menopause* or GSM. This designation replaces older terms like *atrophic vaginitis* and *vulvovaginal atrophy*. Not only is this new nomenclature less disparaging in its implications, but more inclusively reflects the spectrum of problems that the loss of estrogen brings on.

Vaginal changes that occur

The skin lining the vulva and vagina is greatly affected by estrogen. In young girls, the tissue in these areas is very thin. The rise in estrogen that accompanies puberty stimulates the cells to multiply and enlarge. This transforms the genital tissue into a more mature condition which persists throughout the reproductive years. Then, at the time of menopause, if estrogen is not replaced, the tissue reverts back to an almost preadolescent state. When we do a pelvic exam and look into the vagina, these changes in older women are very obvious. Instead of the accordion-like surface texture (known as *rugae*) seen in younger women, the lining of an estrogen-deficient woman is smooth and appears pale and fragile. It can bleed with even the light brush of a Q-tip.

As women approach menopause and even several years prior, they begin to notice the effects of estrogen loss in their GU systems. The cells in the vagina that secrete mucus, our natural moisturizer, diminish and dryness becomes a major problem. (This keeps the manufacturers of K-Y jelly in business!) Along with this can come itching and burning in the vulvar area and around the urethra. Symptoms gradually get worse with time. This leads to *dyspareunia*, the term for pain and difficulty with intercourse – a problem that affects 40% to 50% of postmenopausal women.[3]

In severe cases, the entire vagina can shrink profoundly, making it impossible to insert even the smallest speculum. This is why performing pelvic exams (or having intercourse) can be very uncomfortable and at times even impossible in some women as they age.

Estrogen has many effects in the vagina. It stimulates cell growth, improves blood flow, and helps fortify the collagen fibers that support the infrastructure and elasticity of the vaginal wall. Estrogen-enriched vaginal cells contain high levels of *glycogen* – a storage form of glucose. A rich supply of glucose feeds the vaginal cells as well as promotes the growth of *lactobacilli*, which are normal inhabitants of the vagina. These are the "good" bacteria found in unpasteurized yogurt. Lactobacilli convert glucose into lactic acid – which makes the vagina more acidic. This acidic environment discourages the growth of yeast and "bad" bacteria that may crawl into the opening of the vagina. In this way, estrogen plays a major role not only in preventing vaginal infections but bladder infections as well.

Options for treating GSM – estrogen

Water or silicone-based moisturizers can help alleviate dryness to some degree, and vaginal lubricants may allow satisfactory intercourse – but none of these over-the-counter products alter the underlying physiologic transformation responsible for the problems of GSM – which are the changes that have occurred in the cells. This can only be accomplished with hormone replacement.

Systemic estrogen therapy (meaning standard doses of oral or transdermal estrogen) taken by women for treatment of their hot flashes is generally very effective for both preventing and treating GSM symptoms. However, some women are reticent to take these larger doses of estrogen and only want to address their GU symptoms. For these women there are there are low-dose estrogen products designed specifically to be applied to the vagina and intended exclusively to treat GSM symptoms. These include estrogen creams (Estrace, Premarin, and generic estradiol) or small pellet-like estradiol suppositories (such as Vagifem) which are inserted with applicators into the vagina several times a week. There is also a vaginal ring, Estring, which is placed up in the vagina where it slowly releases estradiol over a three-month period. Every 90 days it needs to be removed and replaced. I started emphasizing this to my patients after I had a big surprise one day when I inserted a speculum to do a PAP smear and found myself staring at three of these rings packed inside a patient's vagina. (She thought they were supposed to dissolve!)

The changes due to GSM progress over time. If left untreated for many years, the lining of the vagina and other tissues in the genital area becomes so thin and fragile that the tissue may not be able to respond to the hormones.

237

Treating these women can help this situation to some degree, but generally a woman can't expect the vagina to return to its previous supple state.

The estrogen in low-dose vaginal products is absorbed into the vaginal cells where it exerts an effect. However, some estrogen does seep into the bloodstream. The small rise in the estrogen level in the blood that occurs shortly after insertion is transient and for all intents and purposes, not much estrogen is delivered elsewhere in the body.[4] This means that these low-dose vaginal preparations cannot be expected to help hot flashes nor prevent bone thinning to any significant degree. In the same vein, these products should not cause any negative estrogen effects. However, there is a debate among oncologists about the safety of allowing women being treated for breast cancer to use these low-dose estrogen products. This is a dilemma for these patients because they suffer a great deal from GSM. Not only do many of these women go through premature menopause from their cancer treatments, but ongoing therapy with strong anti-estrogen drugs causes extremely severe vaginal aging. This is not good for anyone, especially young women.

Although the debate continues, recently some of the major societies have come out with position statements about this situation. The North American Menopause Society[5] and the American College of Obstetricians and Gynecologists[6] recommend that low-dose vaginal estrogen be offered to women with a history of breast cancer if other options have not been helpful. However, for women being treated with drugs like Arimidex, vaginal estrogen is not recommended because, under treatment with these drugs, the amount of estrogen absorbed can be much higher than acceptable.

Low-dose vaginal estrogen is not believed to have a significant effect on the uterus, so most experts concur that it is not necessary for women to take progestogen therapy, as is necessary when taking full-dose estrogen replacement therapy.[7,8] It is also generally believed that women who have had a hysterectomy for uterine cancer can safely take low-dose vaginal estrogen, especially if it was a low-grade malignancy.[5]

Even though low-dose vaginal estrogen therapy is very safe and effective for GSM, many women are hesitant to consider it. One problem that many physicians have encountered is sending a patient home with a prescription only to get a frantic call from her after hours wanting to be reassured that what was ordered is safe. This is because the patient information inserts that come with these products are identical to the ones that come with the full-dose oral or transdermal estrogen products. The printout warns of an increased risk of breast cancer, uterine cancer, heart attacks, and even dementia. This sort of warning is unwarranted because there is a negligible risk of cancer from these formulations, and a number of studies have concluded that they do not increase the risk of heart attacks or clots.[9] Even long-term data from the WHI studies is consistent with this.[10] The major menopause societies are fighting with the FDA to amend the inserts to more accurately reflect the true safety status of these low-dose hormones, but their efforts are apparently running up against bureaucratic sluggishness.

The first low-dose vaginal estrogen product to be approved was Premarin vaginal cream. It is still available today and, although it is a very low dose, even lower-dose vaginal estrogen products are available, which contain roughly one quarter the amount of estrogen as in the older products. They appear to be equally effective in controlling most women's symptoms. Interestingly, it wasn't until 2008 that the FDA approved any of the low-dose products to treat dyspareunia (painful intercourse). And the only product receiving approval is Premarin. However, I think most menopause experts would agree that any of the products approved for treating GSM are effective in treating dyspareunia as they all improve the thickness and elasticity of the vaginal tissue.

Once a woman decides to initiate treatment with vaginally-applied estrogen it usually takes about six to twelve weeks to obtain the full benefit – although some women can see some decrease in symptoms within a few weeks. Usually, daily treatment is recommended for the first two weeks and then a maintenance dose, anywhere from one to three times weekly, keeps the tissue in good shape. Topical moisturizers or lubricants can be used as necessary. All of the various low-dose estrogen products are effective and the choice is up to a woman based on such things as cost, convenience, and personal preference.[11] Some women who have a great deal of dryness or irritation of the vulvar area may prefer a cream, which can be applied to these areas as well as inside the vagina.

Generally it is recommended that women abstain from intercourse for twelve hours after inserting an estrogen product, although the risk of any significant adverse effect on one's partner is trivial.[12] Once women reengage in intercourse, studies have shown regular sexual activity helps keep the vulvar and vaginal tissues in a more "youthful" condition, probably through improved circulation from stimulation. (I guess this is where the phrase "*use it or lose it*" comes from!)

Systemic estrogen therapy, in the form of oral estrogen pills or transdermal estrogen, is usually adequate to control most women's GSM symptoms. However, some women who have continued symptoms may benefit from the addition of low-dose vaginal estrogen.

Options for treatment of GSM – non-estrogen options

Other treatments for vaginal symptoms are being developed. A novel new vaginal preparation, Intrarosa (prasterone) was approved in 2016 for GSM. This contains DHEA (dehydroepiandrosterone). DHEA is a hormone produced in the adrenal glands and is a precursor to both estrogen and testosterone. According to the developers of Intrarosa, after a dose is inserted it is absorbed into the vaginal cells and is converted into estrogen as well as testosterone. The estrogen component should induce the same changes as topical estrogen preparations. Theoretically, the testosterone produced would enhance the effects of topical estrogen.[15] After applying this product, transient elevations of DHEA, testosterone, and estrogen have been noted in the bloodstream.[13,14] This likely would not be expected to cause any worrisome negative effects. However, women who have breast cancer should consult their oncologists regarding the use of this product.

Another recent approach for addressing postmenopausal vaginal problems has been the development of oral SERMs for this purpose. Recall that these are designer drugs that are created to have some positive estrogen effects without some of the negative estrogen effects. A new SERM called *ospemifene* (Osphena) is now available specifically for GSM. This SERM has beneficial estrogen-like effects on the vagina but does not cause negative effects in the breasts or uterus. However, like any new drug, time will tell if it is going to be as safe and successful as initial studies indicate. It is also noted that results may take up to six months – which to me seems like an exceptionally long time to wait! A combination estrogen/SERM product, Duavee, has also been shown to help GSM, but currently is only approved for treatment of hot flashes and osteopenia.

The other innovation causing quite a bit of excitement in gynecology circles is laser therapy. When I first heard about using laser rays in the vagina to treat this condition it sounded screwy – as we generally think of lasers destroying tissue, like removing skin cancers or the LASIK procedures that reshape the cornea to correct poor vision. But what has been discovered is rather than damaging tissue, certain types of laser beams simply heat up the vaginal wall – which promotes an increase in blood flow under the skin. The improvement in circulation stimulates cell growth which thickens the vaginal lining and promotes collagen buildup – creating more support and elasticity to the vaginal wall. Laser therapy is being used in Europe and some research centers in the U.S. but is very early in development. However, clinics are popping up across the country promoting this service to women as a method of vaginal rejuvenation. This technique is not yet approved by the FDA and experts warn women to be cautious about jumping onto this bandwagon too quickly.[16] There is still much unknown about the optimal type of laser beam that should be used and other technicalities, as well as its long-term risks and efficacy.

Other genitourinary problems and how estrogen helps

The lack of estrogen has negative impacts in other areas of the genitourinary tract. It is not uncommon for a woman to experience her first bladder infection shortly after menopause, and this is always an unwelcome surprise. Suddenly you have an urge to go to the bathroom every 30 minutes, feel like you're peeing glass crystals, and then in many cases are horrified to see the toilet bowl filled with bloody red urine. Other terms used to designate these pesky infections you may be familiar with are *UTIs* (urinary tract infections) and *cystitis*.

Why do we get these UTIs and why are they common after menopause? I always take time to educate patients about this because it helps them to better understand how to prevent them from recurring. I first explain that there are millions of bacteria in our colons – their role is to break down undigested byproducts from our food. No matter how fastidiously clean we try to be, there are always some of these bacteria milling around the anal area. From there they can crawl into the vagina and then into the bladder. If you have ever seen one of these creatures in an image from an electron microscope – they literally do have little "feet" that can propel them along like a centipede. Once they enter the bladder they multiply like lightning and, when the numbers reach a threshold level (which is about 5,000 bacteria per drop of urine), they cause symptoms.

Women of all ages are susceptible to bladder infections – particularly when there is a lot of activity "down there", such as during intercourse (that's why you may have heard the term *honeymoon cystitis*). While it is not uncommon to have UTIs when younger, they can be particularly troublesome after menopause. During our reproductive years, the vulvar and vaginal tissue is much plusher and thicker due to estrogen effects. This "rough terrain" makes it hard for the bugs to find their way to the bladder. After menopause, the tissue is much thinner and smoother so the bacteria can skate along that much easier to their destination. In addition, without estrogen's acidifying effects, the normal inhabitants of the vagina, the lactobacilli, disappear. The absence of these "good" bacteria makes it easier for the "bad" bacteria, such as E. Coli (the most common bug causing UTIs) to invade.

The conduit from the bladder that empties the urine is the urethra. The opening of the urethra is located at the twelve o'clock position of the vaginal entrance. As the vaginal and vulvar tissues get thinner the urethra protrudes out more and is more susceptible to being irritated and becomes an easier target for the bacteria to sneak in. Treating women with estrogen improves the condition of this structure which helps ward off these UTIs.

Some women are confused about the difference between bladder infections and vaginal infections. Bladder infections are due to bacteria or other infectious agents that find their way into the bladder. Vaginal infections are caused by organisms that grow on or invade the vaginal lining or cervix.

There are many types of vaginal infections. The infecting organisms can be introduced through sexual contact. These can be caused by bacteria (such as gonorrhea or chlamydia), viruses (such as herpes or HPV), or parasites (such as trichomonas). Vaginal infections can also be due to an overgrowth of certain bacteria normally present in the vagina, such as gardnerella. An infection from this organism, also referred to as *bacterial vaginosis* (BV), is characterized by a discharge and "fishy" odor.

An extremely common vaginal infection in postmenopausal women is due to an overgrowth of yeast, such as Candida. The lack of lactobacilli and the change in the acid-base balance in the vagina that occurs with estrogen deficiency makes a perfect environment for yeast to grow. These infections typically cause itching and sometimes a whitish ("cottage cheesy") discharge. They can be easily treated with a single-dose oral antifungal pill or an intra-vaginal cream. However, yeast infections frequently reoccur.

Estrogen therapy helps prevent both bladder and vaginal infections through its effects on improving the integrity of the tissues of the vagina and around the urethra. Any form of estrogen treatment can be very effective in preventing them.[17]

Urinary incontinence is another common problem women encounter as they age. Incontinence is the term we use to describe unplanned urinary leakage. There are several ways this appears. It may be just a dribble when you cough or sneeze. At other times, it is a sudden urge to urinate, coming out of the blue, causing a little or a lot of urine to escape.

Many factors related to menopause contribute to incontinence problems. A lack of estrogen weakens and widens the opening of the urethra, so there is less resistance to retard the leakage of urine. Estrogen therapy can correct this laxity by increasing the circulation to the tissues around the urethra, thus promoting cell growth, which thickens the tissue within the urethra to better hold back the urine. In addition, it is believed that estrogen's effects on the muscles around the bladder may help calm some of the unwanted contractions that can cause an involuntary leakage of urine.

So while these observations suggest that HRT should improve incontinence problems, studies have not consistently borne this out. Some have shown improvement with vaginal estrogen therapy.[18,19] Others have not demonstrated any benefit,[20] and the WHI concluded that oral HRT worsened incontinence! However, many of the urologists and gynecologists I have worked with feel that estrogen treatment is helpful. It certainly is a fairly simple measure to try a course of vaginal estrogen therapy before prescribing other drugs (which frequently have significant side effects) or embarking on more invasive measures such as surgery.

Finally, another major complaint of women as they age is a general weakness of the pelvic muscles that hold up the bladder, uterus, and vagina – which is known as *pelvic laxity*. This weakness allows the pelvic organs to sink down lower in the abdomen than they are supposed to. Some women may not even be aware of this, but many feel a sensation of heaviness and fullness especially if they bear down. Pelvic laxity is usually very obvious to a doctor when performing a pelvic exam. The walls of the vagina literally collapse against each other and the entire vaginal sack sags. This is particularly common in women who have had multiple children and/or large babies. Gaining excessive amounts of weight also puts pressure on the lower pelvic muscles and predisposes women to this condition.

If there is significant weakness, we use the term *pelvic prolapse* to describe this condition. Women with pelvic prolapse frequently feel as if things are going to "fall out." In my practice, I encounter one or two patients a year who come in for an urgent visit after suddenly noticing a protuberance or bulge coming out of the vagina. This is understandably quite alarming. The protrusion invariably turns out to be the cervix hanging down and sticking out of the vagina. After reassuring them that their uterus will not suddenly drop out while they were grocery shopping, I explain their treatment options.

Mild cases of pelvic laxity can be improved by doing exercises to strengthen the pelvic muscles. Women can learn these by consulting a physical therapist who specializes in this type of treatment and frequently biofeedback therapy is utilized. Other cases can be helped by using a *pessary*. Basically, pessaries are soft plastic cubes or other geometric shapes that a woman inserts into her vagina to prop up the uterus. There are dozens of different types of these things and I always wonder who comes up with the crazy designs that you can choose from. Severe cases of pelvic prolapse generally require surgery, frequently along with a hysterectomy.

Because estrogen has so many beneficial effects on the tissues in our pelvic area, you would think HRT could help with problems of pelvic laxity, but studies have not been definitive. Estrogen treatment has a positive effect on collagen so it may help ward off this problem to some extent – but taking them once the condition is established hasn't been shown to be of any benefit.

What about sex?

I include the topic of sex in this chapter because the consequences of estrogen deficiency in the vagina obviously impact sexual functioning. Dryness and other GSM symptoms can cause pain with intercourse, and women are obviously not going to look forward to having sex if it is uncomfortable. But is there more to it than that? How do menopause and HRT affect sexual interest and sexual satisfaction? I find that most of my patients, if they are having problems, want reliable information about this subject as well as any treatment options that may be available to them.

Although sexual function declines with age, various surveys show that 50% to 80% of people over age 60 engage in sexual intercourse once a month, and many couples continue to be sexually active well into their 70s and 80s.[21,22,23] Many more women may be open to more physical intimacy if some of the age-related hurdles can be overcome – particularly changes that occur in the genital region. The thinning of the lining and loss of elasticity in the vagina can cause significant discomfort when it comes to having sex. Studies show that 44% of postmenopausal women complain of dyspareunia.[24] (And you can imagine that the numbers are likely higher since this is not a topic commonly discussed during your annual physical!)

Estrogen therapy can fortify the vaginal lining making intercourse more comfortable – but does it play a role in other ways? Does it affect libido, the term referring to one's interest and desire to have sex?

It seems the answer is "no" – at least not directly. While estrogen may improve a woman's interest in sex by making intercourse more inviting, it is testosterone that is generally accepted as the driving force of libido. And although women produce male hormones, their levels are much lower than men of comparable ages at every stage in life. Even elderly men at the low end of the testosterone spectrum have levels 20 to 40 times higher than a postmenopausal woman! This is why, as many of my patients have lamented over the years, they don't seem to have the same degree of libido as their husbands. In my experience, the disparity of interest in having sex has been a source of conflict in many marriages (and the array of male performance-enhancing products, such as Viagra, has not helped matters).

Just understanding that there is "nothing wrong with them" has helped many of my patients deal with this dilemma, but it would be nice if there was something else we could offer women who want to boost their desire for sex. Unfortunately, there is no magic bullet to improve a woman's libido. Various drugs, such as Wellbutrin and Buspar, have been prescribed off-label to enhance sexual interest, but are of questionable effectiveness. Some foods (think oysters) have gained the reputation of being aphrodisiacs, but none have been scientifically documented to be truly effective[25] (and historians note it may be more their physical shape than any chemical quality that gives them their notoriety!). Certain plant-based products may have some libido-enhancing qualities, such as yohimbine which purportedly increases blood flow to the genital organs, or Tribulus Terrestris which may increase testosterone levels. However, these supplements are not regulated by the FDA and there is always a question about their purity and safety.

The first drug specifically introduced and approved for enhancing libido in women appeared in 2015 by the name of flibanserin (Addyi). It is a drug that appears to modulate some of the neurotransmitters in the brain that affect sexual desire – principally, it is believed to decrease serotonin activity. Unfortunately, this drug has a number of drawbacks. First of all, it is not currently approved for postmenopausal women – primarily because it has not been studied in the older age groups. Secondly, drinking alcohol is absolutely contraindicated as the combination can cause low blood pressure and fainting. In addition, it needs to be taken daily, can cause frequent side effects such as dizziness and nausea, and has a number of drug interactions. Studies have not been particularly impressive regarding its efficacy. An analysis of several studies has shown only a slight improvement in response – on the order of increasing a woman's "sexually satisfying events" one additional time over a period of two months.[26]

In 2019 bremelanotide (Vyleesi) was approved by the FDA as a drug to enhance sexual desire. It comes as an injection that women must give themselves (similar to an insulin shot) and should be administered within an hour of intercourse. I have no experience with this drug and in clinical trials, up to 40% of women complained of nausea as a side effect.[27] It is not clear the exact mechanism by which this drug increases sexual desire and the actual benefit appears to be modest at best. It is not approved for postmenopausal women, likely due to concerns that it may increase blood pressure. And, like any brand new drug, my advice to patients is to wait until we know more about its safety and side effects before considering it.

What about testosterone?

You may be wondering if women should consider taking testosterone to improve libido. If you polled a hundred primary care doctors, I bet very few would say they have ever prescribed testosterone therapy for their postmenopausal patients. Beside the fact there are no approved testosterone products for women, traditional medical training programs don't advocate male hormones for menopausal management. The general attitude is that giving testosterone to women does not provide any benefit above and beyond estrogen therapy for the issues confronting menopausal women other than (surprise!) her libido. And, there has been controversy about whether it is really beneficial for that. Some researchers have dismissed its effectiveness because they have not found any correlation between testosterone levels and libido.[28] However, measuring testosterone levels in women can be misleading. The current tests are not very accurate when the levels of testosterone are low, and postmenopausal women have extremely low levels.[28]

However, a number of respected studies have found that testosterone therapy does increase libido in women who have gone through either natural or surgical menopause.[29-35] The degree of benefit tends to be proportionate to the amount of testosterone administered. Most of the studies have shown that 300 mcg per day can improve libido. Doses lower than this have not been shown to be very effective. Of note, this is a fraction of the amount of testosterone delivered by products on the market for men. Also, most of the women in these libido studies received both testosterone and estrogen. Thus, we have very little data on the effects and advisability of having postmenopausal women take testosterone alone to improve libido without concurrent estrogen.[36]

An interesting fact to bring to your attention is that oral HRT preparations (or any oral estrogen for that matter, such as birth control pills) actually *decrease* a woman's testosterone level. This occurs because estrogens taken orally have a first-pass effect. This causes the liver to make extra proteins that bind up testosterone and prevent it from attaching to its receptors. This essentially keeps the testosterone from exerting any actions. So it is somewhat ironic that treating a woman with HRT decreases her male hormone levels, which may further decrease her libido. This makes you wonder if we should be thinking more strongly about adding some testosterone to an HRT regimen!

Male hormone use in women can have some negative effects. It can increase acne, as well as stimulate the growth of facial hair, which may not be completely reversible with discontinuation of therapy. In some studies, women taking male hormones noted an increase in aggressiveness (which I guess could be construed as either a good or bad thing!) In addition, there has been some concern about possible negative cardiovascular effects because testosterone may negate some of the beneficial effects of estrogen on the lipid profile and insulin resistance. However, studies have not shown that it adversely affects blood pressure or endothelial function.[37]

Since some of the administered testosterone is converted into estrogen, concern has also been raised about whether testosterone could cause adverse effects on the breast and uterus – although studies have not demonstrated that these complications occur.[38,39,40] In my opinion, the doses are so low that this seems unlikely, but further long-term studies are needed.

Testosterone cannot be taken orally because it undergoes extensive first-pass effects and effective levels are not produced in the bloodstream. To overcome this, a synthetic oral drug called methyltestosterone has been developed. This has been combined with estrogen in a product by the name Estra-Test and approved for use in women. There is a generic version of this drug but it is generally not covered by insurance plans. Methyltestosterone, however, can cause negative effects on cholesterol, and there has been concern that it may cause liver damage (although likely only in higher doses given to men). Therefore, this particular drug is not considered an optimal hormone agent in either men or women.

For men who require hormone treatment, testosterone can be administered by injections into the muscle or under the skin, and there are transdermal and intranasal gels. There is even a buccal system (a product designed to be placed inside the cheek and gum line where it slowly dissolves). There are over 30 different testosterone products designed for men! These products contain much higher concentrations of testosterone than would be appropriate for women.

There are currently no commercial topical testosterone products approved for women in the U.S. or Europe. Two pharmaceutical companies have developed their versions of testosterone patches designed for women, but the FDA is not willing to approve them because of a lack of long-term studies of their safety and efficacy. (There is, however, a female testosterone patch product sold in Australia, if you happen to live down under!)

Many compounding pharmacies, however, do make creams and gels containing low doses of testosterone formulated for women and many naturopathic and longevity clinics routinely prescribe these for their clients as part of a menopausal replacement or anti-aging program. These products require a prescription from a physician. As noted, many menopause experts are leery of compounded preparations because of a lack of FDA oversight and a concern the preparations may not contain the specified doses, and potentially may contain impurities.

Women who desperately want help with their libidos frequently are eager to give testosterone a trial. While most health care providers flat out refuse such requests, many menopause experts acknowledge that a trial of testosterone is not unreasonable once these women have been apprised of the benefits and risks and informed that there are few studies on long-term use.[41] I have prescribed testosterone products (from a compounding pharmacy that I trust) for some of my patients, especially younger women going through premature menopause due to surgical removal of their ovaries. Since the ovaries produce over a third of their male hormones, these women, in particular, have a hard time adjusting to their sudden loss of not only estrogen but testosterone. I have found that my patients who have taken testosterone have had good results with few negative effects.

The other male hormone that has been touted as an option for improving libido is DHEA. Women's DHEA levels decline slowly with age and many anti-aging clinics promote it to improve libido and as a means to maintain youthful vigor. It is available over-the-counter in pill form as a "food supplement." As such, it is not regulated by the FDA. Experts have raised concern about the purity and quality of these products and generally don't recommend them for menopausal hormone treatment.[41] DHEA is a relatively weak androgen and a large review of studies did not find it helpful for libido or sexual function in women.[42,43,44] Significant adverse effects were not noted on blood sugar or cholesterol levels, and it did not cause weight gain. However, there was a mild increase in unwanted hair growth and acne.

What about orgasms?

It is difficult to get consistent data on how many women have problems achieving orgasms – either prior to or after menopause. Articles that I have read cite anywhere from 25% to 85% depending on age, ethnicity, and other factors. But generally, it appears that it is more difficult for women to achieve orgasms beyond menopause. Despite this being a significant problem for many women, there are very few options for treatment. Most experts recommend that, as a first step, patients be educated about their anatomy and the orgasmic process. In many cases, consultation with a sex therapist can be beneficial. There are many reputable providers with expertise in this field, such as those certified by the American Association of Sexuality Educators, Counselors, and Therapists (www.aasect.org).

Topical vaginal estrogen, as well as DHEA cream, may help improve a woman's ability to achieve orgasm to some degree simply by improving the integrity of the vulvar and clitoral tissue, and possibly by enhancing blood flow to the area. Similarly, vaginal testosterone may help in the same way[45,46] and it is postulated that it may also have an effect on the small nerve fibers in the vagina that may increase arousal and orgasmic function. Women have generally turned to compounding pharmacies for this option since there are no commercially approved vaginal testosterone products. Some pharmacies dispense a testosterone gel formulated to be applied to the clitoris prior to intercourse, which is intended to improve orgasms. Some of my patients who have used this treatment have reported that it seems to help.

There are no drugs approved to specifically improve orgasmic function. A few studies have tested Viagra-like drugs and have shown mixed results.[47,48] Devices, primarily vibrators, have been shown to be helpful. There has been considerable research, as well as an internet cornucopia of attestations, that the stimulation achieved with clitoral and vaginal vibrators helps women achieve orgasm. There are also personal clitoral vacuum devices that some women have found beneficial. These have been studied in women with spinal cord injuries and neurological diseases such as multiple sclerosis.[49] The bottom line, however, is that as advanced as medical science has become, we have not made much progress in helping women with this aspect of sexual function.

In conclusion

There are many problems involving the genitourinary system that confront menopausal women. There is much we need to learn. At least we can help patients avoid many of the distressing symptoms and problems associated with GSM, and help women, like my patient Ruthie Ann, find an increased level of enjoyment in their late-in-life relationships. You don't often think that those of us, whose practices are predominantly geriatrics, do this sort of pre-marital counseling and treatment!

Decision Making Helper

Key considerations

The genitourinary syndrome of menopause (GSM) is an inevitable consequence of estrogen loss and symptoms will progress gradually with aging.

Estrogen treatment has been shown to prevent many of these changes and decrease symptoms. Treatment works best when started early, at the time of menopause. Delaying treatment after years of estrogen deficiency may not help reverse all of the negative effects that have occurred. Treatment should continue indefinitely because discontinuation will cause the tissue to revert back to its prior condition.

Both oral and transdermal estrogen prescribed for hot flashes, as well as low-dose products designed for vaginal application, are effective to treat most GSM symptoms. Note that it can take six or more weeks to see improvement in symptoms.

It is not felt necessary to take a progestogen when being treated with the low-dose vaginal estrogen products designed specifically to treat GSM symptoms.

Most major menopause societies feel that low-dose vaginal estrogen is safe in almost all patients with a history of breast cancer except those being treated with certain anti-estrogen drugs. Women with a history of breast cancer should consult their breast cancer specialists when considering treatment options.

Topical estrogen inserted in the vagina has not been shown to increase the risk of blood clots or heart disease and, in low doses, should not affect the uterine lining or increase the risk of uterine cancer. Any vaginal bleeding occurring with therapy needs to be promptly and thoroughly investigated.

Low-dose vaginal estrogen products are generally insufficient to help hot flashes or prevent bone density decline.

There is much evidence to show that topical estrogen helps prevent vaginal and urinary infections and may help incontinence.

HRT does not appear to help issues with pelvic laxity or prolapse.

Estrogen does not increase libido directly, but can decrease discomfort with intercourse and thus may promote a greater interest in sexual desire.

A number of studies indicate that treating women with testosterone improves libido and sexual function but there remains controversy regarding its advisability for women. Guidelines do not recommend testosterone therapy as part of an HRT program, but many experts feel a trial in some patients may be appropriate. Although the risks are considered minimal, side effects are likely such as unwanted hair growth and acne.

Oral DHEA may improve libido although studies have been inconclusive. It can cause male hormone side effects. Since it is considered a food supplement it is not regulated by the FDA, and over-the-counter products may have non-standard ingredients. It is not generally recommended as part of an HRT regimen. Vaginal DHEA is available in a commercial product, prasterone, which appears to improve GSM and may improve sexual function.

Neither estrogen nor testosterone clearly improve orgasmic function but may be somewhat helpful through beneficial effects on vaginal and clitoral tissue health.

Current guidelines regarding HRT and the GU system

Estrogen is approved for the treatment of GSM and providers are advised to prescribe low-dose vaginal therapy as the first choice. Estrogen is not approved for the treatment of sexual dysfunction or any urinary health disorders such as infection prevention, incontinence, or pelvic laxity. Testosterone therapy is not approved for menopausal women for any condition.

What the guidelines don't acknowledge

Topical estrogen therapy appears to help prevent bladder and vaginal infections and decrease discomfort with intercourse. Treatment is only beneficial as long as it is continued. Stopping treatment causes the tissue to regress to its previous condition.

Testosterone therapy may help improve libido in women, with minimal risk.

Chapter 17
Estrogen, Your Skin, Joints, Muscles, and More

Whenever I am with a group of women friends around my age there are several subjects that almost always come up. Besides sharing stories about our children and grandkids, we always moan about our aching joints, sagging skin, and other maladies of aging. But even during get-togethers with other female physicians, there is never any discussion about whether taking HRT might have a bearing on what we are experiencing. We seem to accept that it is just aging that makes our skin thinner, our joints stiffer, and our muscles weaker. Yet as we learn more about estrogen receptors, we are finding that they are present in all these areas and therefore, just as in the bones, the loss of estrogen in the postmenopausal period accelerates a lot of this deterioration.

For some reason, there is a dearth of menopause articles that address the relationship between estrogen and a woman's appearance. And, while my personal observations hardly constitute a scientific study, it has always seemed obvious to me which of my patients have been long-term hormone users and which have not. Women on estrogen appear to have more youthful-looking skin and seem to look more vibrant.

One case in my practice particularly stands out. I followed two sisters for over 30 years from the time they first became patients when they were in their early forties. They were both exceptionally attractive women. They were a year apart in age and looked so much alike that many thought they were twins. They both started HRT in their late 40s, but then the younger sister developed breast cancer and reluctantly went off her estrogen at the insistence of her oncologist. Over the years her older sister, who continued estrogen, didn't seem to age as fast and appeared noticeably younger when they stood side by side – so much so that every year the younger sister lamented that she wished she could have stayed on her hormones.

Of course, this is a single anecdote, but it is experiences like these that invite the question – does HRT have anti-aging properties? Across the U.S. there are hundreds of longevity clinics that attract thousands of clients. Most of what they do is dispense hormones, including HRT. Many expert medical societies frown on some of the treatments these clinics provide, but one wonders if some of their appeal is because women notice positive changes in their bodies. I suspect a large part is due to estrogen replacement.

It is not hard to imagine why this may be plausible. Estrogen exerts positive effects on collagen. Collagen is the substance that gives structure and support to our skin and musculoskeletal system as well as to all of our internal organs and vessels. It is a protein that is woven into many forms – creating the rope-like tendons that attach muscles to bones and the elastic sheets that underlie the surface of our skin. Our bones are basically connective tissue that has been fortified with calcium to make it hard. We know how vital estrogen is for bone health. This chapter deals with what we know about how estrogen affects some of the other areas of our body that you don't hear much about.

Estrogen and our skin

Compared to other topics on HRT, there seems to be relatively little research on this subject. Perhaps it is because the benefit of estrogen on our skin is not considered all that important. And while cosmetic issues are not life and death matters like heart disease and cancer, I have always felt that how you look and feel about yourself has an impact on your health. Interestingly, a recent article in a journal of cosmetic dermatology found that estrogen levels correlated positively with not only enhanced skin health but a women's sense of perceived age and attractiveness.[1]

Research has shown that estrogen exerts major effects on our skin – promoting its growth and repair. As far back as 1985, there have been articles in the medical literature presenting data on the association of estrogen loss with skin thinning, skin dryness, and decreased elasticity. Studies have shown that hormone therapy increases skin thickness in mid-life women, presumably due to its effect on the collagen content.[2] In early 2000, a paper came out in the *American Journal of Dermatology* describing how estrogen treatment benefited the skin by restoring the loss of collagen and improving the capillary blood flow that diminishes after menopause.[3]

The benefits of estrogen have been further supported by other reviews in the dermatologic literature suggesting that estrogen not only helps prevent some of the skin changes that occur after menopause but may reverse skin damage that has occurred.[4,5] Other studies have shown that estrogen helps skin heal after a wound – possibly through its effects on suppressing inflammation and stimulating the growth of new skin cells.[6]

There clearly is quite a bit of data to verify the observations that many of us in healthcare have noted – that hormone replacement helps retard skin aging. This is not something that is frequently discussed when doctors review the benefits and risks of hormone replacement. But my personal opinion is that we should share this research with our patients.

Estrogen and our joints

The cells that comprise our joints are similar to those in our bones and skin, so it seems logical that estrogen will have some effect on the tissues comprising our joints. Indeed, there is considerable evidence that HRT plays a beneficial role in joint health, but you don't hear much about this. While effects on the skin may seem like a purely cosmetic issue, if estrogen has a protective effect on our joints this should not be lightly dismissed. Arthritis affects millions of aging women.

To better understand how estrogen affects our joints it is helpful to review some anatomy. A joint refers to the connecting point between two bones. On each end of the bone is a pad of cartilage that acts as a cushion protecting the bones from banging into each other. Enveloping each of these articulations is a tough capsule that contains a thick, jelly-like fluid that bathes and lubricates the joint. This arrangement allows our skeletons to move and bend smoothly and comfortably.

When we are young, the cartilage pads on our bones are "brand new." Whenever I prepare a fresh chicken and make a surgical cut between the thigh and the drumstick I marvel at how smooth and pristine the cartilage appears – wishing my own cartilage was in such good shape! With aging – starting as early as in our twenties – the work and play we do causes the surface of the cartilage to become eroded and irregular. At some point, this damage can cause a joint to become inflamed, causing fluid accumulation within the joint capsule creating pain, warmth, and swelling over the affected area. Over the years, repetitive trauma gradually wears away the cartilage and leads to aching joints, stiffness, and decreased mobility. These are the hallmarks of the most common type of arthritis, known as *osteoarthritis*. This is also referred to as *DJD* or *degenerative joint disease* or as I like to describe it: "wear and tear" arthritis.

Any of our joints can be affected by this type of arthritis, but the most common sites are the hips, knees, and hands. Both men and women develop osteoarthritis, but after menopause, twice as many women as men develop osteoarthritis despite the fact that men traditionally engage in more activities that strain the joints, such as rough sports and manual labor. In fact, the minute women start losing their hormones, osteoarthritis progresses very rapidly. One study showed that the majority of women being treated by a large arthritis clinic had developed symptoms within four years of going through menopause.[7]

We prescribe anti-inflammatory drugs to calm the pain and inflammation, but despite all our medical breakthroughs, there still are no drugs that can prevent the progression of osteoarthritis. Over time, the cartilage wears completely away. Since cartilage can't replace itself, the only treatment for advanced arthritis is a joint replacement.

Estrogen receptors are present in our joints. Studies in animals have shown that estrogen administration helps protect cartilage from deteriorating.[8] Unfortunately, the data for humans is very scanty because we don't have long-term, large studies to show conclusive benefits of HRT on osteoarthritis. [9,10] However, it has been shown that some SERMs, known to have estrogen-like effects on the joints, appear to help prevent arthritis.[11]

The exact mechanism of how estrogen protects the cartilage is unclear, but it is probably due to its beneficial effects on the maintenance of collagen and its anti-inflammatory properties. In addition, estrogen has a positive impact on the bone just beneath the cartilage. It is known that if the bone next to a joint remains healthy, it helps maintain healthy cartilage.

Though we don't have robust data to claim that estrogen therapy can slow down the development of arthritis, multiple studies have noted that women on estrogen complain of less joint pain than women on a placebo. In fact, one aspect of the WHI study, which you don't hear much about, is that women treated with hormones reported less pain and stiffness in their joints compared to women taking a placebo.[12] And, although the WHI was not designed to directly assess the effects of HRT on arthritis, women not taking HRT went on to have 27% more total hip and 13% more total knee replacements than women on hormones.[13]

Another reason to suspect that estrogen has something to do with helping joint pain is that women placed on drugs that are designed to lower estrogen levels (such as Arimidex) frequently complain of joint pain. Similarly, some of the SERMs which have anti-estrogen properties, such as Tamoxifen, can cause joint pain.

If hormone replacement does help prevent joint damage, this is a huge deal. Disability from arthritis is a major health problem and severely affects quality of life. It greatly limits one's mobility and ability to enjoy those long-awaited activities of retirement. In addition, the cost of caring for patients with arthritis is monumental. We are spending not millions but billions of dollars annually on arthritis treatment – medications, bracing, physical therapy; not to mention joint replacement surgery and rehabilitation. Any form of preventative therapy (such as HRT) would yield huge personal and global health benefits. It is disappointing that we do not have more research in this area.

Estrogen and back pain

Back pain is one of the most frequent reasons patients consult a doctor. Most of the time, especially with aging, this is due to cartilage damage. Each vertebra has little arms or protrusions called facets which are coated with cartilage and these can become inflamed. This causes pain and stiffness aggravated by bending and twisting. This type of back pain is usually brought on by activities that stress the back, like too much gardening or housecleaning.

In addition, pain can be caused by a problem with our spinal discs – the thick pads of cartilage between each of our 23 vertebrae. Over time, these discs can dry out and flatten so that the distance between each vertebra gets smaller. I recall looking at many an x-ray and CAT scan where two vertebrae were stacked so closely together there was almost no space between them – indicating there was hardly anything left of the disc. When this occurs between multiple vertebrae, height loss occurs. The average woman can lose two to four inches from this phenomenon over her lifetime! We tend to accept this as just another part of aging, as men also suffer this type of height loss. However, it has been shown that when women go through menopause, they lose disc height faster than men of comparable ages.[14]

Besides losing height, this deterioration of the discs makes them prone to rupturing and herniating. When this occurs, the pushed-out disc puts pressure on the nerves in the spinal cord causing nerve damage such as sciatica. Furthermore, as the discs deteriorate, they are unable to provide cushioning for the vertebrae on either side of them – making them more susceptible to fractures. Many health care providers don't realize this "double whammy" that untreated menopausal women face – weakened bones plus weakened discs sets them up for spinal compression fractures.

Is HRT helpful to maintain disc health? Since discs contain abundant estrogen receptors, it would be expected that estrogen treatment would promote healthy collagen deposition within the discs.[15] There is strong evidence supporting this. Radiologic studies have shown that women taking estrogen have thicker discs than women not on HRT.[16] In addition research has shown that estrogen increases water retention within the discs, which would keep them more hydrated and less prone to deterioration and rupturing.[17]

It is unfortunate that these impressive benefits of estrogen on our discs are not better appreciated – particularly regarding their effect on the vertebrae. If women at risk for osteoporosis were treated with estrogen, they would be receiving this additional fracture prevention benefit – something not afforded by other bone-building drugs, like Fosamax. And even though estrogen is approved for osteoporosis prevention, almost every guideline you read reminds us that HRT is *not considered first-line treatment for this condition.*

Estrogen and other types of arthritis

I have thus far discussed degenerative arthritis, but there are other forms of arthritis. The other major type is called *inflammatory arthritis.* This type of arthritis occurs when the body's immune system turns on itself and starts attacking the cartilage in the joints. The main type of arthritis in this category is rheumatoid arthritis (RA). Other diseases of this nature include lupus, psoriatic arthritis, Sjogren's syndrome, and polymyalgia rheumatica. How hormones affect these conditions is a complicated topic. Since women tend to have higher rates of lupus and rheumatoid arthritis, it was thought that estrogen may play a role in the development of these diseases. This led to recommendations that these patients avoid oral contraceptives (which are much more potent than hormones used for HRT). However, studies don't consistently find that hormone treatment aggravates either lupus or RA or increases the risks of acquiring them.[18] In fact, studies show that going through menopause earlier than expected increases the risk of rheumatoid arthritis.[19] Furthermore, some studies have shown that the estrogen-suppressing drugs used to treat breast cancer patients may actually increase a woman's risk of developing one of these inflammatory forms of arthritis.[20]

Gout also causes arthritis. Gout occurs when the uric acid level in the blood gets too high and then seeps into the joints and forms crystal deposits. (Just imagine what tiny bits of glass in the joint fluid would feel like!) Men are more prone to gout than women, but after menopause a woman's risk of this rises substantially. Women on HRT have been found to have lower uric acid levels and thus less of a chance of having a gout attack. It appears that hormone treatment, particularly progestogen administration, facilitates the elimination of uric acid.[21,22]

What about our muscles?

This brings us to muscles. At a recent conference presented by the North American Menopause Society, Dr. Neil Binkley from the University of Wisconsin School of Medicine presented a lecture on the topic of *sarcopenia*. I learned of this term only recently and it is one you may be hearing more about in the future. Basically, it means *muscle wasting*.

His talk was about what happens to muscles with aging and specifically what happens to postmenopausal women's muscles. We lose muscle mass as we age and this equates to a loss of strength. Decreased strength leads to a host of negative consequences. Besides not being able to hike and bike and keep up with the grandkids, there is a greater chance of falling and, worse, not being able to get up after it happens. I don't need to add that a fall frequently carries the risk of a fracture which often leads to terrible downstream consequences.

Muscles are loaded with estrogen receptors. This implies that estrogen plays an important role in our muscle cells.[23] After menopause, a woman's strength and performance on muscle tests declines at a faster rate than in a man of comparable age.[24,25] It is not clear exactly how the loss of our female hormones leads to diminished muscle function but appears to be partly due to a decrease in mitochondrial activity, which is the energy-producing mechanism in our cells.[26,27] Maintaining an adequate supply of estrogen should help preserve our muscle integrity and prevent the development of sarcopenia. Studies have shown that postmenopausal women on HRT perform better on strength testing and other muscle performance tests than women not on HRT.[28,29] Adding a regular exercise and strength training program on top of hormone treatment improves the results even more.[30]

Does the timing of initiation of hormones make a difference in preventing sarcopenia? After a finite period of estrogen deprivation, it appears that

259

muscles, like some of the other tissues in our bodies, lose their receptors.[31] This suggests there may be a critical window for women to initiate hormone treatment in order to preserve muscle strength. This would be analogous to what happens to our bones when we lose our estrogen – a rapid and dramatic decline can occur within ten years after menopause that may be difficult to recover from.

Is estrogen good for our eyes, ears, mouth . . . and anything else?

Research has shown that when women go through menopause there can be a substantial decrease in blood flow to the retina. This is the lining inside the eyeball comprised of specialized cells that relay the images that we see to the vision parts of our brain. In one study, estrogen was demonstrated to improve retinal blood flow.[32] The authors speculated that this potentially could decrease the risk of *macular degeneration* in postmenopausal women – which is the most common irreversible condition of vision loss in this age group. Giving further credence to this research, a study by the National Eye Institute showed a decreased risk of wet macular degeneration in women treated with hormone therapy.[33] Wet macular degeneration is the most severe form of this disorder. It is difficult to treat and frequently results in blindness.

There are also studies that suggest that postmenopausal hormone use may decrease cataracts and the risk of glaucoma.[34,35,36] These eye diseases are major sources of disability as we age, and anything that may help prevent them is much needed. I am hopeful that more research on HRT will be done in this area.

The decline in hormone levels after menopause is known to trigger hearing loss.[37] It is believed that estrogen plays an important role in the production of certain proteins that are needed to maintain the integrity of the tiny hairs in the inner ear that convert sound waves into nerve impulses. Studies in rats have demonstrated that removing their ovaries results in hearing loss and that administration of estrogen can restore this.[38]

Taking hormones may also be good for our oral health. There are some interesting studies dealing with HRT and our teeth and gums. Women taking HRT have been shown to have less periodontal disease than women not taking hormones.[39] This benefit could be partially explained by anti-inflammatory effects that have been associated with estrogen use.

Better oral health helps prevent tooth disease, which would decrease extractions. Several studies have shown that women on HRT have a greater chance of retaining their teeth longer than women not taking HRT.[40] This was demonstrated in the Leisure World study – the study where thousands of women living in a retirement community were followed for over twenty years. Estrogen users required dentures less frequently and the longer women took HRT, the less they needed them.[41] Similarly, in the Nurses Study, there was a lesser degree of tooth loss in estrogen-treated women.[42] In some respects, this makes sense, since the beneficial effects of estrogen on our bones should translate into healthier bone around the tooth sockets.[43]

In conclusion

Whenever I open a new edition of *Menopause* or *Climacteric*, the two scholarly journals that report on menopause issues, I'm amazed at the burgeoning amount of research attesting to the negative consequences of estrogen loss and the positive effects of estrogen replacement. While I have enough training to know that large clinical studies are needed to solidify research findings and translate them into patient management guidelines, after reading so many of these articles, it seems it would not be a leap of faith to accept that estrogen replacement is more our friend than our enemy just about everywhere in our bodies.

Decision Making Helper

Key Considerations

Collagen provides the structure and support for our skin, joints, discs, bones, blood vessels, and almost all other organs. Collagen fibers weaken with aging and estrogen has been shown to promote collagen health.

Studies have shown that estrogen improves skin thickness, skin hydration, and wound healing.

Estrogen receptors are present in joints. Women taking HRT have less joint pain. It has not conclusively been shown that HRT prevents osteoarthritis, but many studies indicate women on HRT develop less arthritic changes particularly in the hands, hips, and knees, and may require fewer joint replacement surgeries. At a minimum, HRT does not appear to negatively affect joints.

HRT appears to help prevent disc disease and arthritis of the back and this effect of estrogen on the discs may contribute to HRT's known ability to decrease the risk of vertebral fractures.

Hormone therapy, particularly progestogen therapy, appears to decrease the risk of gout in women after menopause.

Women lose muscle mass and strength as they age and this deterioration occurs at an accelerated rate after menopause. Estrogen therapy has been shown to help prevent this decline, especially when combined with exercise.

HRT may help prevent some of the common eye conditions that occur with aging such as macular degeneration, cataracts, and glaucoma.

There is evidence that HRT helps prevent tooth loss and periodontal/gum disease.

Current guidelines concerning HRT and skin, joints, muscles, eyes, ears and mouth

HRT is not approved for preventative treatment for skin aging, skin disease, arthritis, disc disease, muscle deterioration, eye problems, hearing loss, or dental health.

What the guidelines don't acknowledge

Estrogen therapy has a beneficial effect on the skin, decreases joint pain, and possibly may decrease the risk of arthritis. It may help prevent disc deterioration. In this way, it may further contribute to a decreased risk of back pain and spinal fractures. Estrogen has been shown to have beneficial effects in preventing muscle weakness, eye disease, hearing loss, and tooth loss.

Chapter 18
Estrogen and Your GI Tract

When doctors discuss the risks and benefits of HRT with patients, one of the body systems not getting much attention is the gastrointestinal (GI) system. This consists of the esophagus, stomach, intestines, colon, and the ancillary organs important in digestion – the liver, gallbladder, and pancreas. Hormone replacement therapy has many beneficial effects on these organs. This may come as a surprise to you because many women think just the opposite – that estrogen causes negative GI effects. I think much of this stems from the assumption that morning sickness is caused by high hormone levels. However, the truth of the matter is that we really don't know what causes those terrible first trimester GI symptoms and, in fact, nausea is an uncommon side effect of hormone therapy. In this chapter, I describe what we know about HRT and this often-neglected system.

Estrogen and colon cancer

Colorectal cancer is the third leading cause of all cancer deaths. It is the fourth most common type of cancer in women. However, men have a higher incidence of colon cancer than women.[1] So it makes one wonder if there is something about our female hormones that may be protective. Some interesting studies in mice support this.[2] There are certain strains of mice that have a mutation that makes them prone to grow colon cancers. If the ovaries from these mice are removed, they develop cancer at a more rapid rate. However, if they are treated with estradiol, the rate of occurrence of cancer goes down – indicating that estrogen plays a role in preventing these tumors.

A number of studies in humans have supported this protective benefit. The Nurses Study reported that women who used hormones post menopause had a decreased risk of colorectal cancer.[3] Recall that this was the observational study that followed over 40,000 nurses from 1980 to 1994. A 1999 meta-analysis of a number of other studies came to the same conclusion – that women on HRT had lower rates of colon cancer than women not taking hormones.[4]

Even in the WHI, women in the branch of the study who were taking combined estrogen and progestogen developed fewer colon cancers than women on a placebo. It astounds me that the media focused on the fact that HRT increased breast cancer in this branch of the study, yet no one touted that HRT prevented colon cancer. While there were eight more cases of breast cancer per 10,000 women per year, there were six fewer cases of colon cancer per 10,000 per year!

Interestingly, this same benefit did not show up for the women in the second branch of the WHI, who were taking only estrogen. While this seems puzzling, the answer may be due to a couple of issues. There was an exceptionally high number of colon cancers in the older women between the ages of 70 and 79 who were on estrogen only.[5] This aberration may have skewed the results. In addition, it is possible that the progestogen may have played a role in preventing colon cancer.[6] Other evidence supports this possibility. Investigators have taken human colon cancer cells and grown them in a culture. They found that subjecting these cancer cells to medroxyprogesterone (Provera) slowed their growth.[7] Natural progesterone did not have this effect, but it should be noted that it is much less potent than medroxyprogesterone.

Other studies following the WHI have continued to show that HRT appeared to prevent colon cancer. A huge observational study published in 2016 reported on the health conditions of over a million Danish women between the ages of 50 and 79.[8] Some of the interesting findings from this study were that there was a decreased risk of colon cancer in both estrogen-only users and estrogen-progestogen users, and that women using transdermal estrogen benefited more than women taking the oral forms. The type of progestogen or whether the women were taking it daily or on a cyclic basis did not make a difference. The investigators also noted the benefit was greater for long-term hormone users and that women using HRT were at a lower risk of being diagnosed with more advanced stages of colon cancers.

Subsequently, a nationwide study of the risks and benefits of hormone use was published in Sweden. In this study hormone users had lower rates of colon cancer as well as decreased rates of liver and esophageal cancers compared to non-hormone users.[9] In 2018, the results of a large study that looked at cancer rates and death from cancer in over 75,000 women were published.[10] The investigators found that women who took HRT had a significant decrease not only in the rate of developing colon cancer, but also a lower risk of dying from it, compared to women who had never been on hormones.

Despite these findings, HRT has not been promoted as a preventative intervention for colon cancer. There are still uncertainties. As noted, women in the estrogen-only study arm in the WHI, the gold standard study on HRT, did not benefit from hormone therapy. An additional concern was these women had more advanced forms of cancer compared to women on a placebo. (However, long-term follow-up studies did not show that they died any sooner from these cancers.)

Estrogen and the liver and the biliary system

The liver plays many roles in the body and is truly an amazing organ. An important function it performs is to process drugs as they pass through it – making chemical modifications to detoxify them or convert them into different forms that have different biological actions. This is the first-pass phenomenon, which affects many drugs, including hormones. The liver also makes a myriad of important proteins, stores vitamins and iron, breaks down red blood cells, helps fight infections, and is involved in regulating blood sugar. It is also the site of cholesterol synthesis and where the lipoprotein particles LDL and HDL are processed. The liver is where bile is made. So it is not surprising that a healthy liver is critical for good health.

Many things can cause liver damage – such as excessive alcohol use, toxic substances (like those mushrooms in your yard you're not supposed to eat!), and viruses (such as hepatitis). Genetic disorders, cancers, and circulation problems can also injure the liver. In addition, a problem that is becoming increasingly common is a condition known as a *fatty liver*. We are seeing more of this because more people are becoming obese. When people gain weight, the extra fat gets deposited everywhere, including in the liver.

A fatty liver is a common incidental finding on an ultrasound study or a CAT scan – and while radiologists who interpret these tests note that there is a *fatty appearance* of the liver in their reports, many doctors don't pay much attention to this. This is partly because we used to think this was a relatively innocuous finding, and in many cases it is. However, in some people, these fatty deposits trigger inflammatory reactions that cause damage to the liver cells. This condition is called *NASH,* or *nonalcoholic steatohepatitis*. As more and more of the liver tissue becomes damaged, the liver starts malfunctioning.

Eventually, the cells die causing the liver to shrink and become scarred – which leads to cirrhosis and liver failure.

Not everyone who gains weight develops a fatty liver because some people tend to be more susceptible than others. The good news is that if people can lose weight, the fat in the liver can dissipate and the condition can resolve as long as permanent damage has not occurred.

A fatty liver can develop at any age but is more common in women after menopause.[11,12] It is difficult to sort out whether estrogen deficiency per se causes this, but it likely plays a major role. It has been shown that younger women who have their ovaries removed prior to natural menopause have an increased risk of developing fatty liver disease.[13]

Whether estrogen treatment will help prevent a fatty liver is unclear as there has been relatively little research in this area, but data is accumulating to suggest it does. Studies in mice have shown that estrogen treatment prevents fat accumulation in the livers of obese mice.[14,15] And, observational studies have suggested that this may be the case in women as well.[16] Furthermore, estrogen treatment has been shown to lower liver enzyme levels in estrogen-deficient young women and diabetic women with fatty livers who have enzyme levels above normal.[17,18] It is speculated that the anti-inflammatory and anti-oxidant properties of estrogen play a significant role in helping damaged liver cells heal.[17]

Occasionally women develop adenomas in the liver. These are benign growths that generally do not cause symptoms or problems, but rarely can transform into cancer. In the 1970s, doctors began noting increased numbers of these developing in women on birth control pills. The incidence of these lesions was about one in 1,000,000 in the general population, but women on birth control pills demonstrated a rate at thirty to forty incidents per 1,000,000 women.[19] It was suspected that hormones played a role in the development of these adenomas. The risk appeared to be greater in women who used higher doses and for longer durations. However, it should be noted that the potency of the birth control pills during those years was two times higher than those used in today's contraceptives and five times more potent than the hormones used in postmenopausal women. Thus, it is unclear whether or not HRT may cause these lesions.

One of the many jobs of the liver is to make bile. This is produced by the liver cells and discharged into a network of ducts that drain the bile into the gallbladder where it is stored until a meal is eaten. The presence of ingested food triggers the gallbladder to contract and squirt bile into the stomach. There, bile acts like a detergent mixing with the food to help break down fatty particles into smaller molecules so they can be absorbed.

Bile consists almost exclusively of cholesterol. Sometimes, when the conditions in the gallbladder are not quite right, some of the cholesterol crystallizes and grows into gallstones. A person can have just one or two gallstones or the gallbladder can be packed with them. They can be tiny nuggets or the size of a jawbreaker. Most people with gallstones never know they have them because they may never cause symptoms. However, if they interfere with the release of bile this leads to intermittent bloating or indigestion, especially after a fatty meal.

If a stone is just the right size (about ¼-inch diameter), it can be squirted out along with some bile and get stuck in the duct that goes from the gallbladder to the stomach. This is what causes a gallbladder attack. The blockage causes pain, nausea, and vomiting that can last for a number of hours until the stone finally passes into the stomach (and then out with the stool). If the stone remains stuck in the duct for longer than that – pressure builds up behind it, which is transmitted to the liver and sometimes the pancreas. This causes inflammation and damage to these organs, which can be very serious and even life-threatening. In these situations, surgery needs to be performed to remove the stone (usually along with gallbladder).

One of the adverse effects of estrogen that you hear about is that it increases gallstone formation. Birth control pills and even pregnancy have long been associated with this risk. Therefore, it is not surprising that in many studies over the years, women on HRT developed more gallstones than women who did not take them. This was noted in the Nurses Study as well as in the WHI.[20,21] In the WHI there were an additional 47 more cases of gallbladder problems per 10,000 women per year in the estrogen-progestogen group and 58 more cases per 10,000 women per year in women on estrogen alone compared to women on a placebo. Subsequent studies continue to show this association. The results of a large study published in 2013 that reviewed the health status of over 45,000 women in France found an increased incidence of cholecystectomy (removal of the gallbladder) in women on HRT.[22]

Most of the studies addressing this issue involved women taking *oral* estrogen. It is now becoming apparent that women taking transdermal estrogen do not have an increased risk of gallbladder issues.[23,24] The reason for this once again seems to be due to the first-pass effect. Oral estrogen causes the bile to be supersaturated with cholesterol – a condition that promotes the gallstones to form.[25]

The role of progestogens in gallbladder disease is unclear. It is known that progestogens appear to slow gallbladder emptying.[26] This would tend to further promote the formation of gallstones.

Decision Making Helper

Key Considerations

There is abundant data that suggests HRT decreases the risk of colon cancer. It is unclear whether estrogen or progestogen, or both, contribute to a decrease in risk. However, natural progesterone may not have an impact on the risk of colon cancer.

After menopause the risk of developing a fatty liver increases. Estrogen therapy helps protect against a fatty liver in animal studies and probably prevents this in women, but there is a lack of definitive studies in this area.

Oral estrogen, and probably most progestogens, increase the risk of developing gallstones. Transdermal estrogen appears to pose less of a risk.

Current guidelines regarding HRT and the GI tract

HRT is not recommended for prevention of any gastrointestinal cancers or to help protect against liver disease. Package inserts for estrogens advise that estrogen therapy may increase the risk of developing gallstones.

What the guidelines don't acknowledge

HRT may decrease the risk of colon cancer as well as the risk of developing a fatty liver. The risk of developing gallstones may only occur with oral estrogen.

Chapter 19
Estrogen and Your Life Expectancy

I think most of us try not to dwell on our life expectancies – but people diagnosed with a terminal illness wake up every morning thinking about how long they have to live. Like these patients' friends and families, we physicians frequently feel awkward discussing this delicate subject with them, in part, because we think about how it must feel to have this reality resting so heavily in the forefront of their minds.

Our reluctance to think about life expectancies carries into other realms of our lives – like putting off making that appointment with an attorney to create a will, or not wanting to buy a burial site. It also comes into play when patients don't seem to be motivated to change a behavior that is known to improve their life expectancies – such as quitting smoking or taking their blood pressure medications diligently – even though studies show that these measures prevent deaths from heart disease. We know that screening for various cancers, like colon cancer, can reduce the risk of an early death, yet patients often avoid these exams.

The purpose of including a chapter on estrogen and longevity is to explore the question of whether or not taking hormone replacement therapy has a bearing on life expectancy. I will bet when most doctors have a discussion with a menopausal patient about the risks and benefits of HRT there is no mention whether taking hormones will have any effect on how long she may live. I would also bet most women assume taking estrogen probably *decreases* their life expectancies. And why wouldn't they think that? Ever since the WHI study came out, women have been advised they should only take the lowest dose of hormones for the shortest period of time – and only if nothing else works to control their hot flashes. They have been warned that estrogen increases the risks of breast cancer, heart disease, blood clots, and strokes. So it is not surprising that most women probably assume that taking HRT equates to dying prematurely from one of these afflictions.

But the truth of the matter is that this is not the case. For women just entering menopause (and likely for women later in life) taking HRT actually *increases* life expectancy! I know this sounds unbelievable and I suspect that many health care providers are not aware of the data and studies that support this. So, let's review what has been discovered.

Sex hormones and life expectancy

Life expectancy is a pretty straightforward term – it is an estimate of how long we are expected to live. Women have longer life expectancies than men. Why is this? There are all sorts of theories and possible explanations – such as whether men simply "work themselves to an earlier grave" or more frequently engage in unhealthy behaviors, such as smoking. But more and more evidence is pointing to the basic difference in our genetic makeup – primarily that women have two X chromosomes and men have only one. A major consequence of this is that the main sex hormone produced in women is estrogen, whereas in men it is testosterone. There is quite a bit of evidence to support the theory that sex hormones play a major role in longevity. In situations where men lose their testosterone at a young age, such as with castration, they have longer life expectancies.[1] Women who lose their estrogen prematurely, such as having their ovaries removed, have shorter life expectancies.[2]

Does this imply that male hormones somehow have detrimental health effects, whereas estrogen is protective? We don't know the answers to these questions definitively, but there is considerable data that indicates that the longer a woman has female hormones circulating in her body, the longer her life expectancy. Women who go through menopause later in life tend to live longer and have a greater chance of making it to age 90 than those who are exposed to estrogen for shorter periods of time.[3] Conversely, the younger a woman is when she goes through menopause, the shorter her life expectancy.[4]

Why estrogen and testosterone would have opposite effects on mortality is up for speculation. It likely has a lot to do with how these hormones affect our cardiovascular system. Male hormones tend to create more visceral fat, whereas estrogen tends to inhibit this type of fat. This central fat predisposes individuals to traits that are bad for the heart, such as high cholesterol and triglycerides, insulin resistance (which leads to diabetes), and inflammation (which is bad for the arteries). These adverse cardiac risk factors can appear early in life and promote plaque, steering a man into the fast lane for an earlier death; whereas the lack of these attributes sets up a woman for a longer healthier life – starting way before menopause. These differences in how sex hormones behave accounts for why men get heart disease much earlier than women, by at least ten years on average

HRT effects on life expectancy and mortality

Mortality is a term synonymous with death. If a certain behavior, such as heroin use, increases one's risk of dying, we say that heroin addiction increases mortality. In this situation, calculating mortality risk is relatively straightforward because death is primarily due to a single event – a drug overdose. However, in other areas, assessing mortality risks can be challenging, because it is hard to control the many factors that may contribute to death. For example, when researchers attempt to measure the mortality risk caused by being obese, there are many other factors that may contribute to one's death other than just being severely overweight – such as diabetes, high blood pressure, lack of exercise, sleep apnea, use of weight-loss drugs, etc.

When we try to determine if taking HRT affects mortality, the same difficulty arises because obtaining information that eliminates confounding factors is difficult. But, thanks to a number of studies, it appears fairly certain that hormone use can prolong life expectancy.

Several studies appearing between 1980 and 1995 noted a positive association between hormone therapy and life expectancy.[5,6] This was primarily due to lower cardiovascular deaths in women taking HRT. In addition, the results of the Nurses Study were published during this period. Recall that this was the large observational study that followed over 40,000 nurses from the time of menopause through two decades of postmenopause. The investigators reported that women taking HRT had lower mortality rates from not only heart disease but other causes.[7,8]

Further support for the benefits of HRT on longevity came from the Leisure World project – the study that began in 1981 where investigators followed over 8,000 retired women in a retirement community. After 22 years of follow-up, mortality data was published.[9] Women who had taken HRT lived longer than women who had not used hormones, and the longer the duration of use the longer their life expectancies.

The first large-scale, randomized trial regarding HRT was the WHI study. Because the two branches went on for only five and seven years, respectively, we can't really expect this study to give us meaningful data on mortality. But the encouraging news was that, like several other short-term studies during that period of time, women taking hormones did not die any sooner than women on a placebo.[10,11] In other words, their mortality rates were similar.

However, of more interest is that after the WHI study ended in 2002 and women no longer were treated with HRT, the WHI researchers continued to follow many of the women who had been in the study to monitor their health status. A paper was published in 2017 giving an update.[12] It was noted that 27% of the women who had been in the study had died. (Note that the average age of the women enrolling in the WHI was 63, so that would put many of these women well past age 78 in 2017.) In this paper, the authors reported that there was no difference in the death rates from any cause in either the women who had taken HRT during the study or the women who were on a placebo. An editorialist in the *Journal of the American Medical Association*, where this article was published, called the findings *"compelling and reassuring,"* concluding that *"for women with troubling vasomotor symptoms, premature menopause, or early-onset osteoporosis, hormone therapy appears to be both safe and efficacious."*[13]

Data such as this indicates that taking HRT, at least for up to five years, doesn't appear to have a negative impact on a woman's longevity. But, do hormones prolong life expectancy as suggested by the earlier studies? The answer may come down to the time when HRT is initiated. Recall that the women in the WHI study were considerably older than the age when women typically begin taking hormones. Are we dealing once again with the Timing Hypothesis? Does the age when HRT is initiated affect longevity? To address this, we need to consider more information.

Between 2004 and 2009 several studies were published that included over 26,000 women treated with HRT. The authors once again concluded that women on HRT were not at a higher risk of dying prematurely by taking hormones. And, of more significance, younger women starting hormone treatment around age 50 had lower mortality rates than women initiating HRT at older ages.[14,15,16] Other studies have supported the timing factor as an important issue. A randomized trial published in 2012 demonstrated that women who started HRT shortly after menopause had lower risks of death due to cardiovascular events than women on a placebo.[17] In addition, when you drill down into the data from the WHI update described above, women who started HRT between the ages of 50 to 59 lived longer than their counterparts who did not take hormones.

In 2015, an extensive review of many published studies analyzed the effects of hormone therapy and mortality.[18] Their findings concluded that *"women who started hormone therapy within ten years of menopause had 30% lower mortality rates."* In the same year, a huge observational study of almost 500,000 women in Finland, analyzing hormone use and outcomes over many years, was published.[19] The researchers found that women who had initiated HRT early had substantially longer life expectancies than women not taking it.

The important takeaway from this information is that taking hormone replacement therapy will not shorten a woman's lifespan and, if initiated at the time of menopause, will likely prolong it. Women should be aware of this information when they are making decisions about whether or not to take HRT.

What is it about estrogen therapy that may increase longevity?

The keys to longevity are multidimensional, including factors related to lifestyle, environment, caloric intake, health status, genetics, and – pertinent to this discussion – hormones. The role that hormones play in anti-aging is being extensively studied as well as being exploited by the thousands of longevity clinics that exist throughout the world. Sex hormones, including estrogen therapy for women, are universally prescribed in these clinics – whose providers claim that replacing those hormones that decline over time will keep their clients' bodies and minds working better and longer.

There is no question that estrogen plays a powerful role in preventing heart disease, which has historically been, and continues to be, the number one cause of death in women. So, most of the studies demonstrating HRT's benefit on longevity undoubtedly reflect estrogen's effects in preventing or delaying death from heart attacks and strokes. As described in Chapter 12, estrogen retards the root cause of these maladies – the formation of plaque.

However, estrogen has effects on other organs that contribute to longevity. In summary:

- Estrogen has anti-oxidant and anti-inflammatory effects that prevent cellular damage and promote cellular repair. In the brain, these properties help mitigate the damage caused by the accumulation of toxic debris that leads to Alzheimer's dementia – a disease that has been shown to shorten life expectancy.[20]

273

- Estrogen prevents cell loss in our bones and muscles. Loss of function in these systems leads to weakness, falls, fractures, and frailty – conditions that lead to premature death.

- Estrogen favorably affects fat distribution and fat cell metabolism in ways that decrease the risk of diabetes – a condition that leads to many health complications that can shorten one's lifespan.

All of these attributes of estrogen have the effect of decreasing the risk of the major chronic diseases that affect longevity.

What about estrogen and cancer?

Cancer accounts for one-third of all deaths. Evading cancer clearly is one path to a longer life. So a major question to address in this discussion is the effect of estrogen on cancer. Many women fear that taking HRT will not only increase their risk of breast cancer but increase their risk of dying from it. While it may be that taking estrogen, with or without a progestogen, increases a women's risk of being diagnosed with breast cancer, what has become clear is that women who develop breast cancer have lower risks of dying from it if they have taken hormones![21,22] A large review published in 2017 encompassing over one and a half million women has substantiated this.[23] It is unclear why taking hormones would have this seemingly paradoxical effect, but it probably has something to do with how estrogen affects the immune system or the way hormones modify cancer cells.

Another cancer that has been associated with HRT is uterine cancer. The FDA-mandated literature that accompanies prescriptions for estrogen contains this warning. However, as discussed previously, this risk is essentially negated if women take adequate doses of a progestogen along with estrogen. Combination treatment may even decrease the risk of developing uterine cancer.

To finish the discussion whether HRT impacts cancer mortality, women should be aware of the studies that indicate hormone use may actually decrease the risks of other forms of cancer. As presented in Chapter 18, women on HRT may be at lower risk of colon cancer as well as other cancers of the GI tract. The take-home point here is that, overall, HRT may actually decrease cancer mortality deaths.

Are there consequences of estrogen avoidance?

Another issue to discuss is whether *not* taking HRT has any consequences that may affect longevity. Following the WHI, HRT use dropped dramatically and continues to be used only by a minority of postmenopausal women.[24] Overall it is estimated that less than 10% of postmenopausal women in the U.S. take HRT compared to up to 40% prior to the WHI.[25,26] Older women, in particular, have gone off HRT.[27] There continues to be an ongoing decline in the number of women initiating hormone treatment as they enter menopause, even women who are having hot flashes.[28] Pharmacy claims for estrogen prescriptions in women 50 years or older have shown a downward trend. In 2015 there were 42 prescriptions per 1,000 women dispensed compared to 83 per 1,000 in 2007.[29]

The growing number of women *not* being treated with hormones raises concern that the current guidelines, which essentially discourage HRT, are actually harming postmenopausal women. Articles have appeared that suggest that women may be dying sooner than expected because of this. In one paper it was estimated that "estrogen avoidance" in women aged 50 to 59 years from 2003 to 2009 resulted in as many as 91,610 excess deaths in women who stopped HRT or never started HRT.[30]

There obviously is much controversy about this sort of analysis. Other articles have appeared claiming just the opposite – that the decline in hormone use attributable to the WHI has improved a woman's longevity because there has been a downward trend in breast cancer and heart disease mortality since the study was published. However, these claims have been dismissed with counter-arguments noting that survival rates for these conditions started way before the WHI and can be attributed to other factors[31] – such as improved cancer screening programs, more aggressive treatment of high blood pressure, cholesterol, and diabetes, and more effective drugs and devices to prevent fatal heart rhythm disorders.

However, despite an overall decrease in the rate of heart-related deaths, women are not faring as well as men.[31] In Europe, for instance, in 2014 the proportion of deaths attributable to cardiovascular disease in women was 51%, whereas in men it was 42%.[32] This makes me wonder if estrogen avoidance is playing a role in why women have been lagging behind men in the downward trend in cardiovascular disease deaths. Is it possible that many women, discouraged from taking HRT following the publication of the WHI study, have been quietly building up plaque on their arteries and are now reaching the age where heart disease is showing up? It's alarming to think that we may be on the verge of a major uptick in the number of heart attacks in women who were not encouraged to take HRT when they went through menopause.

An additional issue to reflect on is that more and more aging adults are being diagnosed with diabetes. Although much of this is attributed to the fact that we are seeing more people becoming obese, is it possible that estrogen avoidance is contributing to this epidemic? Many studies, including the WHI, have shown that women who don't take HRT have an increased risk of diabetes. Diabetics face higher rates of mortality not only from heart disease, but from kidney failure and other complications.

Another major area where estrogen avoidance may rear its ugly head is osteoporosis. One of the many benefits of taking HRT is that it very effectively halts the rapid bone loss that occurs when women go through menopause. I suspect that the thousands of women who abandoned their hormones after the WHI were not cognizant of the fact that their actions unleashed the bone-dissolving osteoclasts that had been kept in check by the presence of estrogen. Even women with known osteopenia were not automatically placed on other osteoporosis-preventing drugs, and, if alternate drugs were prescribed, there was a high rate of discontinuation.[33-36] In addition, following the WHI, millions of women have not initiated hormones. As a result, we have an entire generation of women who have been silently losing bone mass and may be on the verge of osteoporosis.

The end result of this would lead us to predict that we would be seeing a rise in hip fractures since the WHI study came out. And indeed, this has occurred.[37,38] Does this impact mortality? It clearly does, particularly in the elderly. A number of studies have shown that a hip fracture portends a shortened life span.[39,40,41] A study from Denmark analyzed data on 170,000 women whose medical records indicated they had had a fracture and found that their mortality rate was twice as high as women who had not suffered one.[42] Other studies have shown that one in four women suffering a hip fracture die within the next year.[43] Those who survive frequently experience a dramatic worsening of their quality of life – including a decrease in mobility and impairment in self-care activities. For many, this is the life event that moves them from independent living into a nursing home. This change in lifestyle can impact one's will to live.

In the future, more information will come forth about the downstream negative consequences of our current reluctance to prescribe hormones. While

I was writing this book, an article appearing in the Center for Disease Control's newsletter, the *Morbidity and Mortality Weekly Report* (MMWR), caught my eye reporting an increase in the incidence of uterine cancer.[44] The authors relate that the reason for this is unclear, but possibly could be due to the rising rates of obesity. Excess fat promotes higher estrogen levels and we know that women with higher estrogen levels have an increased risk of uterine cancer. You probably wonder where I'm going with this – but I suspect that most of these women are not taking HRT. If they were, they would also be on a progestogen. By doing so, this would neutralize their cancer risk not only by negating any adverse effects on the uterus caused by taking estrogen therapy but also from any excess natural estrogen produced by their fat cells. Although this is pure speculation on my part, I am concerned that as time goes on, we may learn of other adverse trends in women's health related to estrogen avoidance.

How long should/can women continue hormone therapy?

It seems appropriate to address this important question in this chapter on longevity because, while data indicates that taking HRT appears to increase a woman's life expectancy, we don't know if the duration of hormone use makes a difference. Is this a situation where "more is better"? This is very difficult to say. Certainly, the prevailing opinion since the WHI study was published has been that "less is better". Many health care providers strictly follow guidelines generated from the outcomes of the WHI and advise women to take hormone replacement therapy *only for the shortest period of time to control symptoms*. This cautionary use of hormones has been further reinforced by the 2017 report from the USPSTF (the preventative services task force described in Chapter 8), which states that *HRT should not be used for preventative therapy*. In many patients' and providers' minds this has been interpreted to mean *don't use hormones at all*.

The impression that HRT should be limited to short-term use because of risks is widespread, particularly among providers who graduated from medical school after the WHI was published in 2002. Recently I visited my old friend Kim, a retired psychologist and former patient. She moved from the city to rural Eastern Washington and was thoroughly enjoying the rustic life. We hadn't seen each other for over a year, and the first thing she said to me was, "Dr. Sandy, you were so right!" She was referring to the conversation we had just before she moved. I had warned her that in light of the aftermath of the WHI she may have trouble finding a physician to renew her estrogen prescription. She went on to relay, "On my first visit with this young doctor,

he held up my estrogen bottle and asked, 'Why are you still taking these?' "
Kim said he delivered his question with a definite reprimanding tone.
Fortunately, Kim and I had had extensive discussions not only about the
benefits and risks of taking HRT but about the benefits and risks of continuing
vs. discontinuing therapy. She had had a hysterectomy at an early age and
started HRT when she went through menopause.

Kim was thin, trim, and had no history of blood clots, hypertension,
diabetes, or other heart risk factors. There was no breast cancer in her family,
but her mother had had colon cancer. Her bone density was that of a 35-year-
old. In addition, Kim had just married the love of her life and was enjoying
frequent sexual relations in their bucolic new home. Despite all of this, her
new doctor still insisted that she stop her hormones. She acquiesced, but
within weeks she started having hot flashes, vaginal dryness, pain with
intercourse, sleep disturbance, and felt sluggish and even a little blue. At 64
years old she had been feeling great until this medication change.

The message being delivered to women today is very different than the one
prior to the WHI, when it was not uncommon for women to continue hormone
treatment indefinitely as long as there were no contraindications or adverse
events. In my practice, I followed hundreds of women on HRT well into their
70s, 80s, and even 90s. Today, women are being advised to stop hormones
once their hot flashes abate. Thousands of women have systematically been
taken off their hormones, regardless of whether they were like my friend Kim
who was not having any negative effects and believed estrogen substantially
improved her quality of life.

This raises some pertinent questions. Does a decision to continue
hormones beyond the age of 60, 65, or longer put women in jeopardy? Does
the length of time a woman takes hormones after menopause have any bearing
on future health events or life expectancy?

A number of studies have given us some insight into these issues. The
cardiovascular protection afforded by HRT continues even with long-term
treatment. A study published prior to the WHI enrolled 9,000 women who
were age 65 or older and followed them for the ensuing six years. The authors
found that women who had been taking hormones at the time of the study had
lower rates of death, primarily due to less cardiovascular disease.[45] Similarly,
in the Leisure World study, where hormone use reduced the risk of fatal and
nonfatal heart attacks, strokes, and other complications of heart disease by
20% to 40%, the reduction was greatest in long-term and/or current users.[46]

This same study also concluded that women who had used HRT for the longest duration of use had the lowest risks of Alzheimer's disease.

Another area where long-term therapy provides benefit is for bone health. Initiating estrogen therapy at the time of menopause not only prevents the rapid bone loss that occurs within the first few years after menopause, but ongoing treatment effectively preserves bone density as long as it is being taken, even well into older age.

On the flip side of the coin, are there downsides to long-term treatment? In considering whether or not to take HRT for longer durations, women should examine this side of the equation. As discussed previously, while it is unclear if estrogen "causes" breast cancer, or primarily "promotes" its growth once it develops, the longer a woman is on HRT, the more likely it is that she may be diagnosed with breast cancer. However, as discussed in Chapter 10, if a woman who has been on HRT develops breast cancer, her prognosis is actually better than if she had not taken hormones.

The other known risk of taking hormones is an increased chance of developing a blood clot. Theoretically, as long as a woman is on hormones, she is at risk for one of these as well as the more serious complication of a clot, which is a pulmonary embolism. However, it has been noted that most of these blood clots occur within the first six months of hormone treatment, so it is probable that women who escape this complication early may be at minimal risk down the line, even with long-term use. Furthermore, we are learning that transdermal estradiol therapy may not increase the risk of blood clots.

The bottom line is there is not a clear-cut reason to advise women to arbitrarily stop HRT. We don't have a major clinical study to guide us. The recommendation to take hormones for only the shortest period of time comes from the concerns generated by the WHI study. However, as you know from earlier chapters of this book, the WHI was a short-term study and its conclusions should only apply to older women who initiated hormones well past menopause. There is plenty of data that indicates that starting hormone treatment at the time of menopause and continuing it for long durations can be beneficial. More and more menopause experts concur with this belief – so much so that there has been a trend toward more liberal recommendations for prescribing HRT. The North American Menopause Society states in its 2017 position statement:

"Hormone therapy does not need to be routinely discontinued in women aged older than 60 or 65 years and can be considered for continuation beyond age 65 years for persistent vasomotor symptoms, quality of life issues, or prevention of osteoporosis after appropriate evaluation and counseling of benefits and risks." [50]

The International Menopause Society likewise recommends that *there are no reasons to place mandatory limitations on the duration of HRT.*[51]

The key message that both of these organizations are trying to disseminate is that women need to be educated and informed about the benefits and risks of HRT and how these apply to their personal health situations and treatment goals. I believe there needs to be more emphasis on the benefits and not just on the risks. We have plenty of evidence to attest to the fact that long-term treatment with HRT can offer substantial benefits and that the actual risks are fairly minimal.

What happens after discontinuing HRT?

Women who are arbitrarily advised to stop HRT should be aware of what to expect. For many women, hot flashes may resume, particularly the closer a woman is to menopause. These may last a few months or even years. And, while they may or may not be bothersome, recall that hot flashes appear to correlate with an elevated risk of heart disease.

Within weeks of going off estrogen, almost all women will gradually notice changes in the vaginal area. The tissue will become thinner and more fragile. These changes will get progressively worse over time and may lead to discomfort with intercourse and an increased risk of vaginal and bladder infections.

While the effects of estrogen on maintaining bone strength will persist up to several years, without estrogen bone density will start to decline. The risk of fractures will increase and there is likelihood that a non-hormone, osteoporosis-preventing drug will be recommended. However, these drugs carry their own array of side effects and potential risks.

In addition, a relatively new revelation is that women who discontinue HRT may face a rapid increase in heart-related problems.[47] The abrupt decrease in estrogen presumably leads to decreased levels of nitric oxide within the arteries. This would lead to constriction of arterial flow, which would be harmful to the heart. And, the loss of estrogen may trigger an increase in adrenaline activity that could cause dangerous heart rhythm irregularities.[48,49]

It is not clear whether stopping hormones abruptly or tapering them gradually is the best way to go off HRT. In my practice, it has seemed that women are more likely to get a resurgence of their hot flashes if they don't gradually decrease their dose, but studies haven't consistently shown that this is the case. In light of the more recent research that shows that abrupt discontinuation may impact the cardiovascular system, it may be wise to taper them off over several weeks.

Some final thoughts . . .

Whenever I visit one of my patients at a retirement facility and pass by the dining room or peak into an exercise class, one thing is always very obvious. Women outnumber the men, by quite a few. In fact, in most of the facilities I frequent, the arrival of a new male resident is always a hot topic of conversation – as there's always a certain degree of novelty having a man join the ranks.

It has occurred to me that most of the women that I encounter in these retirement homes likely went through menopause well before the WHI and likely had been on HRT for a good part of their postmenopausal years. It makes me wonder what things will look like in the next 10 to 15 years when the generation of post-WHI women enter retirement age. Will the ratio of men to women increase because women who have opted out of taking HRT experience higher mortality? I know this sounds far-fetched, but it is interesting to reflect on. Time will tell.

Decision Making Helper

Key Considerations

There is very strong evidence from multiple large studies that taking HRT prolongs longevity, particularly when initiated at the time of menopause.

An article published in 2017, which reported on the status of the women who had been in the WHI study, concluded that taking HRT for up to five years was not linked to a shortened life expectancy or premature death from any cause compared to women who did not take HRT.

281

HRT appears to decrease mortality through its beneficial effects in preventing many chronic diseases known to limit life span, including heart disease, diabetes, and fractures.

There is considerable evidence that HRT does not increase a woman's risk of dying from cancer, including breast cancer, and that taking HRT may even decrease the risk of dying from cancer.

A number of studies have shown that long-term HRT therapy provides considerable benefits with minimal risks.

Current guidelines regarding HRT and longevity

Current guidelines do not address HRT's effects on longevity and mortality, and HRT is not recommended as a preventative therapy for any chronic conditions that are the principal causes of a shortened life span, such as heart disease, cancer, Alzheimer's disease, or diabetes.

Current guidelines recommend that women take hormones only for the shortest duration needed to control symptoms.

What the guidelines don't acknowledge

Women who take HRT, particularly when initiated at the time of menopause, can expect longer life spans and less risk of developing heart disease, osteoporosis, diabetes, and other chronic health conditions.

The recommendation to stop HRT is not based on definitive clinical studies. The two major medical societies (NAMS and IMS) endorse a more liberal use of HRT for women with hot flashes – recommending adequate doses of HRT for as long as necessary to achieve treatment goals and noting that there are no mandatory limitations on the duration of hormone treatment.

Since current guidelines recommend that HRT be prescribed only for women with hot flashes, women not experiencing them are likely missing opportunities to improve their long-term health and longevity.

Chapter 20
The Estrogen Question – It's Your Decision

It isn't often that I disagree with guidelines that have been developed to help physicians provide the best medical care for their patients. But when it comes to HRT, I do. Knowing the important role that estrogen plays in women's bodies since the moment of conception, it simply doesn't make sense that we should spend a third or more of our lives without it. Yet that is where things have stood since 2002 when the results of the WHI essentially curtailed the routine use of hormone replacement in menopausal and postmenopausal women. Based on this one pivotal landmark study, guidelines were created that have discouraged women from taking HRT. A whole generation of women has been told that taking estrogen and progesterone may be dangerous and that further studies are needed before the medical community can assure women that HRT is advisable.

Should women simply accept this? I don't believe this is wise for a number of reasons. It should be apparent to you that accepting the WHI's conclusions as the final word on how to best manage menopausal patients is problematic. The women in the study were not representative of the typical women going through menopause and the hormones used in the study were not the formulations being recommended today. Yet, the WHI findings have been applied to all menopausal women, regardless of age, and to all hormones regardless of the type. We now know that the risks of HRT depend on the woman's age when hormones are first initiated, and that synthetic progestogens may cause more adverse effects than natural progesterone. But, despite an awareness of these important discrepancies, hormone replacement therapy continues to receive a thumbs down for *all* menopausal women and all hormone preparations. This is a case of the best available science being inappropriately applied.

A new "definitive" study that specifically addresses the outcomes of treating younger women entering menopause with hormones is not likely to occur any time soon, if ever. It would need to be a large, double-blind, randomized study the caliber of the WHI. A study of this nature would take years to complete and cost millions of dollars. It is doubtful that any pharmaceutical company would be interested in funding such a study since the hormones that would be used are all available today in generic forms. And, I am afraid that another study of menopausal women is probably a low priority for government funding given other pressing needs.

Given this, what should women do? Sitting on the sidelines, waiting for a change in the guidelines, is not without consequence. Women who forego HRT may face an increased risk of fractures, heart attacks, diabetes, strokes, and even shorter life spans by not taking estrogen.

Having knowledge is power and the goal of this book is to provide women with the information they need to empower themselves to make decisions that are right for them. In order to do so, I believe they should have a clear understanding of the body systems and diseases where estrogen plays a role. Just being told that *"taking estrogen can prevent osteoporosis"* is not as meaningful as understanding what osteoporosis is and how estrogen suppresses the bone-eating osteoclasts. Similarly, in order for women to assess whether HRT is "good" or "bad" for their hearts, they should understand the role estrogen plays in preventing plaque development. Knowing that estrogen positively affects cholesterol and stimulates the powerful artery-opening chemical nitric oxide should help women better appreciate how estrogen lowers the risk of a heart attack.

Once women realize the important role that estrogen plays in so many organ systems, the next step is for them to decide if it makes sense to replace estrogen when their ovaries quit making it. Can we assume that HRT will continue to provide beneficial effects? I believe so, and that is why I have described the many studies that have compared outcomes between women who took hormones and women who did not. These studies, while not considered as definitive as the WHI study, collectively present a compelling case that taking HRT improves a woman's long-term health.

The WHI-generated guidelines have truly handcuffed those of us in the medical profession for nearly two decades. As physicians, do we strictly follow the guidelines and prescribe estrogen only at *the lowest doses for the shortest period of time?* Or, do we spend time with our patients discussing how taking or not taking hormone replacement will affect their bodies and future health?

It has occurred to me that when a woman consults her doctor for hormone management, the experience is somewhat analogous to going to a financial planner for advice about managing her money. There is no single plan suitable for every person. A good financial advisor should have a discussion with her to learn about her personal financial goals and objectives, how nervous she is about taking financial risk, what sorts of companies she wants to invest in, and a host of other issues. If this financial planner simply tells her that he or she will invest her life savings for her without all this background, she should grab her money and run.

A discussion with your health care provider should be equally thorough. Your personal medical situation, your goals and objectives, and a number of other factors pertinent to your willingness or reluctance to take HRT should be taken into account. Hopefully, as you have been reading this book, you have been assessing how the loss of estrogen impacts you, and whether there may be some issues unique to you that may have a bearing on the advisably of taking HRT. To help you make a final determination about how you feel about HRT, I think that reflecting on the following questions and discussion will aid in your decision-making process and help prepare you for a visit with your health care provider.

How do you view menopause?

We don't understand why women go through menopause. Some women believe they should "let nature take its course," and not take any medication to treat a natural life transition. Some of my patients have expressed this sentiment and have decided not to take HRT. This is certainly a path women can take. This would not have much impact on a woman's health if she did not live much longer than after she has gone through menopause – which was the case until a hundred years ago. However, now that women are living much longer the lack of hormones carries much more significance and we are recognizing that many of the medical problems that occur with aging, such as osteoporosis, are closely linked to the loss of estrogen and that estrogen replacement can lessen their impacts.

Is age an issue when it comes to taking HRT?

There's convincing evidence that initiating HRT at the time of menopause carries more benefits than risks. However, based on the WHI and other studies, it appears that delaying HRT more than ten years beyond menopause may have more risks than benefits in some women. I want to emphasize, however, that I am talking about when women *start* taking hormones. Women who are older than sixty who have been taking hormones since the time of menopause are in a different situation and, as discussed in Chapter 19, under these circumstances continuous long-term hormone therapy can provide many benefits.

What are your health issues that HRT might impact?

Clearly, women with some health conditions may benefit from HRT more than others – such as women who are at high risk for osteoporosis. Estrogen may be particularly beneficial for women who have severe hot flashes, as well as for women at high risk for heart disease and diabetes because estrogen promotes a favorable cholesterol pattern and decreases insulin resistance.

However, there are some medical conditions where estrogen therapy has been shown to be an aggravating factor and this will obviously affect decision making. Women who are being treated for uterine or breast cancer and women who have severe liver disease or active blood clots are not considered candidates for HRT. Therefore, it is important to have regular health check-ups and mammograms to make sure that you do not unknowingly have any of these conditions before making your decision about HRT.

What are your treatment goals and personal preferences?

Is getting rid of those awful hot flashes and night sweats your singular goal? In this case, the current guidelines – taking the lowest dose of hormones for the shortest period of time – would suffice as a treatment plan. Similarly, if your only desire is to alleviate vaginal dryness and reduce sexual discomfort, then treatment with topical low-dose estrogen vaginal creams or suppositories may be the best course for you.

However, after reading this book, you may have other goals. If you are in perimenopause and are having issues with depression, would a trial of HRT appeal to you more than something like Prozac? Does the information presented in Chapter 11 on how early estrogen treatment prevents bone loss strike you as a paramount goal? Do the studies that show that estrogen may prevent a heart attack or diabetes impress you enough that you would consider treatment for those reasons? Currently, the guidelines do not advocate HRT for the prevention of any of these disorders, but if the study findings that I have presented in this book appear convincing to you, then you may be inclined to consider HRT.

The 2017 Position Statement published by the North American Menopause Society stresses that hormone therapy *should be individualized – taking into account a woman's personal health risks and preferences.* I believe this recommendation is tremendously relevant. Once you understand the magnitude of the various risks and benefits as they apply to you – you should make your decision based on what is important to you. If you absolutely fear doing anything that may increase your risk of breast cancer or if the specter of a breast biopsy terrifies you, then you likely should not consider HRT. However, if you've watched osteoporosis cripple your grandmother and can't bear to see that scenario in your future, you may be more enthusiastic about taking early estrogen replacement. In each of my chapters I have described the diseases and conditions that HRT might impact in an effort to provide information to help you sort out your personal health risks and preferences.

What is your risk tolerance?

When you participate in any activity where you are asked to sign a waiver, do you question the absolute risk? In low-risk activities, such as renting a bike while on vacation, probably not. If you decided to sign up for a hot air balloon ride, however, you probably would want to know the risks. If the absolute risk of something going wrong was one in 100, odds are you would say, "No thanks!" But what if the absolute risk was one in 1,000? Would you still hop into the basket? The answer would depend on a number of factors, including your risk tolerance. Is this something that you have dreamt of doing forever and it will be a once-in-a-lifetime opportunity? In that case, you might take the risk – you believe the thrill and memory of the experience are worth the chance of a bad outcome.

Similarly, it is imperative to put the potential risks regarding HRT into perspective. Early in the book, I discussed how the results of medical studies can be presented in ways that can be misleading – making the risks seem much higher than they really are. I discussed how important it is to look at the *absolute risks* of any given treatment – meaning the risk in actual numbers.

Taking estrogen may increase your risk of one or more adverse events. In examining the data from the WHI, which is considered the most definitive study of HRT, the absolute risks for almost any adverse event, such as a heart attack or breast cancer, was on the order of one in 1,000 (and, of note, these events rarely resulted in death). You should think about these absolute numbers and balance them against the benefits of taking estrogen.

How do you feel about alternatives to HRT?

Odds are, if you choose not to take hormones, you may be advised to consider some other medication at some point during menopause or postmenopause. For instance, if you are having troublesome hot flashes, your provider may suggest herbal remedies, an antidepressant drug, or even one of the novel new drugs vying for FDA approval. Later, in postmenopause, there is a good chance that if you don't take HRT you will be faced with a need to consider a drug to prevent osteoporosis, or find yourself in a situation where you are advised to take medications for high cholesterol or diabetes – conditions which might have been prevented by taking hormones. All of these products have their own set of side effects and risks and knowing this type of information should be factored into your decision regarding hormone treatment.

Are you ready to talk to your health care provider?

After reading this book and pondering on the issues above, you should be prepared to have a productive visit with your health care provider. This visit deserves a dedicated block of time and can't be accomplished during a brief appointment. Hopefully, your provider has an open mind and is willing to listen to your concerns. If he or she disagrees with a request for HRT, ask for an explanation. If you do not have a satisfying outcome during such a visit you should consider a second opinion. One source for referrals is the North American Menopause Society's website (www.menopause.org), which lists practitioners well versed in updated menopause treatment.

In conclusion

I can't help but be frustrated that there has been such a negative attitude about HRT when in some respects estrogen almost seems a miracle drug. Why do we think it is preferable to place a woman on Paxil for her hot flashes, Fosamax for her bones, Lipitor for her cholesterol, metformin for her blood sugar, and a SERM for her vaginal dryness rather than consider HRT? Estrogen can address all of these issues! This situation brings to mind a quote from the famed physician considered to be the father of internal medicine, Dr. William Osler:

> *"The young physician starts life with 20 drugs for each disease,*
> *and the old physician ends life with one drug for 20 diseases."*

I guess I'm admitting that I am an old physician, but from my perspective, I have always looked for the simplest and most effective plan of treatment for my patients. I don't quite understand why we keep trying to find other solutions to help menopausal women when we have an obvious natural choice: estrogen.

One of my friends, knowing I was writing this book, handed me her May 2019 Harvard newsletter that had the headline, *Sex Hormones and Your Heart*.[1] I appreciated this as I was interested in seeing what sort of advice academia was relaying to their readership regarding HRT, and I was hoping that attitudes were shifting to embrace hormone therapy more enthusiastically. Unfortunately, this was not the case. The article didn't report on any of the recent studies showing that HRT, taken at the time of menopause, can decrease a woman's risk of heart disease. While the author acknowledged that *"hormone therapy is an option"* for women with hot flashes, only women *"without high cardiovascular risk"* should consider them, and only *"take the lowest possible dose for the shortest period of time"*. Sound familiar?

After reading the article it was apparent to me that the author was not going to promote any advice that strays too far from the WHI-generated guidelines. I see this same reluctance in almost every article I read in publications for women, and even in many medical journals written for nurses and primary care doctors.

Most of the 6,000 women entering menopause each day are either afraid to take hormones or discouraged from taking them. This concerns me because not only are women needlessly suffering from their symptoms but may be putting themselves at risk for several preventable medical conditions. Even though many experts in menopause believe that the benefits of initiating HRT at the time of menopause appear to outweigh the risks, this message is just not getting disseminated. By not encouraging HRT, I feel this is a disservice to our patients.

Just before receiving my diploma from medical school, my fellow graduates and I recited the Hippocratic Oath, or at least a variant of this famous Greek pledge. It basically invokes a commitment to practice in a manner that will *"benefit my patients according to my greatest ability and judgment, and I will do no harm or injustice to them."* [2] We often paraphrase this by using the expression, *"first do no harm"* when treating patients. In my opinion, discouraging hormone replacement at the time of menopause causes more harm than good for most women. I don't have a crystal ball to know if and when we will see this formally acknowledged by the medical community but I believe women need to know as much as they can about the benefits of estrogen. That is why I wrote **The Estrogen Question – Know Before You Say "No" to HRT.**

Glossary

A

Absolute risk – the probability or chance of an event occurring. It is usually determined by taking the number of events that occur (such as the number of breast cancers diagnosed) divided by the total number of people in the group studied.

Acetylcholine – one of the chemical neurotransmitters the brain and other nerve cells use to communicate with each other.

Activella – the brand name for a fixed combination HRT product that contains estradiol and a synthetic progestogen, norethindrone.

Adipose tissue – another name for fatty tissue, which is composed of adipose cells, or fat cells.

Alpha estrogen receptor – one of the two different types of estrogen receptors that have been identified. The other type has been named the beta receptor. Different reactions can occur in a cell depending on which type of receptor combines with estrogen.

Alzheimer's disease – one of the most common causes of dementia.

Amyloid – this refers to a collection of proteins that stick together and form fiber deposits and when they accumulate they can cause damage to the surrounding tissue. Amyloid can be caused by a number of diseases and can be deposited in many different organs. Amyloid deposits in the brain are a feature of Alzheimer's disease.

Androgen – any of the male-type hormones including testosterone, androstenedione, DHEA, and DHEAS.

Angina – the term used to describe pain coming from the heart. It usually is perceived as an ache or deep pain on the left part of the chest, but can feel like heartburn, chest tightness, throat or arm pain, or other less characteristic symptoms.

Angiogram – a diagnostic test where dye is inserted into a blood vessel and then x-rays are taken. The dye outlines the vessels in an organ or an extremity allowing doctors to determine if there are any blockages in the arteries in those areas.

Anti-Mullerian hormone – a hormone made by the follicular cells which are the cells that accompany an egg in the ovary. The level of this hormone correlates with the number of eggs remaining in the ovary.

APOE gene – the APOE gene provides instructions for making a protein called apolipoprotein E. There are three slightly different versions of the APOE gene called e2, e3, and e4. The most common type is e3, which is found in more than half of the general population.

Apolipoprotein – proteins that bind fatty acids and cholesterol to form lipoproteins. Many of these have been identified and have names such as apolipoprotein E, which is involved in brain chemistry, and apolipoprotein B, which is the main protein found in LDL (low-density lipoprotein).

Apoptosis – a term that refers to the programmed cell death which occurs as a normal and controlled part of an organism's growth or development. It is a genetically directed process of cell self-destruction and is a way an organism removes damaged or unwanted cells.

Aromatase inhibitor – a type of drug that inhibits the enzyme that converts male hormones into estrogen.

Arrhythmia – a term used to denote an abnormal heart rhythm.

Artery – a blood vessel that carries blood away from the heart and differs in structure from a vein in that it has thicker walls composed partly of a circular layer of muscle.

Atherosclerosis – the medical term for "hardening of the arteries" which is a disease where arteries have developed plaque along their walls.

Atrial fibrillation – a type of abnormal heart rhythm characterized by an irregularly irregular pattern and is usually extremely rapid with a pulse rate over 130.

Atrophy – the term used to describe a wasting away of tissue or an organ, usually due to disease, disuse, or aging. In gynecological discussions, atrophic vaginitis is the term used to describe the thinning and shrinkage of the lining of the vagina and surrounding tissues.

B

Beta estrogen receptor – one of the two different types of estrogen receptors that have been identified. The other type has been named the alpha receptor. Different reactions can occur in a cell depending on which type of receptor combines with estrogen.

Bilateral – means both sides, a bilateral mastectomy means having both breasts removed.

Biologicals – a term used to describe a pharmaceutical agent that is made from a living organism or its products and is used in the prevention, diagnosis, or treatment of various diseases. The drug denosumab (Prolia) used for osteoporosis treatment is an example of a biological drug and is a monoclonal antibody.

Biopsy – refers to obtaining a sample of tissue, usually through a needle aspiration or excision, and then examining the cellular structure microscopically to detect for the presence of cancerous cells or other diseases.

Bisphosphonates – a class of drugs used to prevent and treat osteoporosis. There are oral forms such as alendronate (Fosamax) and injectable forms of bisphosphonates such as zoledronic acid (Reclast).

BMI – *body mass index*. This is a calculated number used to assess a person's physical size and to classify if a person is normal weight, overweight, or obese. It is obtained by taking a person's weight (in kilograms) divided by the square of the height (in meters). A normal BMI is between 18.5 and 24.9.

BRCA gene – a gene that encodes a protein that helps prevent tumor growth. An abnormal BRCA gene increases a woman's risk of breast cancer and ovarian cancer.

Bruit – a noise that can be heard over an artery when using a stethoscope and usually indicates turbulence in the artery caused by some obstruction such as from plaque, or a kink in the artery.

C

Calcium score – a number derived from a CAT scan or EBCT scan of the heart, which measures the amount of calcium present in the arteries that lay on the outside of the heart (the coronary arteries). The score correlates with the amount of plaque buildup on an artery. A calcium score of zero generally implies that there is no significant plaque buildup.

Cancellous bone – also referred to as trabecular bone, is the type of bone that is located in the internal part of a bone that consists of a honeycomb structure that houses the marrow.

Capillary – the tiniest of blood vessels which form a network that connects the arteries and veins.

Carcinogen – an agent that leads to or causes cancer.

Carotid artery – one of the two arteries that carry blood from the heart to the brain. They lay on either side of the the front of the neck.

Castration – the removal of the testicles from a male (human or animal).

CAT scan – stands for *computerized axial tomography* and is also referred to as a CT scan. These are sophisticated x-ray exams that render detailed three-dimensional images of the interior of the body. Sometimes an iodine dye, called a contrast, is injected prior to the exam to enhance the detail of the images.

CEE – *conjugated equine estrogen, see* Premarin

Central fat – also referred to as abdominal fat or visceral fat. This is fat that accumulates around the abdomen, or belly, and also within the abdominal cavity. This type of fat is considered unhealthy fat as it increases the risk of heart disease, insulin resistance, and diabetes.

Cerebrovascular disease – the term used to refer to atherosclerosis, or plaque buildup, in the arteries going into and inside the brain.

Cervix – the lowermost section of the uterus which connects the rest of the uterus to the vagina.

CHF – *see congestive heart failure.*

CIMT – *carotid intima-media thickness*, a non-invasive test where an ultrasound machine is used to measure the thickness of the carotid artery. If thickening is detected, this indicates that some plaque has developed on the lining of the artery.

Cirrhosis – a condition of advanced, severe liver disease where the liver has shrunk in size and is composed of extensive scar tissue.

Clitoris – the small sensitive part of the female sex gland located at the top and front part of the vulva.

Collagen – a type of protein that the body produces that can have variable properties – such as fibrous or elastic qualities. It composes the infrastructure of essentially all our tissues and organs and is the main component of our tendons, cartilage, and bones (where it becomes hardened by calcification).

Compression fracture – a type of fracture where the bone collapses within itself, usually in one of the vertebrae of the back.

Congestive heart failure – a condition that occurs when the heart muscle weakens and is unable to effectively pump blood through the lungs and body such that the blood gets "backed-up" leading to congestion in the lungs and swelling of the legs. It can be caused by various diseases that damage the heart muscle such as damage from a heart attack, long-standing high blood pressure, heart valve damage, or diseases that affect the heart muscle.

Conjugation – the process where a substance is chemically modified to give it different properties. In the body, this usually occurs in the liver. For instance molecules such as sulfate are added to an estrone molecule to make estrone sulfate. Conjugated compounds like these then may pass easier into the urine to get eliminated or be more easily absorbed when taken orally.

Conjugated estrogens – estrogen products that have been conjugated.

Contraceptives – birth control pills or devices.

Coronary artery – an artery that lays on the outside of the heart and delivers blood to the heart muscle.

Coronary artery disease – the term that refers to a buildup of plaque in the coronary arteries.

Corpus luteum – a tiny mass of cells derived from the follicle after an egg is released; it remains in the ovary and becomes the area where progesterone is produced.

Cortical bone – the "hard" exterior part of a bone.

CRP – stands for *C-reactive protein*, one of many proteins that are involved in the immune system. Elevated levels correlate with high levels of inflammation somewhere in the body, and are elevated in diseases such as rheumatoid arthritis.

CT scan – also referred to as a CAT scan, defined above.

CTX test – *carboxy-terminal collagen crosslinks* test, which is a test used to indicate how fast bone is being broken down and can indicate, but not diagnose, if a person is at risk for osteoporosis. High CTX levels indicate that bone is being broken down at a fast rate. The CTX test is helpful in determining if a medication being taken to prevent osteoporosis is working.

Cystitis – another name for a urinary tract infection (UTI) or bladder infection.

D

Dementia – the general term used to denote a severe decline in mental function. Most cases are due to Alzheimer's disease. Multiple small strokes are also a common cause of dementia and this form of dementia is called multi-infarct dementia.

Denosumab – generic name for Prolia, a medication used to prevent and treat osteoporosis.

DEXA – stands for *Dual-energy X-ray absorptiometry*, a test used to measure the density or strength of a bone to assess the risk of osteoporosis.

DHEA – *dehydroepiandrosterone*, one of the male-like hormones found in both men and women.

DHEA-S – refers to a DHEA molecule that has a sulfate molecule attached to it. DHEA-S and DHEA are converted back and forth to each other and essentially have similar effects in the body.

Diabetes – a disease where the blood sugar in the bloodstream runs abnormally high. This leads to multiple medical complications.

Diuretic – the medical term for a "water pill" which is a drug that eliminates salt and water from the body. These are commonly used as blood pressure pills.

DJD – stands for *degenerative joint disease*, the most common form of arthritis which is also known as osteoarthritis. This typically occurs in multiple joints as people age.

Dopamine – one of the neurotransmitters or chemical messengers in the brain.

Duavee – a combination drug containing conjugated estrogens and a SERM, bazedoxifene, indicated for the treatment of hot flashes.

DVT – *deep venous thrombosis*, a blood clot in one of the deep inner veins, usually in the legs.

Dyspareunia – the medical term for pain with intercourse.

E

EBCT – *electron beam computerized tomography*, a type of CAT scan used to detect plaque buildup on the heart. Like a heart CAT scan, this test gives a calcium score, which correlates with the amount of plaque buildup on an artery.

E. coli – short for *Escherichia coli*, a common bacterium found throughout nature particularly in the colons of humans and other animals. They most commonly cause urinary tract infections. There are multiple strains, some of which have properties that can cause severe illnesses.

EKG or ECG – *electrocardiogram*, which is a heart tracing that records the electrical activity of the heart.

Embolism – the term describing the lodging of an embolus that causes blockage inside a blood vessel.

Embolus – a blood clot, air bubble, fatty deposit, or other object which has been carried in the bloodstream to lodge in a vessel and cause an embolism.

Embryo – the term used to describe the bundle of cells that is produced after an egg is fertilized and starts dividing, and is the earliest phase of pregnancy prior to the development of a fetus.

Encode – a term used to describe the process of how the information from a gene in a DNA molecule is converted into a protein.

Endocrine gland – one of the organs in the endocrine system, such as the pituitary gland, adrenal gland, thyroid gland, ovary, and testicle.

Endometrial biopsy – a procedure where a thin straw-like tube is inserted through the cervix to obtain some tissue from the inner cavity of the uterus. The specimen is then examined microscopically to determine if there are any abnormal cells, such as cancer cells, present. This procedure is usually performed as an office procedure.

Endometrium – the tissue lining the inside of the uterus. This is the site where most uterine cancers develop.

Endorphins – chemicals produced by the body to relieve stress and pain. They work similarly to a class of drugs called opioids and when released in the brain can produce a feeling of euphoria.

Endothelium – the term that denotes the single layer of cells lining various organs and cavities of the body, especially the blood vessels. The endothelium maintains the proper dilation and constriction of an artery by producing nitric oxide. This function determines on a moment-to-moment basis how much blood is received by the body's various tissues. The endothelium on the arteries also protects the deeper layers of the artery from various toxic substances, interacts with the blood clotting mechanism, and controls fluid, electrolytes, and numerous other substances that pass back and forth between the bloodstream and the surrounding tissues.

Endothelial dysfunction – refers to a condition in which the endothelial layer (the inner lining) of the small arteries fails to function normally. As a result, it cannot continue to perform the functions listed above. This can lead to a number of problems, including plaque formation, circulatory problems, and an increased risk of a heart attack.

Equilin estrogens – estrogens produced by horses.

Estradiol or E2 – the primary female sex hormone and is produced by the ovaries. Preparations used for HRT are labeled 17-beta-estradiol, which is the same as the estradiol produced in the ovaries.

Estring – a small ring containing estradiol which is inserted into the vagina and releases a small amount of estrogen over a three-month period. It is designed to treat vaginal dryness.

Estriol or E3 – the primary estrogen produced during pregnancy and is a very weak estrogen.

Estrogen – any of the female hormones including estradiol, estrone, estriol and their related compounds.

Estrone or E1 – a form of estrogen that can be converted into estradiol and is the most prominent form of estrogen produced after menopause.

Ethinyl estradiol – a potent synthetic estrogen compound that is found in essentially all estrogen-containing birth control pills.

F

Factor V Leiden mutation – a mutation of one of the genes that is responsible for one of the clotting factors in the blood. This mutation causes the blood to clot more readily, thus increasing the risk of developing blood clots, which most commonly occur in the legs.

Fallopian tube – the tube on either side of the uterus which connects the ovaries to the uterus.

Fatty liver – a condition where fat accumulates within the liver, usually developing when people become overweight or obese.

Femur – the long bone of the upper leg between the knee and the pelvic bone.

First-pass effect – a phenomenon where drugs are processed by the liver after being taken orally. The drugs are absorbed by the stomach into the bloodstream and immediately are routed to the liver. This process affects the way the drugs behave in the body and frequently results in a rapid inactivation of the drug so that higher doses are required compared to drugs applied onto the skin. The consequence of this leads to differences in the way the drugs behave in the body. Oral estrogen stimulates the liver to produce other proteins that may have adverse effects in the body.

Flow-mediated dilation – the term that refers to the dilation of an artery when blood flow increases in that artery. The primary cause of flow-mediated dilation is the release of nitric oxide by endothelial cells and is a technique used to indirectly measure nitric oxide production.

Follicle – refers to the fluid-filled sac within the ovary that contains an egg. The cells surrounding the egg are called follicular cells and produce hormones, and are the main source of estradiol production.

Forteo – the brand name for the drug teriparatide which is an injectable drug used to treat advanced cases of osteoporosis.

FRAX test – an online *Fracture Risk Assessment tool*, used to calculate the risk of an osteoporotic fracture.

Free radical – the term used to describe an atom or a molecule that possesses a chemical charge that can cause damage to other molecules. An example is a water molecule (H_2O) that is missing one hydrogen atom (H) and this HO particle causes "oxidative" damage to cells and tissues, particularly to the lining of the arteries which leads to plaque development.

FSH – *follicle-stimulating hormone*. This is a hormone produced by the pituitary gland and released into the bloodstream where it acts on the ovary to stimulate an egg to become mature and be released. Once the eggs have disappeared at the time of menopause, the FSH level rises in an attempt to make the ovary release an egg. High levels of FSH are an indication that a woman is in postmenopause.

G

GSM – *Genitourinary Syndrome of Menopause* – a term used to describe all the changes affecting the vagina, bladder and other organs in the lower female pelvic region that are affected by the loss of estrogen at the time of menopause.

Genitourinary system – the system that includes the vulva, vagina, urethra, bladder, and other organs in the lower pelvic region.

Gestation – the process of carrying a fetus in the womb from the time of conception to birth.

Glucagon – a hormone produced by the pancreas that acts to raise blood sugar.

Glucose – the technical name for the form of sugar that circulates in our bloodstream.

Glycogen – basically a form of starch which our cells store for energy; glycogen can be rapidly broken down into glucose molecules.

Gonad – refers to a sex gland that produces either eggs or sperm, i.e., an ovary and a testes.

H

HDL – *high-density lipoprotein*, which is a compound that circulates in the bloodstream and is composed of cholesterol and proteins. It is considered the "good cholesterol" because high levels are associated with a lower risk of heart disease.

Hematoma – a localized collection of blood outside of a blood vessel, such as a bruise and is usually caused by an injury that damages a blood vessel.

Hepatosteatosis – or hepatic steatosis, is a term that refers to a liver containing fatty deposits.

HPV – *human papillomavirus* – a virus that causes genital warts in both women and men. It is passed back and forth from sexual contact. There are multiple strains and several strains have been found to cause cancer, particularly cervical cancer in women, but HPV can also cause cancer in other parts of the body.

HRT – short for *Hormone Replacement Therapy*. This usually refers to regimens that include estrogen and progestogen or just estrogen alone. Sometimes the abbreviations ERT is used to refer to estrogen-only therapy. MRT which stands for Menopausal Replacement Therapy is also used interchangeably with HRT.

Hs-CRP – *highly-sensitive CRP (C-reactive protein)*. C-reactive protein is elevated in conditions where there is inflammation. The highly sensitive test measure very small levels of inflammation and correlates with an increased risk of developing heart disease.

Hypercoagulable state – a term used to describe a condition in the body that makes a person prone to forming blood clots. A hypercoagulable state can be caused by a genetic mutation in the blood clotting system, cancer, drugs, and other causes.

Hypothalamus – an area of the brain that coordinates the autonomic nervous system and regulates many functions including body temperature, thirst, hunger, and other systems. The hypothalamus is the area of the brain that is involved in sleep, arousal, memory, and emotional activity. It sends signals to the pituitary to release FSH, LH, and other hormones involved in the endocrine system.

Hysterectomy – the term to indicate the surgical removal of the uterus (which includes the cervix).

5-hydroxytryptamine (5-HT) – the chemical name for serotonin.

I

Insulin – the hormone produced by specialized cells in the pancreas, whose role is to keep the blood sugar (glucose) in the bloodstream from getting too high.

Insulin resistance – a term used to refer to the condition where the cells in the body do not respond to insulin. This leads to increased levels of blood sugar in the bloodstream and is the main mechanism that leads to Type 2 Diabetes.

Intravaginal – applying or inserting something inside the vagina, such as a suppository or hormone cream applied with an applicator.

Isoflavones – naturally-occurring compounds that are considered to be a type of phytoestrogen. The most common source of isoflavones come from soy products.

IUD – stands for *intrauterine device*, which is a small plastic device that is inserted into the uterus by a health care provider. An IUD can be impregnated with progestogen hormones which are slowly released inside the uterus over a several year period. Progestogen-containing devices, such as the Mirena IUD, are typically used as a means of birth control, but are approved to control heavy menstrual bleeding. This type of device is also used to provide a progestogen for women on HRT, but using the device in this manner is not approved by the FDA.

K

Ketoacidosis – a serious condition that can occur when the blood sugar level becomes extremely high, leading to high levels of ketones in the blood stream. This causes the blood to become acidic and usually occurs in diabetics due to a lack of insulin.

Kyphoplasty – a technique similar to vertebroplasty, where a surgeon inserts cement into a collapsed vertebra to build it up as a means of treating a compression fracture of a vertebra.

Kyphosis – the term used to describe a forward bowing of the spine, usually due to multiple compression fractures.

L

Laparoscopy – a surgical procedure in which a fiber-optic instrument is inserted through a small incision into the abdominal wall to view the organs in the abdomen or to permit a surgical procedure. The scope used is called a laparoscope. Small surgical instruments are inserted through other incisions to perform the surgery while viewing the inside of the abdomen on a video screen.

LDL – *low-density lipoprotein*. The cholesterol particle that is considered the "bad cholesterol" because high levels of LDL increase the risk of heart disease.

Leptin – a hormone made predominantly by fat cells that is released into the bloodstream and inhibits hunger, which leads to a decrease in caloric intake.

LH – *luteinizing hormone*, a hormone produced by the pituitary gland. In women, its primary roles are to stimulate the release of the egg, transform the follicle into the corpus luteum, and stimulate the production of progesterone.

Libido – refers to one's sex drive, the term that denotes a desire for sexual activity.

Lipoprotein – particles that are composed of a core of fat and cholesterol surrounded by proteins called apolipoproteins. The outer protein has the chemical characteristics to make them soluble in water which allows them to be transported within the bloodstream and into the fluid around the cells.

Longevity – long duration of life.

Lumbar spine – the portion of the spine that sits just on top of the pelvic bones, composed of the lower five lumbar vertebrae.

M

Macular degeneration – an eye disease that causes damage to the retina. There are two forms. The most common form is a milder form called dry macular degeneration. The more severe form, wet macular degeneration, is characterized by an overgrowth of blood vessels on the retina which can bleed. Both forms can progress over time and cause blindness.

Mastectomy – removal of a breast.

Medroxyprogesterone – the generic name for the synthetic progestogen, Provera. This is also used in the long-acting birth control shot, depo-Provera.

Meta-analysis – a statistical analysis that combines the results of multiple studies in an effort to resolve uncertainty when reports disagree.
Metabolic syndrome – refers to a cluster of conditions that occur together that have been shown to increase the risk of heart disease, stroke, and Type 2 diabetes. These conditions include elevated blood pressure, high blood sugar, excess body fat around the waist, high triglyceride levels, and low levels of HDL.

Metastasis – the term to denote the development of a malignant tumor that has spread from the original site of a cancer.

Methyltestosterone – a synthetic male hormone, formulated to be able to be taken orally.

Micronize – a process that breaks down a substance such as a drug into fine particles so that it may be more easily absorbed.

Microvascular angina – a term that refers to chest pain that develops from constriction of blood flow in very small arteries on the heart.

Mitochondria – the tiny organelles or structures inside a cell that are responsible for producing the energy the cell requires to live.

Monoclonal antibodies – antibodies produced from a single type of white cell. Antibodies are proteins whose job is specifically to seek and attach to substances in the body, such as bacteria. Monoclonal antibodies can be made in the lab by cloning a particular white cell which then produces large numbers of antibodies. These can then be given to a patient to treat a specific condition. Monoclonal antibodies have been developed to treat some types of cancer, autoimmune diseases, osteoporosis, asthma, and other conditions.

Morbidity – refers to having a disease or a symptom of a disease. It is also a term to describe the amount of a disease within a population.

Mortality – refers to the state of being mortal (destined to die). In medical studies it is a term used in reporting death rates, such as the number of deaths in a certain group of people in a certain situation.

MRI scan – *magnetic resonance imaging* scan, which is similar to a CAT scan, but instead of radiation a strong magnetic field and radio waves are used to create detailed images of the organs and tissues within the body.

Multi-infarct – refers to having multiple infarcts, which are areas of damaged tissue caused by a lack of blood. Multi-infarct dementia is a form of dementia caused by multiple, small strokes.

Murmur – a sound coming from the heart that can be heard by using a stethoscope placed on the chest. It is a swooshing noise heard between heartbeats, and usually is caused by the sound of blood going through an abnormal heart valve.

N

NASH – *nonalcoholic steatohepatitis*. This term refers to a type of liver disease, called steatohepatitis, that is caused by conditions other than alcohol toxicity.

Neuron – a nerve cell. Nerves and the brain are composed of neurons.

Neurotransmitter – a chemical messenger produced by brain cells that is released into the synapses and travels from one neuron to another. This is the biochemical mechanism that allows nerve cells to communicate with each other.

Nitric oxide – a colorless gas consisting of one nitrogen atom and one oxygen atom. It is produced in the endothelium and rapidly causes blood vessels to relax and dilate, which allows an increase in blood flow.

NTX test – *N-terminal telopeptide*, is a fragment released when bone is being broken down. Measuring the level of these fragments in the blood or urine assesses the rate of bone breakdown. A high level indicates a rapid loss of bone. This test is not used to diagnose osteoporosis, but is helpful in predicting if a woman is at risk, and is also helpful in assessing if a medication being taken for osteoporosis is working.

Nucleus – the structure inside a cell that contains DNA.

O

Observational study – a type of study where individuals are observed or certain outcomes are measured, but no treatment is given. Observational studies are helpful in many ways but cannot determine cause and effect.

Oncologist – a doctor who is a specialist trained in the treatment of cancer.

ONJ – *osteonecrosis of the jaw*, *see* osteonecrosis.

Oophorectomy – refers to the surgical removal of an ovary; bilateral oophorectomy means the removal of both ovaries; unilateral oophorectomy means the removal of one ovary.

Osteoarthritis – also referred to as degenerative arthritis, which is the "wear and tear" arthritis that occurs with aging.

Osteoblast – the cells within the bones that are responsible for building bone.

Osteoclast – the cells within the bones that are responsible for removing bone.

Osteonecrosis – also known as avascular necrosis. It is a disease where a segment of bone dies because it has been deprived of blood.

Osteopenia – a condition of the bone where it has become thinner than expected for a young adult, but not to the point of being osteoporotic.

Osteoporosis – a term that means the bones have become so thin that they are at an extremely high risk of being fractured.

Ovulation – the term used to denote when a mature egg is released by the ovary. This normally occurs once a month in women of reproductive age. The egg floats into the fallopian tube where it may or may not become fertilized before it is transported into the uterus.

Oxidation – a normal chemical reaction that occurs in the body that is important in producing energy. Free radicals are produced in this process, which are normally neutralized. If there is an imbalance in this process, excessive oxidation occurs, causing oxidative stress which can damage cells, proteins and DNA.

P

PAC – *premature atrial contraction*, an "extra beat" originating from the atrium, or top part of the heart; PACs tend to be benign and are perceived as "skipped beats" and are not generally associated with worrisome heart problems.

Patent foramen ovale – a hole between the two upper chambers of the heart (the atria). This hole normally closes before birth but can remain open in some individuals.

Pelvic bones – the bones that make up the "bowl" where the femurs (upper legs) attach and where the spinal column rests. The pelvic skeleton is composed of the sacrum, the ischium, and the ilium.

Pelvis – the lowest part of the abdominal area enclosed by the pelvic bones, containing the uterus, bladder, ovaries and the bottom section of the intestines.

PET scan – *positron emission tomography* scan. A scan performed after a small dose of a radioactive chemical is injected into the bloodstream where it is absorbed by specific organs or tissues. Areas of high uptake demonstrate increased biologic activity. PET scans can locate where the body is fighting an infection, where a cancer is growing, or where other metabolic processes are occurring.

PFO – *see patent foramen ovale.*

Phlebitis – refers to an inflammation in a vein. It is usually due to a blood clot and this is termed thrombophlebitis.

Phytoestrogen – a substance that occurs naturally in plants that has mild estrogen-like properties but does not have the same chemical skeleton as estrogen.

Placebo – a "sugar pill" or harmless substance or procedure. In medical studies it is used as a control to assess the efficacy of a treatment.

Plaque – this has several meanings in medicine (such as a small lesion or dental plaque) but when discussing heart disease it refers to the buildup of a substance on the wall of an artery that is composed of fat, cholesterol, calcium, and other substances. Plaque formation and progression is the underlying feature that causes atherosclerosis.

Polycystic ovarian syndrome – or PCOS, a condition characterized by multiple ovarian cysts, infrequent ovulation, problems with fertility, and irregular menstrual periods. It is also characterized by excessive levels of testosterone which cause hair growth and acne. It is also associated with insulin resistance and other metabolic abnormalities.

Premarin – the brand name for the estrogen product known as conjugated equine estrogens (CEE) which is a drug derived from pregnant horses' urine. It contains estrone plus several conjugated estrogens unique to horses.

Progesterone – a hormone produced in the body which plays many roles and is a precursor hormone that is converted into a number of other hormones.

Progestin – a term used to refer to a synthetic progestogen.

Progestogen – a term that refers to any agent that has progesterone-like effects. This includes natural progesterone as well as a number of synthetic drugs, such as those used in birth control pills and HRT.

Prolia – the brand name for denosumab, a monoclonal antibody drug used to prevent and treat osteoporosis.

Prothrombin mutation – a mutation in a gene that encodes for a blood-clotting protein (Factor II) that can increase a person's risk of a blood clot.

Provera – the brand name for a synthetic progestogen, medroxyprogesterone.

Pulmonary embolism – a blockage of one of the arteries in the lungs, usually caused by a blood clot that has traveled from the legs (from deep venous thrombosis), through the heart and then out into the pulmonary artery. The area of the lung beyond the blockage becomes damaged due to the lack of blood flow.

PVC – *premature ventricular contraction*, an "extra beat" originating from the lower part of the heart, or ventricle. These types of beats are more worrisome than PACs and can lead to ventricular fibrillation which can cause sudden death.

R

Randomized controlled trial – a study in which people are allocated at random (by chance alone) to receive one of several treatments. One group receives a "non-treatment" (placebo) and serves as a control group. The participants in each group are matched for like characteristics. The participants are followed closely over a period of time, and then the outcomes of each group are compared. These types of studies are considered the most reliable way of determining whether a cause-effect relation exists between treatment and outcome, and are considered the "gold standard" type of studies.

Receptor – the term used to refer to a special site on a cell that uniquely combines with an entity circulating in the blood. When this entity combines with its receptor, it triggers some actions in the cell. Receptors are specific for certain compounds, such as estrogen or progesterone, although molecules with nearly identical features may interact with them. Hormones and other drugs cannot exert their effects unless they can latch onto a receptor.

Relative risk – in medical studies is the ratio of the probability of an outcome in a treatment group to the probability of an outcome in a non-treatment group. This ratio compares these two groups to each other rather than to the whole of the group and so is much different than absolute risk.

Romosozumab – the generic name for a new type of osteoporosis drug called Evenity.

Rugae – means "ruglike" – a term to describe an accordion-like surface of a tissue layer, such as inside the vagina.

S

Salpingectomy – refers to the surgical removal of a fallopian tube.

Sarcopenia – refers to the loss of muscle mass and strength.

SERD – *selective estrogen receptor down-regulator*. These drugs block estrogen production and are used in breast cancer treatment.

SERM – *selective estrogen receptor modulator*, which is a drug created to be able to attach to an estrogen receptor and cause estrogen-like effects, or estrogen-blocking effects.

Serotonin – one of the neurotransmitters in the brain involved primarily in regulating mood, but is involved in other brain functions.

Sham procedure – a "fake" procedure performed as part of a study to act as a placebo treatment.

Soft plaque – a form of arterial plaque that may be more prone to rupturing that does not contain very much calcium.

SSRIs – stands for *selective serotonin reuptake inhibitors*, which are drugs used to treat depression. They work by increasing serotonin levels in the brain synapses.

Standard deviation – a statistical term used to indicate how far above or how far below a value is from the average value.

Steatohepatitis – a term that refers to inflammation in the liver caused by fat accumulation.

Stroke – the term that describes an area where the brain has been damaged. This is usually caused by a blockage in an artery in the brain due to a blood clot (usually arising from a clot in the heart) or a fragment of plaque (usually broken off from plaque on a carotid artery), but can be due to a broken blood vessel within the brain (usually from a ruptured aneurysm), or a tumor, or other cause.

Superficial phlebitis – an inflamed vein usually caused by a blood clot in one of the small veins on the surface of the leg.

Surrogate marker – a substitute measure in a scientific study. In research, frequently it may take many years to determine if a treatment is effective. For instance, studying whether cholesterol lowers the risk of a heart attack may take years. It has been shown that people who are at risk of having a heart attack develop hardening of the arteries. A test that detects for the presence and progression of hardening of the arteries, such as an ultrasound-based CIMT test, can be used as a surrogate marker to correlate with the risk of developing a heart attack.

Synapse – the small gap between nerve cells.

T

T-Score – the score determined by a bone density test (DEXA scan) that tells how a person's bone density compares to that of a 35-year old person, whose T-score is considered to be a normal value.

Tau protein – a protein normally present in the brain that can accumulate in certain conditions and cause damage and is believed to be a factor in Alzheimer's disease.

Thoracic spine – the mid-portion of the spine consisting of 12 vertebrae that sit below the cervical (neck) vertebrae and above the lower (lumbar) vertebrae.

Thrombophlebitis – inflammation in a vein caused by a blood clot.

Thrombosis – a blood clot that develops inside a blood vessel.

TIA – *transient ischemic attack*, an episode characterized by temporary neurologic symptoms similar to those caused by a stroke, such as weakness, numbness, or speech problems. In a TIA, the symptoms last less than 24 hours and then resolve. TIAs are frequently warning signs of a stroke.

Trabecular bone – also called cancellous bone, is honeycomb-like bone that is present in the interior of most bones.

Transdermal – refers to the application of a liquid or a patch onto the skin. A transdermally applied medication penetrates the skin and then enters the blood circulation.

Transient ischemic attack – *see* TIA.

Transsexual female – refers to a transgender female (who is a biologic male who identifies as a female) who has usually proceeded with medical therapy to acquire female attributes.

U

Ultrasound – an imaging technique that uses sound waves to identify structures inside the body and provide images of these structures.

Unilateral – means on one side; a unilateral mastectomy means having one breast removed.

Urethra – the tube that drains urine out of the bladder. In women, the urethral opening is located at the 12:00 position at the entrance of the vagina.

Uric acid – a chemical derived from the breakdown of organic compounds in the body. It is eliminated in the urine as a waste product, but can be deposited in various tissues and joints, causing gout and other problems.

USPSTF – *United States Preventative Services Task Force*, a government agency consisting of a panel of experts who systematically review the evidence of the effectiveness of preventative health services and makes recommendations on the advisability of performing them.

V

Vaginitis – a disease where the vagina is infected or inflamed.

Vein – a blood vessel in the circulatory system that carries blood back to the heart.

Venous insufficiency – refers to a condition where the veins, usually in the legs, aren't functioning to assist in propelling the blood back to the heart. This results in swollen veins, such as varicose veins, and leg swelling. Over time this can cause pain and redness in the legs.

Venous thrombosis – refers to a blood clot within a vein.

Vertebra – refers to one of the bones that make up the spine. There are 7 in the neck known as the cervical vertebrae, 12 in the mid-back known as the thoracic vertebrae, and 5 in the lower back called the lumbar vertebrae.

Vertebral artery – one of two arteries located in the back of the neck. They carry blood from the heart to supply the cerebellum, which is the part of the brain that controls balance and coordinates muscular activity.

Vertebroplasty – a procedure, similar to kyphoplasty, where cement is inserted into a vertebra to shore it up following a compression fracture.

Vertigo – a type of dizziness characterized by a sensation of the surroundings spinning or moving; usually caused by an inner ear problem but can originate from problems in the brain.

Viscera – a term referring to our internal organs; primarily those in the abdomen.

Visceral fat – fat located within the abdominal cavity which is stored around organs such as the liver and intestines. This type of fact is associated with adverse health risks such as heart disease and diabetes.

Vulva – a part of a woman's genitals that includes the labia, clitoris, vaginal opening, and the opening to the urethra (the tube that drains the bladder).

Z

Z-Score – the score derived by a bone density test (DEXA scan) that compares a person's bone density to a person of the same age and sex.

Bibliography

Chapter 2: What is Menopause?

2-1 Amundsen D, et al. The age of menopause in classical Greece and Rome. Human Biology. 1970;4(2):79.

2-2 Nelson L. Clinical Practice - Primary ovarian insufficiency. New England Journal of Medicine. 2009;360(6):606.

2-3 Siddle N, Sarrel P, Whitehead M. The effect of hysterectomy on the age at ovarian failure: identification of a subgroup of women with premature loss of ovarian function and literature review. Fertil Steril. 1987;47(1):94.

2-4 Farquhar C, Sadler L, et al. The association of hysterectomy and menopause: a prospective cohort study. BJOG. 2005;112(7):956.

2-5 Rosendahl M, Simonsen K, Kier, J. The influence of unilateral oophorectomy on the age of menopause. Climateric. Sept. 2017; 20(6):540-5.

2-6 De Bruin J, Bovenhuis H, et al. The role of genetic factors in age at natural menopause. Hum Reprod. 2001;16(9):2014.

2-7 Stolk L, Perry J, et al. Meta-analyses identify 13 loci associated with age at menopause and highlight DNA repair and immune pathways. Nat Genet. 2012;44(3):260.

2-8 Forman M, Mangini L, et al. Life-course origins of the ages at menarche and menopause. Adolesc Health Med Ther. 2013; 4:1-21.

2-9 Mondul A, et al. Age at natural menopause and cause-specific mortality. Am. J. Epidemiol. 2005;162:1089-1097.

2-10 Farnham A. Uterine disease as a factor in the production of insanity. Alienist Neurologist. 1187:8:532.

2-11 Barnabei V, Grady D, et al. Menopausal symptoms in older women and the effects of treatment with hormone therapy. Obstet Gynecol. Dec 2002;100(6):1209-18.

2-12 Mann E, Hunter M. Concordance between self-reported and sternal skin conductance measures of hot flushes in symptomatic perimenopausal and postmenopausal women: a systematic review. Menopause. 2011;18:709-722.

2-13 Utian W. Psychosocial and socioeconomic burden of vasomotor symptoms in menopause: a comprehensive review. Health Qual Life Outcomes. 2005;3:47.

2-14 Gartoulla P, Bell R, Worsley R, Davis S. Moderate-severely bothersome vasomotor symptoms are associated with lowered psychological general wellbeing in women at midlife. Maturitas. 2015;81:487-492.

2-15 Franco O, et al. Use of plant-based therapies and menopausal symptoms: a systematic review and meta-analysis. JAMA. June 2016;315(23):2554-63.

2-16 Ee C, French S, Xue C, et al. Acupuncture for menopausal hot flashes: clinical evidence update and its relevance to decision making. Menopause. August 2017;23(8):980-987.

2-17 Ee C, Xue C, et al. Acupuncture for menopausal hot flashes: a randomized trial. Ann Intern Med. Feb. 2016;2:146-154.

2-18 Hu X, Bull S, Hunkeler E, et al. Incidence and duration of side effects and those rated as bothersome with selective serotonin reuptake inhibitor treatment for depression: patient report versus physician estimate. J Clin Psychiatry. 2004;65(7):959.

2-19 Cheshire W, Fealey R. Drug-induced hyperhidrosis and hypohidrosis: incidence, prevention and management. Drug Saf. 2008;31(2):109.

2-20 Prague J, Roberts R, Comninos A, et al. Neurokinin 3 receptor antagonism as a novel treatment for menopausal hot flushes: a phase 2, randomised, double-blind, placebo-controlled trial. Lancet. 2017;389(10081):1809-1820.

2-21 Biglia N, Cagnacci A, Gambacciani M, et al. Vasomotor symptoms in menopause: a biomarker of cardiovascular disease risk and other chronic diseases. Climacteric. 2017;20:306-12.

2-22 Herber-Gast G, Brown W, Mishra G. A longitudinal study of over 11000 women followed for 14 years: hot flushes and night sweats are associated with coronary heart disease risk in midlife: a longitudinal study. BJOG. 2015;122:1560-7.

2-23 Thurston R, Chang Y, Barinas-Mitchell E, et al. Physiologically assessed hot flashes and endothelial function among midlife women. Menopause. Aug. 2017;24(8):886-893.

2-24 Thurston RC, Aizenstein HJ, Derby CA, et al. Menopausal hot flashes and white matter hyperintensities. Menopause. 2016;23:27-32.

2-25 Kravitz H, Ganz P, Bromberger et al. Sleep difficulty in women at midlife: a community survey of sleep and the menopausal transition. Menopause. Jan. 2003;10(1):19-28.

2-26 Keefe, D. Hormone replacement therapy alleviated sleep apnea in menopausal women. Menopause. 1999;6:196-200.

2-27 Peccei, J. A critique of the grandmother hypotheses: old and new. Am. J. Hum. Biol. 2001;13:434-452.

2-28 Brent LJ, Franks DW, Cant M, et al. Ecological knowledge, leadership, and the evolution of menopause in killer whales. Current Biology. 2015. http://dx.doi.org/10.1016/j.cub.2015.01.037

2-29 Blurton-Jones N, Hawkes K, O'Connell, J. Antiquity of postreproductive life: are there modern impacts on hunter-gatherer postreproductive life spans? Am. J. Hum. Biol. 2002;14:184-205.

Chapter 3: Our Hormones, Drugs and Menopause

3-1 Sicotte N, Liva S, Klutch R, et al. Treatment of multiple sclerosis with the pregnancy hormone estriol. Ann Neurol. 2002;52:421-428.

3-2 Coelingh B, Herjan J, et al. Pharmacodynamic effects of the fetal estrogen estetrol in postmenopausal women: results from a multiple-rising-dose study. Menopause. June 2017;24(6): 677-685.

3-3 Prestwood K, Kenny A, et al. Ultralow-dose micronized 17beta-estradiol and bone density and bone metabolism in older women: a randomized controlled trial. JAMA. 2003;290(8):1042.

3-4 Ettinger B, Ensrud K, Wallace R, et al. Effects of ultralow-dose transdermal estradiol on bone mineral density: a randomized clinical trial. Obstet Gynecol. 2004;104(3):443.

3-5 Stuenkel CA, Manson JE. Compounded bioidentical hormone therapy. Does the regulatory double standard harm women? JAMA Intern Med. 2017;177(12):1719-1720.

3-6 Yuksel N, Treseng L, et al. Promotion and marketing of bioidentical hormone therapy on the internet: a content analysis of websites. Menopause. October 2017;24(10):1129-1135.

3-7 Eden J, Hacker N, Fortune M. Three cases of endometrial cancer associated with "bioidentical" hormone replacement therapy. Med J Aust. 2007;187:244-245.

3-8 Gass M, et al. Use of compounded hormone therapy in the US: Report of the North American Menopause Society survey. Menopause. Dec 2015;12:1276-84.

3-9 US Food and Drug Administration. Evamist (Estradiol Transdermal Spray): Drug Safety Communication - Unintended Exposure of Children and Pets to Topical Estrogen. Available at http://www.fda.gov/Safety/MedWatch/ SafetyInformation/SafetyAlertsforHumanMedicalProducts/ucm220548.htm.

3-10 Stanczyk FZ, Paulson RJ, Roy S. Percutaneous administration of progesterone: blood levels and endometrial protection. Menopause. 2005;12:232-237.

3-11 Elshafie Q, et al. Transdermal natural progesterone cream for postmenopausal women: inconsistent data and complex pharmacokinetics. J Obstet Gynaecol. 2007;27(7):655-9.

3-12 Valshisht S. Bleeding profiles and effects on the endometrium for women using a novel combination of transdermal oestradiol and natural progesterone cream as part of a continuous combined hormone replacement regime. BJOG. 2005;112(10):1402-6.

3-13 Stute P, Neulen J. The impact of micronized progesterone on the endometrium: a systematic review. Climacteric. August 2016;19(4):316-28.

3-14 Wakatsuki A, Okatani Y, Ikenoue N, Fukaya T. Effect of medroxyprogesterone acetate on endothelium-dependent vasodilation in postmenopausal women receiving estrogen. Circulation. 2001;104(15):1773.

3-15 Mather K, Norman E, Prior J, Elliott T. Preserved forearm endothelial responses with acute exposure to progesterone: a randomized cross-over trial of 17-beta estradiol, progesterone, and 17-beta estradiol with progesterone in healthy menopausal women. J Clin Endocrinol Metab. 2000;85:4644-4649.

3-16 Prior J. Progesterone as a bone-trophic hormone. Endocr Rev.1990;11(2):386.

3-17 Liu R, Muse K. The effects of progestins on bone density and bone metabolism in postmenopausal women: a randomized controlled trial. Am J Obstet Gynecol. April 2005;192(4):1316-23.

3-18 The Writing Group for the PEPI. Effects of hormone therapy on bone mineral density: results from the Postmenopausal Estrogen/Progestin Interventions (PEPI) trial. JAMA. 1996;276(17):1389.

3-19 Gallagher J, Kable W, et al. Effect of progestin therapy on cortical and trabecular bone: comparison with estrogen. Am J Med. 1991;90(2):171.

3-20 Munk-Jensen N, Pors Nielsen S, et al. Reversal of postmenopausal vertebral bone loss by oestrogen and progestogen: a double blind placebo controlled study. Br Med J (Clin Res Ed). 1988;296(6630):1150.

3-21 Gruber C, Huber J. Differential effects of progestins on the brain. Maturitas. 2003;46(Suppl 1):S71-S75.

3-22 Ruana X, Mueck A. Systemic progesterone therapy—oral, vaginal, injections and even transdermal? Maturitas. Nov 2014;79(3):248-55.

3-23 Montplaisir J, et al. Sleep in menopause: differential effects of two forms of hormone replacement therapy. Menopause. 2001; 8: 10-16.

3-24 Taylor J. Plasma progesterone, oestradiol 17 beta and premenstrual symptoms. Acta Psychiatr Scand. 1979;60(1):76.

3-25 Canonico M, Oger E, Plu-Bureau G, et al. Estrogen and Thromboembolism Risk (ESTHER) Study Group. Hormone therapy and venous thromboembolism among postmenopausal women: impact of the route of estrogen administration and progestogens: The ESTHER Study. Circulation. 2007;115:840-845.

3-26 Speroff L. Transdermal hormone therapy and the risk of stroke and venous thrombosis. Climacteric. 2010;13:429-432.

3-27 Sturdee D. Are progestins really necessary as part of a combined HRT regimen? Climacteric. August 2013;16 (Suppl 1):79-84.

3-28 Moorjani S, Dupont A, et al. Changes in plasma lipoprotein and apolipoprotein composition in relation to oral versus percutaneous administration of estrogen alone or in cyclic association with utrogestan in menopausal women. J Clin Endocrinol Metab. 1991;73(2):373-9.

3-29 Stevenson JC; Chines A, Pan K, et al. A pooled analysis of the effects of conjugated estrogens/bazedoxifene on lipid parameters in postmenopausal women from the selective estrogens, menopause, and response to therapy (SMART) trials. J Clin Endocrinol Metab. June 2015;100(6):2329-38.

3-30 Komi J, Lankinen KS, DeGregorio M, Heikkinen J, et al. Effects of ospemifene and raloxifene on biochemical markers of bone turnover in postmenopausal women. J Bone Miner Metab. 2006;24(4):314.

3-31 Portman D, Bachmann G, Simon J. Ospemifene, a novel selective estrogen receptor modulator for treating dyspareunia associated with postmenopausal vulvar and vaginal atrophy. Menopause. 2013;20(6):623.

3-32 Archer D, et al. Ospemifene's effects on lipids and coagulation factors: a post hoc analysis of phase 2 and 3 clinical trial data. Menopause. October 2017;24(10):1167-1174.

3-33 Formoso G, Perrone E. Short-term and long-term effects of tibolone in postmenopausal women. The Cochrane Database of systematic reviews [Cochrane Database Syst Rev]. Oct 12 2016;CD008536.

3-34 Bennetts H, Underwood E, Shier F. A specific breeding problem of sheep on subterranean clover pastures in western Australia. Australian Veterinary Journal.1946;22:2-12.

3-35 Roberts H, Lethaby A. Phytoestrogens for menopausal vasomotor symptoms: A Cochrane review summary. Maturitas. 2014;78:79-81.

3-36 Liu J, Ho S, Su Y, et al. Effect of long-term intervention of soy isoflavones on bone mineral density in women: A meta-analysis of randomized controlled trials. Bone. 2009;44:948-53.

3-37 Ricci E, Cipriani S, Chiaffarino F, et al. Soy isoflavones and bone mineral density in perimenopausal and postmenopausal western women: a systematic review and meta-analysis of randomized controlled trials. J Womens Health (Larchmt). 2010; 19:1609.

3-38 Elraiyah T, Sonbol M, Wang Z, et al. Clinical review: the benefits and harms of systemic dehydroepiandrosterone (DHEA) in postmenopausal women with normal adrenal function: a systematic review and meta-analysis. J Clin Endocrinol Metab. 2014; 99:3536-3542.

Chapter 4: Medical Studies 101

4-1 Yu EW, Bauer SR, et al. Proton pump inhibitors and risk of fractures: a meta-analysis of 11 international studies. Am J Med. 2011;124(6):519.

4-2 Frieden Thomas R. Evidence for health decision making - beyond randomized, controlled trials. NEJM. August 2017;377: 465-475.

4-3 Average cost per patient in biopharmaceutical clinical trials in the United States in 2013, by phase; The Statistics Portal; https://www.statista.com/statistics/645490/per-patient-clinical-trial-costs-in-us/.

4-4 Roth JA, Etzioni R, Waters TM, et al. Economic return from the Women's Health Initiative estrogen plus progestin clinical trial: a modeling study. Annals of Internal Medicine. 2014;160(9):594-602.

4-5 The History of Malaria, an Ancient Disease; CDC website: www.cdc.gov/malaria/about/history/index.html.

Chapter 5: Estrogen Therapy – A Brief History

5-1 Wilson, RA. Feminine Forever. New York, NY: J.B. Lippincott Co; 1966.

5-2 Green TH. Gynecology Essentials of Clinical Practice. 2nd edition. Boston, MA: Little Brown and Company; 1971.

5-3 Goldstein, F, Stampfer MJ. Role of hormone replacement in cardiovascular disease. In: Treatment of the Menopausal Woman. New York,NY: Raven Press; 1994: 223-233.

5-4 Stampfer MJ, Colditz GA, et. al. Postmenopausal estrogen therapy and cardiovascular disease. Ten-year follow-up from the Nurses' Health Study. NEJM. Sep 1991;325(11):756-62.

5-5 Paganini-Hill A, Corrada MM, Kawas CH. Increased longevity in older users of postmenopausal estrogen therapy: the Leisure World Cohort Study. Menopause. Jan-Feb 2006;13(1):12-8.

5-6 Barrett-Connor E, Slone S, Greendale G, et al. The Postmenopausal Estrogen/Progestin Interventions Study: primary outcomes in adherent women. Maturitas. July 1997;27(3):261-74.

5-7 Hodis HN, Mack WJ, Lobo RA, et al. Estrogen in the prevention of atherosclerosis. A randomized, double-blind, placebo-controlled trial. Ann Intern Med 2001;135:939-953.

5-8 Hammond CB, Nachtigall LE. Is estrogen replacement therapy necessary? Journal of Reproductive Medicine. 1985:30(10 Suppl):797-801.

5-9 Hulley S, Grady D, Bush T, et al. Randomized trial of estrogen plus progestin for secondary prevention of coronary heart disease in postmenopausal women: Heart and Estrogen/Progestin Replacement Study (HERS) research group. JAMA 1998; 280:605-613.

5-10 Rossouw J, Anderson G, et al. Writing Group for the WHI Investigators. Risks and benefits of estrogen plus progestin in healthy postmenopausal women: principal results from the WHI Randomized Controlled Trial. JAMA. 2002;288(3):321.

5-11 Pines A. Women's Health Initiative and rate of hormone use: a study that impacted a whole generation. Menopause. June 2018;25(6):586-588.

Chapter 6: The WHI – The Good, the Bad, and the Ugly

6-1 Rossouw J, Anderson G, et al. Writing Group for the Women's Health Initiative Investigators. Risks and benefits of estrogen plus progestin in healthy postmenopausal women: Principal results from the Women's Health Initiative Randomized Controlled Trial. JAMA. 2002;288(3):321.

6-2 Anderson G, Limacher M, et al. Women's Health Initiative Steering Committee. Effects of conjugated equine estrogen in postmenopausal women with hysterectomy: The Women's Health Initiative Randomized Controlled Trial. JAMA. 2004;291(14):1701.

6-3 From The New York Times: Gina Kolata with Melody Petersen, JULY 10, 2002; and Francie Grace CBS July 9, 2002, 2:32 AM.

6-4 Keating N, Cleary P, et al. Use of hormone replacement therapy by postmenopausal women in the United States. Ann Intern Med. 1999;130:545-553.

6-5 Steinkellner A, Denison S, et al. A decade of postmenopausal hormone therapy prescribing in The United States: long term effects of the WHI. Menopause. 2012;19:616-621.

6-6 Sprague B, Trentham-Dietz A, Cronin K. A sustained decline in postmenopausal hormone use: results from the National Health and Nutrition Examination Survey, 1999-2010. Obstet Gynecol. 2012;120:595-603.

6-7 Miller VM, Harman SM. An update on hormone therapy in postmenopausal women: mini-review for the basic scientist. Am J Physiol Heart Circ Physiol. August 2017;313:H1013-H1021.

6-8 Council for International Organizations of Medical Science (CIOMS). Benefit-risk balance for marketed drugs: Evaluating safety signals. Report of CIOMS Working Group IV. Geneva, Switzerland: CIOMS; 1998. Available at: www.cioms.ch/publications/g4-benefit-risk.pdf.

6-9 Rossouw JE, Anderson GL et al. Risks and benefits of estrogen plus progestin in healthy postmenopausal women: principal results from the Women's Health Initiative randomized controlled trial. JAMA. 2002;288(3):321.

6-10 Anderson GL, Limacher M, et al. Effects of conjugated equine estrogen in postmenopausal women with hysterectomy: the Women's Health Initiative randomized controlled trial. JAMA. 2004;291(14):1701.

6-11 Manson J, Aragaki A, Rossouw J, et al. Menopausal hormone therapy and long-term all-cause and cause-specific mortality. The Women's Health Initiative Randomized Trials. JAMA. 2017;318:927-938.

6-12 Langer R, Simon J, et al. Menopausal hormone therapy for primary prevention: why the USPSTF is wrong. Climacteric. 2007;20(5):402-413.

6-13 The 2017 Hormone Therapy Position Statement of The North American Menopause Society. Menopause. 2017;24(7):728-753.

Chapter 7: Estrogen Receptors and the Timing Hypothesis

7-1 Grodstein F, Manson JE, Stampfer MJ. Postmenopausal hormone use and secondary prevention of coronary events in the Nurses' Health Study: a prospective, observational study. Ann Intern Med 2001;135:1-8.

7-2 Hulley S, et al. Randomized trial of estrogen plus progestin for secondary prevention of coronary heart disease in post-menopausal women. JAMA. 1998:280:605-13.

7-3 Waters DD, Alderman EL, Hsia J, et al. Effects of hormone replacement therapy and antioxidant vitamin supplements on coronary atherosclerosis in postmenopausal women: a randomized controlled trial. JAMA. 2002;288:2432-2440.

7-4 Merz CN, Kelsey SF, Pepine CJ, et al. The Women's Ischemia Syndrome Evaluation (WISE) study: protocol design, methodology and feasibility report. J Am Coll Cardiol. 1999;33:1453-1461.

7-5 Angerer P, Stork S, Kothny W, et al. Effect of oral postmenopausal hormone replacement on progression of atherosclerosis: a randomized, controlled trial. Arterioscler Thromb Vasc Biol. 2001; 21:262-268.

7-6 Os I, Hofstad AE, Brekke M, et al. The EWA (Estrogen in Women with Atherosclerosis) study: a randomized study of the use of hormone replacement therapy in women with angiographically verified coronary artery disease. Characteristics of the study population, effects on lipids and lipoproteins. J Intern Med. 2000; 247:433-441.

7-7 Rossouw JE, Anderson GL, Prentice RL, LaCroix AZ, Kooperberg C, Stefanick ML, Jackson RD, Beresford SA, Howard BV, Johnson KC, Kotchen JM, Ockene J, Writing Group for the Women's Health Initiative Investigators, Risks and benefits of estrogen plus progestin in healthy postmenopausal women: principal results from the Women's Health Initiative randomized controlled trial. JAMA. 2002;288(3):321.

7-8 Hernan MA, Alonso A, Logan R, et al. Observational studies analyzed like randomized experiments: an application to postmenopausal hormone therapy and coronary heart disease. Epidemiology. 2008;19:766-779.

7-9 Rossouw JE, Prentice RL, Manson JE, et al. Postmenopausal hormone therapy and risk of cardiovascular disease by age and years since menopause. JAMA. 2007;297:1465-1477.

7-10 LaCroix AZ, Chlebowski RT, Manson JE, et al. Health outcomes after stopping conjugated equine estrogens among postmenopausal women with prior hysterectomy: a randomized controlled trial. JAMA. 2011;305:1305-1314.

7-11 Harman SM, Brinton EA, Cedars M, et al. KEEPS: The Kronos Early Estrogen Prevention Study. Climacteric. 2005; 8:3-12.

7-12 Mosekilde L, Hermann AP, Beck-Nielsen H, et al. The Danish Osteoporosis Prevention Study (DOPS): project design and inclusion of 2000 normal perimenopausal women. Maturitas. 1999; 31:207-219.

7-13 Schierbeck LL, Rejnmark L, et al. Effect of hormone replacement therapy on cardiovascular events in recently postmenopausal women: randomized trial. BMJ. 2012;345:e6409.

7-14 Mikkola TS, Tuomikoski P, Lyytinen H, et al. Estradiol-based postmenopausal hormone therapy and risk of cardiovascular and all-cause mortality. Menopause. 2015; 22:976-983.

7-15 Boardman HM, Hartley L, Eisinga A, et al. Hormone therapy for preventing cardiovascular disease in post-menopausal women. Cochrane Database Syst Rev. 2015;CD002229.

7-16 Hodis HN, Mack WJ, Henderson VW, et al. Vascular effects of early versus late postmenopausal treatment with estradiol. New Engl J Med. 2016;374:1221-1231.

7-17 Rosenfeld ME, Kauser K, Martin-McNulty B, et al. Estrogen inhibits the initiation of fatty streaks throughout the vasculature but does not inhibit intra-plaque hemorrhage and the progression of established lesions in apolipoprotein E deficient mice. Atherosclerosis. 2002;164:251-259.

7-18 Clarkson TB et al. Estrogen effects on arteries vary with stage of reproductive life and extent of subclinical atherosclerosis progression. Menopause. 2007;14:373-384.

7-19 Suzuki S, et al. Timing of estrogen therapy after ovariectomy dictates the efficacy of its neuroprotective and anti-inflammatory actions. Proc Natl Acad Sci USA. 2007;104:6013-8.

7-20 Shumaker S, Legault C, Rapp S, et al. Estrogen plus progestin and the incidence of dementia and mild cognitive impairment in postmenopausal women: The Women's Health Initiative Memory Study: A randomized controlled trial. JAMA. 2003;289(20):2651-62.

7-21 Louet JF, LeMay C, et al. Antidiabetic actions of estrogen: insight from human and genetic mouse models. Curr Atheroscler Rep. 2004;6(3):180.

7-22 Pereira RI, Casey BA, Swibas TA, et al. Timing of estradiol treatment after menopause may determine benefit or harm to insulin action. J Clin Endocrinol Metab. 2015;100:4456-62.

7-23 Shang DP, Lian HY, et al. Relationship between estrogen receptor 1 gene polymorphisms and postmenopausal osteoporosis of the spine in Chinese women. Genet Mol Res. 2016 Jun 3;15(2).

7-24 Smith EP, Boyd J, Frank GR, et al. Estrogen resistance caused by a mutation in the estrogen-receptor gene in a man. N Eng J Med. 1994;331(16):1056.

7-25 Schliebs R, Arendt T. The cholinergic system in aging and neuronal degeneration. Behav Brain Res. Aug 2011;221(2):555-63.

7-26 Losordo DW, Kearney M, et al. Expression of the estrogen receptor in normal and atherosclerotic coronary arteries of premenopausal women. Circulation. 1994;89:1501-1510.

7-27 Park YM, Pereira RI. Time since menopause and skeletal muscle estrogen receptors, PGC-1α, and AMPK. Menopause. July 2017;24(7):815-823.

7-28 Tarhouni K, et al. Determination of flow mediated outward remodeling in female rodents: respective roles of age, estrogens and timing. Arterioslcer Thromb Vasc Biol. 2014;34:1281-1289.

7-29 The 2017 Position Statement of the North American Menopause Society. Menopause. 2017;24(7):728-753.

Chapter 8: HRT and the Guidelines

8-1 Menopause. U.S. Food and Drug Administration website. https://www.fda.gov/consumers/womens-health-topics/menopause.

8-2 Speroff, Leon. The Menopause: A Signal for the Future. In: Treatment of the Postmenopausal Woman, edited by Rogerio Lobo. New York. Raven Press; 1994:1-8.

8-3 Paganini-Hill, A. Morbidity and Mortality Changes with Estrogen Replacement Therapy. In: Treatment of the Postmenopausal Woman, edited by Rogerio Lobo. New York. Raven Press; 1994:399-404.

8-4 Langer RD, Simon JA, Pines A, Lobo RA, Hodis HN, Pickar JH, Archer DF, Sarrel PM, Utian WH. Menopausal hormone therapy for primary prevention: why the USPSTF is wrong. Climacteric. 2017; 20 (5):402-413.

8-5 The 2017 Hormone Therapy Position Statement of the North American Menopause Society. Menopause. July 2017;24(7):728-753.

Chapter 9: Estrogen and Your Uterus and Ovaries

9-1 Wright JD, Herzog TJ, Tsui J, et al. Nationwide trends in the performance of inpatient hysterectomy in the United States. Obstet Gynecol. 2013;122:233-247.

9-2 Thakar R, Ayers S, Clarkson P, Stanton S, Manyonda I. Outcomes after total versus subtotal abdominal hysterectomy. N Engl J Med. 2002;347:1318-1325.

9-3 Kuppermann M, Summitt R, Varner R, et al. Sexual functioning after total compared with supracervical hysterectomy: a randomized trial. Obstet Gynecol. 2005;105:1309-1318.

9-4 Brown, D. Laparoscopic or vaginal hysterectomy? Menopause. January 2015; 22(1):9-11.

9-5 FDA Updated Assessment of The Use of Laparoscopic Power Morcellators to Treat Uterine Fibroids. December 2017. https://www.fda.gov/MedicalDevices/ProductsandMedicalProcedures/SurgeryandLife Support/ucm584463.htm.

9-6 Hunter MS. Long-term impacts of early and surgical menopause. Menopause. March 2012;19 (3):253-254.

9-7 Mahal AS, Rhoads, KF, et al. Inappropriate oophorectomy at time of benign premenopausal hysterectomy. Menopause. 2017;24(8):8:947-953.

9-8 Farquhar CM, Sadler L, Harvey SA, Stewart AW. The association of hysterectomy and menopause: a prospective cohort study. BJOG. 2005;112(7):956.

9-9 Laughlin-Tommaso SK, Stewart EA, Grossardt BR, et al. Incidence, time trends, laterality, indications, and pathological findings of unilateral oophorectomy before menopause. Menopause. May 2014;21(5):442-449.

9-10 Chen L, Berek JS. Endometrial carcinoma: epidemiology and risk factors. UoToDate review article, updated July 7, 2017. http://seer.cancer.gov/statfacts/html/corp.html.

9-11 Chlebowski RT, Anderson GL. Continuous combined estrogen plus progestin and endometrial cancer: The Women's Health Initiative Randomized Trial. J Natl Cancer Inst. Dec. 2015 14:108(3) djv350.

9-12 Davey DA. Menopausal hormone therapy: a better and safer future. Climacteric. 2018;21:(5):454-461.

9-13 Ziegler D, Ferriani R, et al. Vaginal progesterone in menopause: crinone 4% in cyclical and constant combined regimens. Reprod. 2000;15 Suppl 1:149.

9-14 O'Donnell RL, Clement KM, Edmondson RJ. Hormone replacement therapy after treatment for a gynaecological malignancy. Curr Opin Obstet Gynecol. 2016; 28: 32-41.

9-15 Manta L, Suciu N, Toader O, et al. The etiopathogenesis of uterine fibromatosis. J Med Life. 2016; 9:39-45.

9-16 Srinivasan, V, Martens, MG. Hormone therapy in menopausal women with fibroids: is it safe? Menopause. August 2018;25(8):930-936.

9-17 Marsden J, Sturdee D. Cancer issues. Best Pract Res Clin Obstet Gynaecol. 2009;23:87-107.

9-18 Baber RJ, Panay A, Fenton A. The IMS Writing Group 2016. Recommendations on women's midlife health and menopause hormone therapy. Climacteric. 2016; 19(2):109-150.

9-19 Li D, Ding CY, Qiu LH. Postoperative hormone replacement therapy for epithelial ovarian cancer patients: a systematic review and metaanalysis. Gynecol Oncol. 2015;139:355-362.

9-20 Gabriel CA, Tigges-Cardwell J, et al. Use of total abdominal hysterectomy and hormone replacement therapy in BRCA1 and BRCA2 mutation carriers undergoing risk reducing salpingo-oophorectomy. Fam Cancer. 2009;8:23-28.

Chapter 10: Estrogen and Your Breasts

10-1 Hsieh C, Trichopoulos D, et al. Age at menarche, age at menopause, height and obesity as risk factors for breast cancer: associations and interactions in an international case-control study. Int J Cancer. 1990;46(5):796.

10-2 Bittner, J. The causes and control of mammary cancer in mice. Harvey Lect. 1948: 42:221.

10-3 Colditz GA, Hankinson SE, Hunter DL, et al. The use of estrogens and progestins and the risk of breast cancer in postmenopausal women. NEJM. 1995;332:1589-1593.

10-4 Collaborative group on hormonal factors in breast cancer. Breast cancer and hormone replacement therapy: collaborative reanalysis of data from 51 epidemiological studies of 52,705 women with breast cancer and 108,411 women without breast cancer. Lancet. 1997; 350(9084):1047.

10-5 Beral V. Million women study collaborators, breast cancer and hormone replacement therapy in the Million Women study. Lancet. 2003;362(9382):419.

10-6 Fournier A, Berrino F, Riboli E, et al. Breast cancer risk in relation to different types of hormone replacement therapy in the E3N-EPIC cohort. Int J Cancer. 2005;114:448-454.

10-7 Lee S, Ross R, et al. An overview of menopausal oestrogen-progestin hormone therapy and breast cancer risk. Br. J. Cancer. 2005; 92:2049-58.

10-8 Farhat G, Parimi N, Chlebowski R, et al. Sex hormone levels and risk of breast cancer with estrogen plus progestin. J Natl Cancer Inst. Oct. 2013;2;105 (19):1496-503.

10-9 National Institutes of Health. NHLBI Stops Trial of Estrogen Plus Progestin Due to Increased Breast Cancer Risk, Lack of Overall Benefit. Press release, July 9, 2002. Available from: http://www.nhlbi.nih.gov/whi/pr_02-7-9.pdf.

10-10 McTiernan A, Martin C, et al. Estrogen-plus-progestin use and mammographic density in postmenopausal women: Women's Health Initiative randomized trial. J Natl Cancer Inst. 2005;97(18):1366.

10-11 Greendale G, Reboussin B, Sie A, et al. Effects of estrogen and estrogen-progestin on mammographic parenchymal density. Postmenopausal Estrogen/Progestin Interventions (PEPI) investigators. Ann Intern Med. 1999;130:262.

10-12 Fournier A, Mesrine S, Dossus L, et al. Risk of breast cancer after stopping menopausal hormone therapy in the E3N Cohort. Breast Cancer Res Treat. 2014; 145:535-543.

10-13 Lignières B, de Vathaire F, Fournier S, et al. Combined hormone replacement therapy and risk of breast cancer in a French cohort study of 3175 women. Climacteric. 2002;5:332-340.

10-14 Yang Z, Hu Y. Estradiol therapy and breast cancer risk in perimenopausal and postmenopausal women: a systematic review and meta-analysis. Gynecol Endocrinol. 2017 Feb;33(2):87-92.

10-15 Fournier A, Berrino F, Riboli E, et al. Breast cancer risk in relation to different types of hormone replacement therapy in the E3N-EPIC Cohort. Int J Cancer. 2005;114:448-454.

10-16 Ruan X, et al. Increased expression of progesterone receptor membrane component 1 is associated with aggressive phenotype and poor prognosis in ER positive and negative breast cancer. Menopause. 2016;24(2):203.

10-17 Chlebowski R, Rohan T, et al. Breast cancer after use of estrogen plus progestin and estrogen alone: analyses of data from 2 Women's Health Initiative randomized clinical trials. JAMA Oncol. June 2015;1(3):296-305.

10-18 Position Statement. The 2017 hormone therapy position statement of the North American Menopause Society. Menopause. July 2017;24(7):728-753.

10-19 Santen RJ. Menopausal hormone therapy and breast cancer. J Steroid Biochem Mol Biol. July 2014;142:52-61.

10-20 Santen RJ, Yue W, Heitjan DF. Modeling of the growth kinetics of occult breast tumors: role in interpretation of studies of prevention and menopausal hormone therapy. Cancer Epidemiol Biomarkers Prev. 2012;21:1038-48.

10-21 Schierbeck L, Rejnmark L, Tofteng C, et al. Effect of hormone replacement therapy on cardiovascular events in recently postmenopausal women: randomized trial. BMJ. 2012;345:e6409.

10-22 Holm M, Olsen A, Kroman N, Tjonneland A. Lifestyle influences on the association between pre-diagnostic hormone replacement therapy and breast cancer prognosis: results from the Danish diet, cancer and health prospective cohort. Maturitas 2014; 79:442.

10-23 Mikkola T, Savolainen-Peltonen H, Tuomikoski P, et al. Reduced risk of breast cancer mortality in women using postmenopausal hormone therapy: a Finnish nationwide comparative study. Menopause. 2016; 23:1199-1203.

10-24 Manson J, Aragaki A, Rossouw J, et al. Menopausal hormone therapy and long-term all-cause and cause-specific mortality: the Women's Health Initiative randomized trials. JAMA. 2017; 318(10):927-938.

10-25 Sener S, Winchester D, et al. The effects of hormone replacement therapy on postmenopausal breast cancer biology and survival. Am J Surg. 2009;197(3):403.

10-26 Bakken K, Fournier A, et al. Menopausal hormone therapy and breast cancer risk: impact of different treatments. The European Prospective Investigation into Cancer and Nutrition. Int J Cancer. 2011;128(1):144.

10-27 Chlebowski R, Anderson G. Changing concepts: menopausal hormone therapy and breast cancer. J Natl Cancer Inst. 2012;104:517-27.

10-28 Prentice R. Postmenopausal hormone therapy and the risks of coronary heart disease, breast cancer, and stroke. Semin Reprod Med. 2014;32:419-425.

10-29 Shah N, Borenstein J, Dubois R. Postmenopausal hormone therapy and breast cancer: a systematic review and meta-analysis. Menopause. 2005;12:668-678.

10-30 Chlebowski R, Anderson G. Menopausal hormone therapy and cancer: changing clinical observations of target site specificity. Steroids. 2014;90:53-59.

10-31 Collaborative Group on Hormone Factors in Breast Cancer. Lancet. 2019;394:1159-1168.

10-32 Eden JA, Bush T, Nand S, et al. A case-control study of combined continuous estrogen-progestin replacement therapy among women with a personal history of breast cancer. Menopause. 1995;2:67-72.

10-33 Dew J, Eden J, Beller E, et al. A cohort study of hormone replacement therapy given to women previously treated for breast cancer. Climacteric. 1998;1:137-42.

10-34 O'Meara ES, Rossing MA, Daling JR, et al. Hormone replacement therapy after a diagnosis of breast cancer in relation to recurrence and mortality. J Natl Cancer Inst. 2001;93:754-62.

10-35 Meurer LN, Lená S. Cancer recurrence and mortality in women using hormone replacement therapy: meta-analysis. J Fam Pract. 2002;51:1056-62.

10-36 Durna EM, Heller GZ, Leader LR, et al. Breast cancer in premenopausal women: recurrence and survival rates and relationship to hormone replacement therapy. Climacteric. 2004;7:284-91.

10-37 Bluming A, Tavris C. Estrogen matters: why taking hormones in menopause can improve women's well-being and lengthen their lives - without raising the risk of breast cancer. New York, NY:Little, Brown Spark. Hachette Book Group;2019.

Chapter 11: Estrogen and Your Bones

11-1 Karim R, Dell R, Greene D, et al. Hip fractures in postmenopausal women after cessation of hormone therapy: results from a prospective study in a large health management organization. Menopause. 2011;18:1172-1177.

11-2 Johnell O, Kanis JA. An estimate of the worldwide prevalence and disability associated with osteoporotic fractures. Osteoporos Int. 2006;17(12):1726.

11-3 Panula J, et al. Mortality and cause of death in hip fractures age 65 and older: a population based study. BMC Musculoskel Disorders. 2011;(12):105.

11-4 Warming L, Hassager C, Christiansen C. Changes in bone mineral density with age in men and women: a longitudinal study. Osteoporosis Int. 2002;13(2):105.

11-5 Finkelstein, JS, Brockwell SE, et al. Bone mineral density changes during the menopause transition in a multiethnic cohort of women. J Clin Endocrinol Metab. March 2008;93(3):861-868.

11-6 Orces CH. In-hospital hip fracture mortality trends in older adults: the national hospital discharge survey, 1988-2007. J Am Geriatr Soc. 2013;61(12):2248.

11-7 Panula J, Pihlajamäki H, Mattila VM, et al. Mortality and cause of death in hip fracture patients aged 65 or older: a population-based study. BMC Musculoskelet Disord. 2011;12:105.

11-8 Empana JP, Dargent-Molina P, Béart G, et al. Effect of hip fracture on mortality in elderly women: The EPIDOS prospective study. J Am Geriatr Soc. 2004;52:685-90.

11-9 International Osteoporosis Foundation. Facts and Statistics. https://www.iofbonehealth.org/facts-statistics.

11-10 Kanis JA. World Health Organization (2007) Assessment of osteoporosis at the primary health care level. Summary report of a WHO scientific group. WHO, Geneva. www.who.int/chp/topics/rheumatic/en/index.html.

11-11 Estrada K, Styrkarsdottir U, et al. Genome-wide meta-analysis identifies 56 bone mineral density loci and reveals 14 loci associated with risk of fracture. Nat Genet. 2012;44(5):491.

11-12 Zhu L, et al. Effect of hormone therapy on the risk of bone fractures: a systematic review and meta-analysis of randomized controlled trials. Menopause. April 2016;23 (4):461-70.

11-13 Villareal D, Binder E, Williams D. Bone mineral density response to estrogen replacement in frail elderly women: a randomized controlled trial. JAMA. 2001;286(7):815.

11-14 Lufkin E, Wahner H, O'Fallon W. Treatment of postmenopausal osteoporosis with transdermal estrogen. Ann Intern Med. 1992;117(1):1.

11-15 The North American Menopause Society. The 2017 Hormone Therapy Position Statement. Menopause. July 2017;24(7):728-753.

11-16 Prior JC. Progesterone for the prevention and treatment of osteoporosis in women. Climacteric. 2018;21(4):366-374.

11-17 Seifert-Klauss V, Schmidmayr M, et al. Progesterone and bone: a closer link than previously realized. Climacteric. 2012;15:sup1: 26-31.

11-18 Benhamou C. Effects of osteoporosis medications on bone quality. Joint Bone Spine. 2007;74:39-47.

11-19 Kalyan S, et al. Systemic immunity shapes the oral microbiome and susceptibility to bisphosphonate associated osteonecrosis of the jaw. J. Transl Med. 2015:13:212.

11-20 Shane E, Burr D, Abrahamsen B, et al. Atypical subtrochanteric and diaphyseal femoral fractures: second report of a task force of the American Society for Bone and Mineral Research. J Bone Miner Res. 2014;29(1):1.

11-21 Khosla S et al. Benefits and risks of bisphosphonate therapy for osteoporosis. J Clin Endocrinol Metab. July 2012;97(7):2272-82 .

11-22 Lamy O, Gonzalez-Rodriguez E, et al. Severe rebound-associated vertebral fractures after denosumab discontinuation: 9 clinical cases report. J Clin Endocrinol Metab. 2017;102(2):354.

11-23 Anastasilakis AD, Polyzos SA et al. Clinical features of 24 patients with rebound-associated vertebral fractures after denosumab discontinuation: systematic review and additional cases. J Bone Miner Res. 2017;32(6):1291.

11-24 Rosen, H. Selective estrogen receptor modulators for prevention and treatment of osteoporosis. From UpToDate Review, updated January 12, 2018. https://www.uptodate.com/contents/selective-estrogen-receptor-modulators-for-prevention-and-treatment-of-osteoporosis.

11-25 Cosman F, Crittenden D, Adachi JD, et al. Romosozumab treatment in postmenopausal women with osteoporosis. N Engl J Med. 2016;375(16):1532.

11-26 Papadakis G, et al. The benefits of menopausal hormone therapy on bone density and microarchitecture persists after its withdrawal. J. Clin. Endocrine Metab. December 2016;12:5004-5011.

11-27 Penning-van Beest FJ, Goettsch WG, Erkens JA. Determinants of persistence with bisphosphonates: a study in women with postmenopausal osteoporosis. Clin Ther. Feb. 2006;28(2):236-42.

11-28 Wang Z, Ward MM, Chan L, Bhattacharyya T. Adherence to oral bisphosphonates and the risk of subtrochanteric and femoral shaft fractures among female Medicare beneficiaries. Osteoporos Int. 2014;25:2109-16.

Chapter 12: Estrogen and Your Heart

12-1 Women's Heart Foundation. Women and Heart Disease Fact Sheet. 2006. Available from: http://www.womensheart.org/content.

12-2 Colditz GA, Willett WC, Stampfer MJ, et al. Menopause and the risk of coronary heart disease in women. N Engl J Med. 1987;316:1105-10.

12-3 Roger VL, Go AS, et al. Heart disease and stroke statistics: 2011 update: a report from the American Heart Association. Circulation. 2011;123e: 18-19.

12-4 Ford ES, Capewell S. Coronary heart disease mortality among young adults in the US from 1980 through 2002. Concealed leveling of mortality rates. J Am Coll Cardiol. 2007;50:2128-2132.

12-5 Stampfer MJ, Colditz GA. Estrogen replacement therapy and coronary heart disease: a quantitative assessment of the epidemiologic evidence. Prev Med. 1991:20:47-63.

12-6 Stampfer MJ, Colditz GA, et al. Postmenopausal estrogen therapy and cardiovascular disease. ten-year follow-up from the Nurses' Health study. NEJM. Sept 1991;325(11):756-62.

12-7 Goff DC, Lloyd-Jones DM, et al. 2013 ACC/AHA guideline on the assessment of cardiovascular risk: a report of the American College of Cardiology/American Heart Association Task Force on Practice Guidelines. J Am Coll Cardiol. July 2014;63(25 Pt B):2935 - 2959.

12-8 Charchar FJ, Bloomer LD, Barnes TA, et al. Inheritance of coronary artery disease in men: an analysis of the role of the Y chromosome. Lancet. 2012; 379:915.

12-9 Rivera CM, Grossardt BR, Rhodes DJ, et al. Increased cardiovascular mortality after early bilateral oophorectomy. Menopause. 2009;16:15-23.

12-10 Shuster LT, Rhodes DJ, et al. Premature menopause or early menopause: long-term health consequences. Maturitas. 2010;65:161-6.

12-11 Wellons M, Ouyang P, et al. Early menopause predicts future coronary heart disease and stroke: the Multi-Ethnic Study of Atherosclerosis. Menopause. 2012;19:1081-7.

12-12 Muka T, Oliver-Williams C, et al. Association of age at onset of menopause and time since onset of menopause with cardiovascular outcomes, intermediate vascular traits, and all-cause mortality: a systematic review and meta-analysis. JAMA Cardiol. 2016;1:767-776.

12-13 Ley SH, Li Y, Tobias DK, Manson JE, et al. Duration of reproductive life span, age at menarche, and age at menopause are associated with risk of cardiovascular disease in women. J Am Heart Assoc. 2017;6. pii: e006713.

12-14 Matthews KA, Crawford SL, Chae CU, et al. Are changes in cardiovascular disease risk factors in midlife women due to chronological aging or to the menopausal transition? J Am Coll Cardiol. 2009; 54:2366-2373.

12-15 El Khoudary SR, Wang L, Brooks MM, et al. Increase HDL-C level over the menopausal transition is associated with greater atherosclerotic progression. J Clin Lipidol. 2016; 10:962-969.

12-16 Issa, Z, Seely, EW. Effects of hormone therapy on blood pressure. Menopause. April 2015;22(4):456-468.

12-17 Pollow DP Jr, Romero-Aleshire MJ. ANG II-induced hypertension in the VCD mouse model of menopause is prevented by estrogen replacement during perimenopause. American Journal of Physiology, Regulatory, Integrative and Comparative Physiology. Dec 2015;309(12):R1546-52.

12-18 Shimbo D, Wang L, Lamonte MJ, et al. The effect of hormone therapy on mean blood pressure and visit-to-visit blood pressure variability in postmenopausal women: results from the Women's Health Initiative randomized controlled trials. J Hypertens. Oct 2014;32(10):2071-81.

12-19 Harman SM, Brinton EA, Cedars M, et al. KEEPS: The Kronos Early Estrogen Prevention Study. Climacteric. 2005;8:3-12.

12-20 Rownley KA, et. al. Cardiovascular effects of 6 months of hormone replacement therapy versus placebo: differences associated with years since menopause. American Journal of Obstetrics And Gynecology. April 2004;190 (4):1052-8.

12-21 Zacharieva S, Shigarminova R, Nachev E, et al. Ambulatory blood pressure monitoring and active renin in menopausal women treated with amlodipine and hormone replacement therapy. The Official Journal of the International Society of Gynecological Endocrinology. July 2004;19 (1):26-32.

12-22 Boschitsch E, Mayerhofer S, Magometschnigg D. Hypertension in women: the role of progesterone and aldosterone. Climacteric. 2010;13:307-13.

12-23 Pu D, Tan, R, et al. Metabolic syndrome in menopause and associated factors: a meta-analysis. Climateric. 2017;20(6):583-591.

12-24 Menke A, Casagrande S, Geiss L, Cowie CC. Prevalence of and trends in diabetes among adults in the United States. JAMA. Sept. 2015;314(10):1021-9.

12-25 Dørum A, Tonstad S, Liavaag AH, et al. Bilateral oophorectomy before 50 years of age is significantly associated with the metabolic syndrome and Framingham risk score: a controlled, population-based study (HUNT-2). Gynecol Oncol. 2008;109:377-83.

12-26 Michelsen TM, Pripp AH, Tonstad S, et al. Metabolic syndrome after risk-reducing salpingo-oophorectomy in women at high risk for hereditary breast ovarian cancer: a controlled observational study. Eur J Cancer. 2009;45:82-9.

12-27 Mauvais-Jarvis F, Manson JE, Stevenson JC, Fonseca VA. Menopausal hormone therapy and type 2 diabetes prevention: evidence, mechanisms and clinical implications. Endocr Rev. 2017;38:173-88.

12-28 Kanaya AM, Herrington D, Vittinghoff E, Lin F, et al. Glycemic effects of postmenopausal hormone therapy: the Heart and Estrogen/Progestin Replacement Study. A randomized, double-blind, placebo-controlled trial. Ann Intern Med. 2003;138(1):1-9.

12-29 Espeland MA, Hogan PE, Fineberg SE, et al. Effect of postmenopausal hormone therapy on glucose and insulin concentrations. PEPI Investigators. Postmenopausal Estrogen/Progestin Interventions. Diabetes Care. 1998;21:1589-95.

12-30 Margolis KL, Bonds DE, Rodabough RJ, et al. The Women's Health Initiative Investigators. Effect of oestrogen plus progestin on the incidence of diabetes in postmenopausal women: results from the Women's Health Initiative hormone trial. Diabetologia. 2004;47:1175-87.

12-31 Bonds DE, Lasser N, Qi L, et al. The effect of conjugated equine oestrogen on diabetes incidence: the Women's Health Initiative Randomized Trial. Diabetologia. 2006;49:459-68.

12-32 Xu Y, Lin J, Wang S, Xiong J, Zhu Q. Combined estrogen replacement therapy on metabolic control in postmenopausal women with diabetes mellitus. Kaohsiung J Med Sci. 2014;30:350-61.

12-33 Sumino H, et al. Effect of transdermal hormone replacement therapy on the monocyte chemoattractan protein 1 concentrations and other vascular inflammatory markers on the endothelial function in postmenopausal women. Am J. Cardio. 2005;96:148-53.

12-34 Yasui T, Maegawa M, Tomita J, et al. Changes in serum cytokine concentrations during the menopausal transition. Maturitas. 2007; 56:396-403.

12-35 Georgiadou P, Sbarouni E. Effect of hormone replacement therapy on inflammatory biomarkers. Adv Clin Chem. 2009; 47:59-93.

12-36 Lakoski SG, Herrington DM. Effects of hormone therapy on C-reactive protein and IL-6 in postmenopausal women: a review article. Climacteric. 2005; 8:317-326.

12-37 Abdi F, Mobedi. Effects of hormone replacement therapy on immunological factors in the postmenopausal period. Climacteric. 2016 Jun;19(3):234-9.

12-38 Njølstad I, Arnesen E, Lund-Larsen PG. Smoking, serum lipids, blood pressure, and sex differences in myocardial infarction. A 12-year follow-up of the Finnmark Study. Circulation. 1996;93(3):450.

12-39 Prescott E, Hippe M, Schnohr P, Hein HO, Vestbo J. Smoking and risk of myocardial infarction in women and men: a longitudinal population study. BMJ. 1998;316(7137):1043.

12-40 He J, Vupputuri S, Allen K, Prerost MR. Passive smoking and the risk of coronary heart disease-a meta-analysis of epidemiologic studies. N Engl J Med. 1999;340(12):920-926.

12-41 Mehta LS, Watson KE, et al. Cardiovascular disease and breast cancer: where these entities intersect: a scientific statement from the American Heart Association and on behalf of the American Heart Association Cardiovascular Disease in Women and Special Populations Committee of the Council on Clinical Cardiology; Council on Cardiovascular and Stroke Nursing; and Council on Quality of Care and Outcomes Research. Circulation. 2018;137:e30-e66.

12-42 Wilson, P. Overview of possible risk factors for cardiovascular disease. From: UpToDate Dec. 2017 https://www.uptodate.com/contents/overview-of-established-risk-factors-for-cardiovascular-disease.

12-43 Hulley S, Grady D, Bush T, et al. Randomized trial of estrogen plus progestin for secondary prevention of coronary heart disease in postmenopausal women: Heart and Estrogen/Progestin Replacement Study (HERS) research group. JAMA. 1998; 280:605-613.

12-44 Rossouw J, Anderson G, et al. Writing Group for the Women's Health Initiative Investigators. Risks and benefits of estrogen plus progestin in healthy postmenopausal women: principal results from the Women's Health Initiative Randomized Controlled Trial. JAMA. 2002;288(3):321.

12-45 Anderson G, Limacher M, Assaf AR et al. Effects of conjugated equine estrogen in postmenopausal women with hysterectomy: the Women's Health Initiative randomized controlled trial. JAMA. 2004: 291:1701-2.

12-46 Hodis HN, Mack WJ et al. Vascular Effects of Early vs. Late Postmenopausal Treatment with Estradiol. New England Journal of Medicine. 2016:374:1221-31.

12-47 Kearney JF and Solomon CG. Postmenopausal hormone therapy and atherosclerosis - time is of the essence. NEJM. 2016;374(13):1279-80.

12-48 Manson JE, Allison MA, Rossouw JE, et al. Estrogen therapy and coronary-artery calcification. N Engl J Med. 2007;356:2591-602.

12-49 E Manson JE, Cheblowski RT, Stefanick ML, et al. Menopausal hormone therapy and health outcomes during the intervention and extended post stopping phases of the Women's Health Initiative randomized trials. JAMA. 2013;310:1353-68.

12-50 Grodstein F, Manson J, Stampfer MJ. Hormone therapy and coronary heart disease: the role of time since menopause and age at hormone initiation. J Womens Health. 2006;15:35-44.

12-51 Rossouw JE, Prentice RL, Manson JE, et al. Postmenopausal hormone therapy and risk of cardiovascular disease by age and years since menopause. JAMA. 2007;297:1465-1477.

12-52 Schierbeck LL; Rejnmark L, et al. Effect of hormone replacement therapy on cardiovascular events in recently postmenopausal women: randomised trial. BMJ. Oct. 2012;9(345): e6409.

12-53 Boardman HM, et. al. Hormone therapy for preventing cardiovascular disease in post-menopausal women. Cochrane Database Syst. Rev 2015;(3):CD002229.

12-54 Gudmundsson A, Aspelund T, Sigurdsson G, et al. Long-term hormone replacement therapy is associated with low coronary artery calcium levels in a cohort of older women: the Age, Gene/Environment Susceptibility-Reykjavik Study. J Am Geriatr Soc. Jan. 2017;65(1):200-206.

12-55 Rosenfeld ME, Kauser K, et al. Estrogen inhibits the initiation of fatty streaks throughout the vasculature but does not inhibit intra-plaque hemorrhage and the progression of established lesions in apolipoprotein E deficient mice. Atherosclerosis. 2002; 164:251-259.

12-56 Clarkson TB, Appt SE. Controversies about HRT: lessons from monkey models. Maturitas. 2005; 51:64-74.

12-57 Schachinger V, Zeiher AM. Prognostic implications of endothelial dysfunction: does it mean anything? Coron Artery Dis. 2001;12:435-44.

12-58 Usselman, CW, Stachenfeld MS et al. The molecular actions of estrogen in the regulation of vascular health. Exp Physiol. 2016;101: 356-61.

12-59 Hu FB, Grodstein F, Hennekens CH, et al. Age at natural menopause and risk of cardiovascular disease. Arch Intern Med. 1999;159(10):1061.

12-60 Mondul AM, Rodriguez C, Jacobs EJ. Age at natural menopause and cause-specific mortality. Am J Epidemiol. 2005;162(11):1089.

12-61 Morselli E. Santos RS, The effects of oestrogens and their receptors on cardiometabolic health. Nat Rev Endocrinol. June 2017;13(6):352-364.

12-62 Herrington DM, Expeland MA, Crouse JR, et al. Estrogen replacement and brachial artery flow-mediated vasodilation in older women. Arterioscler Thromb Vasc. Biol. 2001;21:1955-61.

12-63 Hurtado R, Celani M, et al. Effect of short-term estrogen therapy on endothelial function: a double-blinded, randomized, controlled trial. Climacteric. 2016;19(5): 448-451.

12-64 Miller VM, Duckles SP. Vascular actions of estrogens: functional implications. Pharmacol Rev. 2008; 60:210-241.

12-65 Pinna C. Cignarella A, et al. Prolonged ovarian hormone deprivation impairs the protective vascular actions of estrogen receptor alpha agonists. Hypertension. 2008: 51: 1210-7.

12-66 Bowling MR, Xing D et al. Estrogen effects on vascular inflammation are age dependent: role of estrogen receptors. Arterioscler Thromb Vasc Biol. 2014: 34:1477-85.

12-67 Dorszewska J. Cell biology of normal brain aging: synaptic plasticity-cell death. Aging Clin Exp Res. April 2013;25(1):25-34.

12-68 Losordo DW, Kearney M, Kim EA, et al. Variable expression of the estrogen receptor in normal and atherosclerotic coronary arteries of premenopausal women. Circulation. 1994;89:1501-1510.

12-69 Rosenfeld ME, Kauser K, Martin-McNulty B, Polinsky P, et al. Estrogen inhibits the initiation of fatty streaks throughout the vasculature but does not inhibit intra-plaque hemorrhage and the progression of established lesions in apolipoprotein E deficient mice. Atherosclerosis. 2002;164:251-259.

12-70 Hodgin JB, Krege JH, Reddick RL, Korach KS. Estrogen receptor alpha is a major mediator of 17beta-estradiol's atheroprotective effects on lesion size in Apoe-/- mice. J Clin Invest. 2001;107(3):333.

12-71 Mendelsohn ME, Karas RH. Molecular and cellular basis of cardiovascular gender differences. Science. 2005;308:1583-1587.

12-72 Goffin F, Manaut C, Frankenne F, et al. Expression pattern of metalloproteinases and tissue inhibitors of matrix-metalloproteinases in cycling human endometrium. Biol Reprod. 2003;69:976-984.

12-73 Mikkola TS, Savolainen-Peltonen H. New evidence for cardiac benefit of postmenopausal hormone therapy. Climateric. 2017;20(1):5-10.

12-74 Kim CJ, Min YK, et al. Effect of hormone replacement therapy on lipoprotein(a) and lipid levels in postmenopausal women. Influence of various progestogens and duration of therapy. Arch Intern Med. Aug. 1996;156(15):1693-700.

12-75 Rosano GM, Webb CM, Chierchia S, et al. Natural progesterone, but not medroxyprogesterone acetate, enhances the beneficial effect of estrogen on exercise-induced myocardial ischemia in postmenopausal women. J Am Coll Cardiol. 2000;36:2154-10.

12-76 Gambacciani M, A. Cagnacci A, S. Lello S. Hormone replacement therapy and prevention of chronic conditions. Climacteric. Jan. 2019; DOI:10.1080/ 13697137.2018.1551347.

12-77 Prior JC, Elliott TG, Norman E, et al. Progesterone therapy, endothelial function and cardiovascular risk factors: a 3-month randomized, placebo-controlled trial in healthy early postmenopausal women. PLoS One. JN 2014; 21;9(1):e84698. doi: 10.1371/ journal. pone.0084698. eCollection 2014.

Chapter 13: Estrogen and Your Clotting System

13-1 Simes J, Becattini C, Agnelli G. Aspirin for the prevention of recurrent venous thromboembolism: the INSPIRE collaboration. (International Collaboration of Aspirin Trials for Recurrent Venous Thromboembolism). Circulation. 2014;130(13):1062.

13-2 Pérez Gutthann S, García Rodríguez LA, et al. Hormone replacement therapy and risk of venous thromboembolism: population based case-control study. BMJ. 1997;314(7083):796.

13-3 Miller J, Chan BK, Nelson HD. Postmenopausal estrogen replacement and risk for venous thromboembolism: a systematic review and meta-analysis for the U.S. Preventive Services Task Force. Ann Intern Med. 2002;136(9):680.

13-4 Kujovich JL. Hormones and pregnancy: thromboembolic risks for women. Br J Haematol. 2004;126(4):443.

13-5 Andra H et al. Venous thromboembolism in pregnancy. Arteriosclerosis, Thrombosis, and Vascular Biology. 2009;29:326-331.

13-6 Canonico M, Plu-Bureau G, et al. Hormone replacement therapy and risk of venous thromboembolism in postmenopausal women: systematic review and meta-analysis. BMJ 2008; 336:1227-1231.

13-7 Olié V, Canonico M, Scarabin PY. Risk of venous thrombosis with oral versus transdermal estrogen therapy among postmenopausal women. Curr Opin Hematol. 2010;17:457-463.

13-8 Bergendal A, Kieler H. Risk of venous thromboembolism associated with local and systemic use of hormone therapy in peri- and postmenopausal women and in relation to type and route of administration. Menopause. 2016; 23 (6):593-599.

13-9 Laliberté, F, Dea K. Does the route of administration for estrogen hormone therapy impact the risk of venous thromboembolism? Estradiol transdermal system versus oral estrogen-only hormone therapy. Menopause. Nov. 2018;25(11):1297-1305.

13-10 Simon JA, Laliberté F, Duh MS, et al. Venous thromboembolism and cardiovascular disease complications in menopausal women using transdermal versus oral estrogen therapy. Menopause. 2016;23:600-610.

13-11 Sweetland S, Beral V, Balkwill A, et al. Million Women Study Collaborators: venous thromboembolism risk in relation to use of different types of postmenopausal hormone therapy in a large prospective study. J Thromb Haemost. 2012;10:2277-2286.

13-12 Roach RE, Lijfering WM, Helmerhorst FM, Cannegieter SC, et al. The risk of venous thrombosis in women over 50 years old using oral contraception or postmenopausal hormone therapy. J Thromb Haemost. 2013; 11:124-131.

13-13 The 2017 Hormone Therapy Position Statement of The North American Menopause Society. Menopause. 2017;24(7):728-753.

13-14 Miller VM, Lahr BD, et al. Longitudinal effects of menopausal hormone treatments on platelet characteristics and cell-derived microvesicles. Platelets. 2016;27(1):32-42.

13-15 American College of Gynecologists. ACOG committee opinion no. 556: postmenopausal estrogen therapy: route of administration and risk of venous thromboembolism. Obstet Gynecol. 2013;121:887-890.

13-16 Vickers MR, MacLennan AH, Lawton B, et al. Main morbidities recorded in the Women's International Study of Long Duration Oestrogen After Menopause (WISDOM): a randomised controlled trial of hormone replacement therapy in postmenopausal women. BMJ. 2007;335:239.

13-17 Canonico M, Plu-Bureau G, Scarabin PY. Progestogens and venous thromboembolism among postmenopausal women using hormone therapy. Maturitas. 2011;70:354-360.

13-18 Prior JC, Elliott TG, Norman E, Stajic et al. Progesterone therapy, endothelial function and cardiovascular risk factors: a 3-month randomized, placebo-controlled trial in healthy early postmenopausal women. PLoS One. Jan. 2014;9(1):e84698.

13-19 Canonico M, Fournier A, Carcaillon L, et al. Postmenopausal hormone therapy and risk of idiopathic venous thromboembolism: results from the E3N cohort study. Arterioscler Thromb Vasc Biol. 2010;30:340-345.

13-20 Canonico M, Oger E, Plu-Bureau G, et al. Hormone therapy and venous thromboembolism among postmenopausal women: impact of the route of estrogen administration and progestogens: the ESTHER study. Circulation. 2007;115:840-845.

13-21 Olié, V, Plu-Bureau, G. Hormone therapy and recurrence of venous thromboembolism among postmenopausal women. Menopause. May 2011;18(5):488-493.

Chapter 14: Estrogen and Your Brain

14-1 Lokuge S, Frey B, et al. Depression in women: windows of vulnerability and new insights into the link between estrogen and serotonin. J Clin Psychiatry. 2011:1563-1569.

14-2 Luine V. Estradiol increases choline acetyltransferase activity in specific basal forebrain nuclei and projection areas of female rats. Exp Neurol. 1985;89(2):484.

14-3 Barth C, Villringer A, Sacher J. Sex hormones affect neurotransmitters and shape the adult female brain during hormonal transition periods. Front Neurosci. 2015 Feb 20;1-20.

14- 4 Vargas K, Milic J, Zaciragic A, et al. The functions of estrogen receptor beta in the female brain: a systematic review. Maturitas. 2016 Nov;93:41-57.

14-5 McEwen B. Clinical Review 108: The molecular and neuroanatomical basis for estrogen effects in the central nervous system. J Clin Endocrinol Metab. 1999; 84(6):1790.

14-6 Sárvári M, Kalló I, Hrabovszky E, et al. Hippocampal gene expression is highly responsive to estradiol replacement in middle-aged female rats. Endocrinology. July 2015;156 (7): 2632-45.

14-7 Plassman B, Langa K, et al. Prevalence of dementia in the United States: the aging, demographics, and memory study. Neuroepidemiology. 2007;29(1-2):125-32.

14-8 Murphy D, DeCarli C, et al. Sex differences in human brain morphometry and metabolism: an in vivo quantitative magnetic resonance imaging and positron emission tomography study on the effect of aging. Arch Gen Psychiatry. 1996;53:585-594.

14-9 Lord C, Engert L, et al. Effect of sex and estrogen therapy on the aging brain: a voxel-based morphometry study. Menopause. July 2010;7(4): 846-851.

14-10 Canevelli M. Grande G. et. al. Spontaneous reversion of mild cognitive impairment to normal cognition: a systematic review of literature and meta-analysis. J. Am Med Dir Assoc. Oct 2016;17:948.

14-11 Epperson C, Sammel M, Freeman E. Menopause effects on verbal memory: findings from a longitudinal community cohort. J Clin Endocrinol Metab. 2013;98:3829-3838.

14-12 Berent-Spillson A, Persad C, et al. Hormonal environment affects cognition independent of age during the menopause transition. J Clin Endocrinol Metab. 2012; 97:E1686-E1694.

14-13 Boss L, Kang D, Marcus M, Bergstrom N. Endogenous sex hormones and cognitive function in older adults: a systematic review. West J Nurs Res. 2014; 36:388-426.

14-14 Rentz D, et al. Sex Differences in episodic memory in midlife: impact of reproductive aging. Menopause. November 2017;24(4):400-408.

14-15 Rocca W, et al. Increased risk of cognitive impairment or dementia in women who underwent oophorectomy before menopause. Neurology. Sept. 2007;69 (11):1074-83.

14-16 Shaywitz S, et al. Effect of estrogen on brain activation patterns in postmenopausal women during working memory tasks. JAMA. 1999;281(13):1197.

14-17 Resnick SM, Maki PM, Golski S, et al. Effects of estrogen replacement therapy on PET cerebral blood flow and neuropsychological performance. Horm Behav. 1998;34(2):171.

14-18 Matthews K, Cauley J, Yaffe K, et al. Estrogen replacement therapy and cognitive decline in older community women. J Am Geriatr Soc. 1999;47(5):518.

14-19 LeBlanc E, Janowsky, J. Hormone replacement therapy and cognitive function: systematic review and meta-analysis. JAMA. 2001;285 (11):1489.

14-20 Grady D, Yaffe K, et al. Effect of postmenopausal hormone therapy on cognitive function: the Heart and Estrogen/Progestin Replacement Study. Am J Med. 2002;113:543-548.

14-21 Shumaker S, Legault C, Rapp S, et al. Estrogen plus progestin and the incidence of dementia and mild cognitive impairment in postmenopausal women: the Women's Health Initiative Memory Study: a randomized controlled trial. JAMA. 2003;289(20):2651.

14-22 Yaffe K, Haan M, et al. Estrogen use, APOE, and cognitive decline: evidence of gene-environment interaction. Neurology. 2000;54(10):1949.

14-23 Carlson M, Zandi P, Plassman B, et al. Hormone replacement therapy and reduced cognitive decline in older women: The Cache County Study. Cache County Study Group. Neurology. 2001;57(12):2210.

14-24 Ryan J, Carrière I, et al. Characteristics of hormone therapy, cognitive function, and dementia: the prospective 3C Study. Neurology. 2009;73(21):1729.

14-25 Rice M, Graves A, et al. Postmenopausal estrogen and estrogen-progestin use and 2-year rate of cognitive change in a cohort of older Japanese American women: The Kame Project. Arch Intern Med. 2000;160(11):1641.

14-26 Espeland M, Shumaker S, et al. Long-term Effects on cognitive function of postmenopausal hormone therapy prescribed to women aged 50 to 55 years. WHIMSY Study Group. JAMA Intern Med. 2013;173(15):1429.

14-27 Gleason C, Dowling N, et al. Effects of hormone therapy on cognition and mood in recently postmenopausal women: findings from the randomized, controlled KEEPS-Cognitive and Affective Study. PLoS Med. 2015;12:e1001833.

14-28 Henderson V, St John J, et al. Cognitive effects of estradiol after menopause: a randomized trial of the timing hypothesis. Neurology. 2016;87:699-708.

14-29 Wroolie T, et al. Differences in verbal memory performance in postmenopausal women receiving hormone therapy: 17 beta estradiol versus conjugated equine estrogens. American Journal of Geriatric Psychiatry. Sept. 2011; 19(9):792-802.

14-30 Alzheimer's Association. 2017 Alzheimer's Disease Facts and Figures. Alzheimers Dementia. 2017;13:325-373.

14-31 Holtzman D, Herz J, Bu G. Apolipoprotein E and Apolipoprotein E receptors: normal biology and roles in Alzheimer disease. Cold Spring Harb Perspect Med. 2012;2(3):a006312.

14-32 What APOE means for your health. Alzheimer's Drug Discovery Foundation. Available at: alzdiscovery.org/cognitive-vitality/whatapoe-means-for-your-health. Accessed November 24, 2016.

14-33 Kantarci K, Lowe V, et al. Early postmenopausal transdermal 17β-Estradiol therapy and amyloid-β deposition. J Alzheimers Dis. May 2016;53(2):547-56.

14-34 Pines, A. Alzheimer's disease, menopause and the impact of the estrogenic environment. Climacteric. 2016;19:(5):430-432.

14-35 Jaffe A, Toran-Allerand C, et al. Estrogen regulates metabolism of Alzheimer amyloid beta precursor protein. J Biol Chem. 1994;269(18):13065.

14-36 Paganini-Hill A, Henderson V. Estrogen deficiency and risk of Alzheimer's disease in women. American Journal of Epidemiology. Aug. 1994;140(3):256-261.

14-37 Zandi P, Carlson M, Plassman B, et al. Hormone replacement therapy and incidence of Alzheimer's disease in older women: The Cache County Study. JAMA. 2002;288(17):2123.

14-38 Shumaker S, Legault C, Rapp S, et al. Estrogen plus progestin and the incidence of dementia and mild cognitive impairment in postmenopausal women: The Women's Health Initiative Memory Study: A randomized controlled trial. JAMA. 2003;289(20):2651.

14-39 Bagger Y, Tanko L, et al. PERF Study Group. Early postmenopausal hormone therapy may prevent cognitive impairment later in life. Menopause. 2005;12:12-17.

14-40 Henderson V, Benke K, et al. MIRAGE Study Group. Postmenopausal hormone therapy and Alzheimer's disease risk: interaction with age. J Neurol Neurosurg Psychiatry. 2005;76:103-105.

14-41 Shao H, Breitner J, et al. Cache County Investigators. Hormone therapy and Alzheimer disease dementia: new findings from the Cache County Study. Neurology 2012;79:1846-1852.

14-42 O'Brien J, Jackson J, et al. Postmenopausal hormone therapy is not associated with risk of all-cause dementia and Alzheimer's disease. Epidemiol Rev. 2014;36:83-103.

14-43 Imtiaz B, Tuppurainen M, et al. Postmenopausal hormone therapy and Alzheimer's disease: a prospective cohort study. Neurology. 2017; 88:1062-1068.

14-44 Shumaker S, Legault C, Kuller L, et al. Conjugated equine estrogens and incidence of probable dementia and mild cognitive impairment in postmenopausal women: Women's Health Initiative Memory Study. JAMA. 2004; 291:2947-2958.

14-45 Imtiaz B, Taipale H, Tanskanen A, et al. Risk of Alzheimer's disease among users of postmenopausal hormone therapy: a nationwide case-control study. Maturitas. 2017;98:7-13.

14-46 Berent-Spillson A, Briceno E. Distinct cognitive effects of estrogen and progesterone in menopausal women. Psychoneuroendocrinology. Sept. 2015;59:25-36.

14-47 Asthana S, Baker LD, Craft S, et al. High-dose estradiol improves cognition for women with AD: results of a randomized study. Neurology. 2001; 57:605-612.

14-48 Yoon BK, Kim DK, et al. Hormone replacement therapy in women with Alzheimer's disease: a randomized, prospective study. Fertil Steril. 2003; 79:274-280.

14-49 Cohen L, et al. Risk for new onset of depression during the menopausal transition: the Harvard study of moods and cycles. Arch Of General Psychiatry. 2006;63(4):385-90.

14-50 Rocca W, et al. Long-term risk of depressive and anxiety symptoms after early bilateral oophorectomy. Menopause. 2008;(15):1050-59.

14-51 Hildreth K, Ozemek C. Vascular dysfunction across the stages of the menopausal transition is associated with menopausal symptoms and quality of life. Menopause. 2018;25(9):1-9.

14-52 Berhan Y, Berhan A. Is desvenlafaxine effective and safe in the treatment of menopausal vasomotor symptoms? A meta-analysis and meta-regression of randomized double-blind controlled studies. Ethiop J Health Sci. 2014;24(3):209-218.

14-53 Soares, C. Tailoring strategies for the management of depression in midlife years. Menopause. June 2017;24(6):699-701.

14-54 Schmidt P, Ben D, et al. Effects of estradiol withdrawal on mood in women with past perimenopausal depression: a randomized clinical trial. JAMA Psychiatry. 2015;72:714-726.

14-55 Darmon M, Al Awabdh S, Emerit M, Masson J. Insights into serotonin receptor trafficking: cell membrane targeting and internalization. Prog Mol Biol Transl Sci. 2015;132:97-126.

14-56 Soares C, Almeida O, Joffe H, Cohen L. Efficacy of estradiol for the treatment of depressive disorders in perimenopausal women: a doubleblind, randomized, placebo-controlled trial. Arch Gen Psychiatry. 2001;58:529-534.

14-57 Onalan G, Onalan R, et al. Mood scores in relation to hormone replacement therapies during menopause: a prospective randomized trial. The Tohoku Journal Of Experimental Medicine. Nov. 2005;207(3):223-31.

14-58 Raz L, Hunter L. Differential effects of hormone therapy on serotonin, vascular function and mood in the KEEPS. Climacteric, Feb. 2016;19(1):49-59.

14-59 Gordon J, Rubinow D, et al. Efficacy of transdermal estradiol and micronized progesterone in the prevention of depressive symptoms in the menopause transition: a randomized clinical trial. JAMA Psychiatry. 2018;75(2):149-157.

14-60 Rubinow D, Johnson S, et al. Efficacy of estradiol in perimenopausal depression: so much promise and so few answers. Depress Anxiety. 2015; 32:539-549.

14-61 Zhou C, Fang L, Chen Y, et al. Effect of selective serotonin reuptake inhibitors on bone mineral density: a systematic review and meta-analysis. Osteoporos Int. June 2018;29(6):1243-1251.

14-62 Georgakis M, Thomopolous T, et al. Association of age at menopause and duration of reproductive period with depression after menopause. a systematic review and meta-analysis. JAMA Psychiatry 2016; 73:139-149.

14-63 Campbell K, Dennerstein L, et al. Impact of menopausal status on negative mood and depressive symptoms in a longitudinal sample spanning 20 years. Menopause. May 2017;24(5):490-496 .

14-64 Joffe H, Bromberger J. Shifting paradigms about hormonal risk factors for postmenopausal depression age at menopause as an indicator of cumulative lifetime exposure to female reproductive hormones. JAMA Psychiatry. 2016; 73:111-112.

14-65 Bourque M, Dluzen D, Di Paolo T. Neuroprotective actions of sex steroids in Parkinson's Disease. Front Neuroendocrinol. 2009;30:142-157.

14-66 Faubion S, Kuhle C, Shuster L, Rocca W. Long-term health consequences of premature or early menopause and considerations for management. Climacteric. 2015;18:483-491.

14-67 Phillips S, et al. Effects of estrogen on memory function in surgically menopausal women. Psychoneuroendrcrinology. 1992;17(5):485-95.

14-68 Currie L, et al. Postmenopausal estrogen use affects risk for Parkinson disease. Archive of Neurology. June 2004;61(6):886-88.

14-69 Popat R, Van Den Eeden S, Tanner C, et al. Effect of reproductive factors and postmenopausal hormone use on the risk of Parkinson disease. Neurology. 2005;65:383-390.

14-70 Simon K, Chen H, et al. Reproductive factors, exogenous estrogen use, and risk of Parkinson's disease. Mov Disord 2009;24:1359-1365.

14-71 Bourque M, Dluzen D, Di Paolo T. Neuroprotective actions of sex steroids in Parkinson's disease. Front Neuroendocrinol. 2009;30:142-157.

14-72 Labandeira-Garcia J, Rodriguez-Perez A. Menopause and Parkinson's disease. interaction between estrogens and brain renin-angiotensin system in dopaminergic degeneration. Front Neuroendocrinol. Oct. 2016;43:44-59.

14-73 Ripa P, Ornello R, Degan D, et al. Migraine in menopausal women: a systematic review. Int J Womens Health. 2015;7:773-82.

14-74 Lay C, Broner S. Migraine in women. Neurol Clin. 2009;27:503-11.

14-75 Facchinetti F, Nappi R, et al. Hormone supplementation differently affects migraine in postmenopausal women. Headache. 2002;42:924-9.

14-76 Hipolito Rodrigues M, Maitrot-Mantelet L, et al. Migraine, hormones and the menopausal transition. Climacteric. June 2018;21(3):256-266.

14-77 MacGregor E. Migraine headache in perimenopausal and menopausal women. Curr Pain Headache Rep. 2009;13:399-403.

14-78 Feigin VL, Nguyen G, Cercy K, Johnson CO, Alam T, et al. The GBD 2016 Lifetime Risk of Stroke Collaborators. The Global, regional, and country-specific lifetime risks of stroke, 1990 and 2016. N Engl J Med. Dec. 2018;379(25):2429-2437.

14-79 Lisabeth LD, Beiser AS, Brown DL, et al. Age at natural menopause and risk of ischemic stroke: the Framingham Heart Study. Stroke 2009;40:1044-9.

14-80 Faubion S, Kuhle C, Shuster L, Rocca W. Long-term health consequences of premature or early menopause and considerations for management. Climacteric. 2015;18:483-491.

14-81 Rexrode K, Manson, J. Estrogens and stroke: disentangling a complex relationship. Menopause. March 2012;9(3): 247-249.

14-82 Viscoli CM, Brass LM, Kernan WN, et al. A clinical trial of estrogen-replacement therapy after ischemic stroke. N Engl J Med. 2001;345:1243-1249.

14-83 Paganini-Hill A, et al. Postmenopausal oestrogen treatment and stroke: a prospective study. BMJ. 1988; 297: 519-522.

14-84 Mikkola TS, Tuomikoski P, Lyytinen H, et al. Estradiol-based postmenopausal hormone therapy and risk of cardiovascular and all-cause mortality. Menopause. 2015;22:976-983.

14-85 Mikkola T, Tuomikoski P, Lyytinen H, et al. Increased cardiovascular mortality risk in women discontinuing postmenopausal hormone therapy. J Clin Endocrinol Metab. 2015; 100:4588-4594.

14-86 Rossouw J, Prentice R, Manson J, et al. Postmenopausal hormone therapy and risk of cardiovascular disease by age and years since menopause. JAMA. 2007; 297:1465-1477.

14-87 Boardman H, Hartley L, Eisinga A, et al. Hormone therapy for preventing cardiovascular disease in post-menopausal women. Cochrane Database Syst Rev. 2015.;(3):CD002229.

14-88 Salpeter S, Cheng J, et al. Bayesian meta-analysis of hormone therapy and mortality in younger postmenopausal women. Am J Med. 2009;12:1016-1022.

14-89 Apostolakis S, Sullivan RM, MD, Olshansky B. Hormone replacement therapy and adverse outcomes in women with atrial fibrillation: an analysis from the atrial fibrillation follow-up investigation of rhythm management trial. Stroke. 2014;45:3076-3079.

14-90 Speroff L. Transdermal hormone therapy and the risk of stroke and venous thrombosis. Climacteric. 2010;13:429-432.

14-91 Prema, B, et al. The effect of transdermal estrogen patch use on cardiovascular outcomes: a systematic review. J. Womens Health. 2017;26:1319-1325.

14-92 Mikkola T, et al. Estradiol-based postmenopausal hormone therapy and risk of cardiovascular and all-cause mortality. Menopause. Sept. 2015;22(9): 976-83.

Chapter 15: Estrogen and Your Fat Cells and Diabetes

15-1 Sternfeld B, et al. Physical activity and changes in weight and waist circumference in midlife women: findings from the Study of Women's Health Across the Nation. American J. of Epidemiology. Nov. 2004;160(9):912-22.

15-2 Flegal K, Kruszon-Moran D, et al. Trends in obesity among adults in the United States 2005 to 2014. JAMA. 2016;315:2284-2291.

15-3 Pu D, Tan R, Yu Q, Wu J. Metabolic syndrome in menopause and associated factors: a meta-analysis. Climacteric. 2017;20(6):583-591.

15-4 Rogers N, Perfield J, et al. Reduced energy expenditure and increased inflammation are early events in the development of ovariectomy-induced obesity. Endocrinology. 2009;150:2161-8.

15-5 Davis S, Castelo-Branco C. Understanding weight gain at menopause. Climacteric. 2012;15:419-429.

15-6 Xu Y, Nedungadi T, Zhu L, Sobhani N. Distinct hypothalamic neurons mediate estrogenic effects on energy homeostasis and reproduction. Cell Metab. 2011;14(4):453.

15-7 Gambino YP, Maymó JL, Pérez-Pérez A, et al. 17Beta-estradiol enhances leptin expression in human placental cells through genomic and nongenomic actions. Biol Reprod. 2010;83:42.

15-8 Stubbin R, et al. Oestrogen alters adipocyte biology and protects female mice from adipocyte inflammation and insulin resistance Diabetes. Obesity and Metabolism. Jan. 2012;14(1):58-66.

15-9 Matthews K, Abrams B, Crawford S, et al. Body mass index in mid-life women: relative influence of menopause, hormone use, and ethnicity. Int J Obes Relat Metab Disord. 2001;25:863-873.

15-10 Franklin R, Ploutz-Snyder L, Kanaley J. Longitudinal changes in abdominal fat distribution with menopause. Metabolism. 2009;58:311-315.

15-11 Abdulnour J, Doucet E, Brochu M, et al. The effect of the menopausal transition on body composition and cardiometabolic risk factors: A Montreal-Ottawa new emerging team study. Menopause. 2012;19:760-767.

15-12 Sakuma K, Yamaguchi A. Sarcopenic obesity and endocrinal adaptation with age. Int J Endocrinol. 2013;2013:204:164.

15-13 Karvonen-Gutierrez C, Kim C. Association of mid-life changes in body size, body composition and obesity status with the menopausal transition. Healthcare (Basel, Switzerland). 2016;4:42.

15-14 Shea K, et al. Body composition and bone mineral density after ovarian hormone suppression with and without estradiol treatment. Menopause. 2105; 22(10):1045-52.

15-15 Stefanska A, Bergmann K, Sypniewska G. Metabolic syndrome and menopause: pathophysiology, clinical and diagnostic significance. Adv Clin Chem. 2015;72:1-75.

15-16 Park Y, Zhu S, Palaniappan L, et al. The metabolic syndrome: prevalence and associated risk factor findings in the U.S. population. From the third national health and nutrition examination survey - 1988-1994. Arch Intern Med. 2003;163:427-36.

15-17 Pucci G, Alcidi R, Tap L, et al. Sex and gender-related prevalence, cardiovascular risk and therapeutic approach in metabolic syndrome: a review of the literature. Pharmacol Res. 2017;120:34-42.

15-18 Dørum A, Tonstad S, Liavaag A, et al. Bilateral oophorectomy before 50 years of age is significantly associated with the metabolic syndrome and Framingham risk score: a controlled, population-based study (HUNT-2). Gynecol Oncol. 2008;109:377-83.

15-19 Michelsen T, Pripp A, Tonstad S, et al. Metabolic syndrome after risk-reducing salpingo-oophorectomy in women at high risk for hereditary breast ovarian cancer: a controlled observational study. Eur J Cancer. 2009;45:82-9.

15-20 Hanson R, Imperatore G, Bennett P, Knowler W. Components of the metabolic syndrome and incidence of type 2 diabetes. Diabetes. 2002; 51(10):3120.

15-21 Ford E, Li C, Sattar N. Metabolic syndrome and incident diabetes: current state of the evidence. Diabetes Care. 2008;31:1898-904.

15-22 Pu D, Tan R, Yu Q, Wu J. Metabolic syndrome in menopause and associated factors: a meta-analysis. Climacteric. Dec. 2017;20(6):583-591.

15-23 Kautzky-Willer A, Harreiter J, Pacini G. Sex and gender differences in risk, pathophysiology and complications of type 2 diabetes mellitus. Endocr Rev. June 2016; 37(3): 278-316.

15-24 Janka H, Michaelis D. Epidemiology of diabetes mellitus: prevalence, incidence, pathogenesis and prognosis. Z. Arztl. Fortbild. Qualitätssich, 2002;96:159-165.

15-25 Monterrosa-Castro A, Blumel J, Portela-Buelvas K. Type II diabetes mellitus and menopause: a multinational study: collaborative group for research of the climacteric in Latin America. Climacteric. 2013;16:663-72.

15-26 LeBlanc E, Kapphahn K, Hedlin H, et al. Reproductive history and risk of type 2 diabetes mellitus in postmenopausal women: findings from the Women's Health Initiative. Menopause. 2017;24:64-72.

15-27 Brand J, van der Schouw Y, Onland-Moret N, et al. Age at menopause, reproductive life span, and type 2 diabetes risk: Results from the EPIC-InterAct Study. Diabetes Care. 2013;36:1012-19.

15-28 Anagnostis P, Christou K, et al. Early menopause and premature ovarian insufficiency are associated with increased risk of type 2 diabetes: a systematic review and meta-analysis. European Journal of Endocrinology. Jan. 2019;180(1):41-50.

15-29 Kritz-Silverstein D, Barrett-Connor E, Wingard DL. Hysterectomy, oophorectomy, and heart disease risk factors in older women. Am J Public Health.1997;87:676-80.

15-30 Pirimoglu ZM, Arslan C, Buyukbayrak EE, et al. Glucose tolerance of premenopausal women after menopause due to surgical removal of ovaries. Climacteric. 2011;14:453-457.

15-31 Appiah D, Winters S, Hornung C. Bilateral oophorectomy and the risk of incident diabetes in postmenopausal women. Diabetes Care. 2014;37:725-33.

15-32 Louet J, LeMay C, Mauvais-Jarvis F. Anti-diabetic actions of estrogen: insight from human and genetic mouse models. Curr Atheroscler Rep. 2004;6(3):180.

15-33 Hevener AL, Zhou Z, Moore TM, Drew BG, Ribas V. The impact of ERalpha action on muscle metabolism and insulin sensitivity - strong enough for a man, made for a woman. Mol Metab. 2018;15:20-34.

15-34 Park YM, Pereira R, Rocio I, et al. Time since menopause and skeletal muscle estrogen receptors, PGC-1α, and AMPK. Menopause. July 2017;24(7):815-823.

15-35 Malacara JM, Huerta R, Rivera B, Esparza S, Fajardo ME. Menopause in normal and uncomplicated NIDDM women: physical and emotional symptoms and hormone profile. Maturitas 1997;28:35-45.

15-36 Di Donato P, Giulini NA, Bacchi Modena A, et al. Gruppo di Studio Progetto Menopausa Italia. Risk factors for type 2 diabetes in women attending menopause clinics in Italy: a cross-sectional study. Climacteric 2005;8:287-293.

15-37 Ren Y, Zhang M, Liu Y, et al. Association of menopause and type 2 diabetes mellitus. Menopause. Mar. 2019;26(3):325-330.

15-38 Soriguer, F, Morcillo, S, Hernando, V, et al. Type 2 diabetes mellitus and other cardiovascular risk factors are no more common during menopause: longitudinal study. Menopause. July-August 2009;16(4):817-821.

15-39 Cobin RH, Goodman NF, American Association Of Clinical Endocrinologists and American College Of Endocrinology position statement on menopause-2017 update. Endocrine Practice. July 2017;23 (7):869-888.

15-40 Gallo, M et al. Combination estrogen-progestin contraceptives and body weight: systemic review of randomized controlled trials. Obste Gynecol. 2004;103(2):359-373.

15-41 Margolis K, Bonds D, Rodabough R, et al. Effect of estrogen plus progestin on the incidence of diabetes in postmenopausal women: results from the Women's Health Initiative Hormone Trial. Diabetologia. 2004; 47:1175-1187.

15-42 Norman R, Flight I, Rees M. Oestrogen and progestogen hormone replacement therapy for peri-menopausal and post-menopausal women: weight and body fat distribution. Cochrane Database Syst Rev 2000; CD001018.

15-43 Mattiasson I, Rendell M, Tornquist C, et al. Effects of estrogen replacement therapy on abdominal fat compartments as related to glucose and lipid metabolism in early postmenopausal women. Horm Metab Res. 2002;34:583-588.

15-44 Espeland MA, Stefanick ML, Kritz-Silverstein D, et al. Effect of postmenopausal hormone therapy on body weight and waist and hip girths. Postmenopausal Estrogen-Progestin Interventions Study Investigators. J Clin Endocrinol Metab. 1997;82:1549-1556.

15-45 Chen Z, Bassford T, Green SB, et al. Postmenopausal hormone therapy and body composition—a sub study of the estrogen plus progestin trial of the Women's Health Initiative. Am J Clin Nutr. 2005;82:651-656.

15-46 Mauvais-Jarvis F, Manson J, Stevenson J, Fonseca V. Menopausal hormone therapy and type 2 diabetes prevention: evidence, mechanisms and clinical implications. Endocr Rev. 2017;38:173-88.

15-47 Hevener A, Clegg D, Mauvais-Jarvis F. Impaired estrogen receptor action in the pathogenesis of the metabolic syndrome. Mol Cell Endocrinol. December 2015; 15:306-321.

15-48 Salpeter S, Walsh J, Ormiston T, et al. Meta-analysis: effect of hormone replacement therapy on components of the metabolic syndrome in postmenopausal women. Diabetes Obes Metab. 2006;8:538-54.

15-49 Triusu R, Cowie C, Harris M. Hormone replacement therapy and glucose metabolism. Obstet Gynecol. 2000;96:665-70.

15-50 Manson J, Rimm E, Colditz G, et al. A prospective study of postmenopausal estrogen therapy and subsequent incidence of non-insulin-dependent diabetes mellitus. Ann Epidemiol. 1992;2:665-73.

15-51 Pentti K, Tuppurainen M, Honkanen R, et al. Hormone therapy protects from diabetes: The Kuopio Osteoporosis Risk Factor and Prevention Study. Eur J Endocrinol. 2009;160(6):979-983

15-52 Di Donato P, Giulini N, Bacchi Modena A, et al. Risk factors for type 2 diabetes in women attending menopause clinics in Italy: a cross-sectional study. Climacteric 2005;8:287-93.

15-53 Kanaya A, Herrington D, Vittinghoff E, Lin F, Grady D, et al. Glycemic effects of postmenopausal hormone therapy: The Heart and Estrogen/Progestin Replacement Study. A randomized, double-blind, placebo-controlled trial. Ann Intern Med. 2003;138(1):1-9.

15-54 Rossi R, Origliani G, Modena M. Transdermal 17-B-estradiol and risk of developing type 2 diabetes in a population of healthy, non-obese postmenopausal women. Diabetes Care. 2004;27:645-9.

15-55 Xu Y, Lin J, Wang S, Xiong J, Zhu Q. Combined estrogen replacement therapy on metabolic control in postmenopausal women with diabetes mellitus. Kaohsiung J Med Sci. 2014;30:350-61.

15-56 The 2017 Hormone Therapy Position Statement of The North American Menopause Society. Menopause. July 2017;24(7):728-753.

15-57 Pereira I, Casey B, Swibas T, et al. Timing of estradiol treatment after menopause may determine benefit or harm to insulin action. J Clin Endocrinol Metab. 2015;100:4456-62.

15-58 Manson J, Chlebowski R, Stefanick M, et al. Menopausal hormone therapy and health outcomes during the intervention and extended post stopping phases of the Women's Health Initiative randomized trials. JAMA. 2013;310:1353-68.

15-59 Harman SM, Brinton EA, Cedars M, et al. KEEPS: The Kronos Early Estrogen Prevention Study. Climacteric. 2005;8:3-12.

15-60 Stuenkel, C. Menopause, hormone therapy and diabetes. Climacteric. 2017;20:(1):11-21.

15-61 Brand J, Onland-Moret N, Eijkemans M, et al. Diabetes and onset of natural menopause: results from the European Prospective Investigation into Cancer and Nutrition. Hum Reprod. 2015;30:1491-8.

15-62 Triusu R, Cowie C, Harris M. Hormone replacement therapy and glucose metabolism. Obstet Gynecol. 2000;96:665-70.

15-63 Ferrara A, Karter A, Ackerson L, Liu J, Selby J. Hormone replacement therapy is associated with better glycemic control in women with type 2 diabetes: The Northern California Kaiser Permanente Diabetes Registry. Diabetes Care. 2001;24:1144-50.

15-64 Crespo C, Smit E, Snelling A, et al. Hormone replacement therapy and its relationship to lipid and glucose metabolism in diabetic and non-diabetic postmenopausal women: results from the Third National Health and Nutrition Examination Survey (NHANES III). Diabetes Care. 2002;25:1675-80.

15-65 Mosca L, Benjamin E, Berra K, et al. Effectiveness-based guidelines for the prevention of cardiovascular disease in women—2011 update. A guideline from the American Heart Association. Circulation. 2011;123:1243-62.

15-66 Mackay L, Kilbride L, Adamson KA, Chisholm J. Hormone replacement therapy for women with type 1 diabetes mellitus Cochrane Database Syst Rev. June 2013;(6):CD008613.

Chapter 16: Estrogen and Your Genitourinary System (and Sex)

16-1 Kagan, R. Rivera, E. Restoring vaginal function in postmenopausal women with genitourinary syndrome of menopause. Menopause. Jan. 2018;25:106-108.

16-2 Krychman M, Graham S, Bernick B, Mirkin S, Kingsberg SA. The Women's EMPOWER Survey: women's knowledge of and awareness of treatment options for vulvar and vaginal atrophy remain inadequate. J Sex Med. 2017;14:425-433.

16-3 Bachmann, G, Phillips, N. Local estrogen benefits of postmenopausal women with dyspareunia: data confirming what clinicians already know! Menopause. Feb. 2018;25(2):127-128.

16-4 Santen RJ. Vaginal administration of estradiol: effects of dose, preparation and timing on plasma estradiol levels. Climacteric. 2015;18:121-134.

16-5 The 2017 Hormone therapy position statement of The North American Menopause Society. Menopause. July 2017; 24(7):728-753.

16-6 Farrell R. American College of Obstetricians and Gynecologists' Committee on Gynecologic Practice. ACOG Committee Opinion No. 659: The use of vaginal estrogen in women with a history of estrogen-dependent breast cancer. Obstet Gynecol. 2016;127:e93-e96.

16-7 Lethaby A, Ayeleke RO, Roberts H. Local oestrogen for vaginal atrophy in postmenopausal women. Cochrane Database Syst Rev. 2016; 8:CD001500.

16-8 Pinkerton JV, Kaunitz AM, Manson JE. Vaginal estrogen in the treatment of genitourinary syndrome of menopause and risk of endometrial cancer: an assessment of recent studies provides reassurance. Menopause. 2017;24:1329-32.

16-9 American College of Obstetricians and Gynecologists. ACOG committee opinion no. 556: Postmenopausal estrogen therapy: route of administration and risk of venous thromboembolism. Obstet Gynecol 2013;121:887-890.

16-10 Crandall CJ, Hovey KM, Andrews CA, et al. Breast cancer, endometrial cancer, and cardiovascular events in participants who used vaginal estrogen in the Women's Health Initiative observational study. Menopause. Jan. 2018;25(1):11-20.

16-11 Suckling J, Lethaby A, Kennedy. Local oestrogen for vaginal atrophy in postmenopausal women. Cochrane Database Syst Rev. 2006.

16-12 Hurst BS, Jones AI, Elliot M. Absorption of vaginal estrogen cream during sexual intercourse: a prospective, randomized, controlled trial. Reprod Med. 2008;53(1):29.

16-13 Portman, DJ, Labrie F. Lack of effect of intravaginal dehydroepiandrosterone (DHEA, prasterone) on the endometrium in postmenopausal women. Menopause. Dec. 2015;22(12):1289-1295.

16-14 Ke Y, Labrie F, Gonthier R et al. Serum levels of sex steroids and metabolites following 12 weeks of intravaginal 0.50% DHEA administration. Steroid Biochem Mol Biol. Nov. 2015;154:186-96.

16-15 Melisko ME, Goldman ME, Hwang J et al. Vaginal testosterone cream vs estradiol vaginal ring for vaginal dryness or decreased libido in women receiving aromatase inhibitors for early-stage breast cancer: a randomized clinical trial. JAMA Oncol. Mar 2017;3(3):313-319.

16-16 American College of Obstetricians and Gynecologists. Fractional laser treatment of vulvovaginal atrophy and U.S. Food and Drug Administration clearance: Position statement. www.acog.org/Resources-And-Publications/Position-Statements/Fractional-Laser-Treatment-of-Vulvovaginal-Atrophy-and-US-Food-and-Drug-Administration-Clearance. May 2016.

16-17 Al-Azzawi F, Bitzer J. Therapeutic options for postmenopausal female sexual dysfunction. Climacteric. 2010;13(2):103-120.

16-18 Pinkerton, J, Bushmakin, et al. Most bothersome symptom in women with genitourinary syndrome of menopause as a moderator of treatment effects. Menopause. Oct. 2016;23(10):1092-1101.

16-19 Cody JD, Jacobs ML, Richardson K, et al. Oestrogen therapy for urinary incontinence in post-menopausal women. Cochrane Database Syst Rev. 2012;10:CD001405.

16-20 Santen RJ, Allred DC, Ardoin SP, et al. Postmenopausal hormone therapy: an Endocrine Society scientific statement. J Clin Endocrinol Metab. 2010;95(7 Suppl 1):s1.

16-21 Agronin M. Sexual dysfunction in older adults, UPTODATE Review, Up dated Oct. 24, 2017. https://www.uptodate.com/contents/sexual-dysfunction-in-older-adults?search=sexual%20dysfunction%20 geriatric&source=search.

16-22 Fisher LL. Sex, romance, and relationships: 2009 AARP survey of midlife and older adults. American Association for Retired Persons 2010. https://www.aarp.org/research/topics/life/info-2014/srr_09.html.

16-23 Montenegro XP. American Association for Retired Persons. Sexuality at Midlife and Beyond: 2004 Update of Attitudes and Behaviors. AARP: 2005. https://assets.aarp.org/rgcenter/general/2004_sexuality.pdf.

16-24 Kingsberg SA, Wysocki S, Magnus L, Krychman ML. Vulvar and vaginal atrophy in postmenopausal women: findings from the REVIVE (REal Women's Views of Treatment Options for Menopausal Vaginal Changes) survey. J Sex Med. 2013;10:1790-1799.

16-25 West E, Krychman M. Natural aphrodisiacs – a review of selected sexual enhancers. Sex Med Rev. Oct. 2015;3(4):279-288.

16-26 Jaspers L, Feys F, Bramer WM. Efficacy and safety of flibanserin for the treatment of hypoactive sexual desire disorder in women: a systematic review and meta-analysis. JAMA Intern Med. April 2016;176(4):453-62.

16-27 FDA approves new treatment for hypoactive sexual desire disorder in premenopausal women. United States Food and Drug Administration. https://www.fda.gov/news-events/press-announcements/fda-approves-new-treatment-hypoactive-sexual-desire-disorder-premenopausal-women.

16-28 Davis SR, Davison SL, Donath S et al. Circulating androgen levels and self-reported sexual function in women. JAMA. 2005;294(1):91.

16-29 Davis SR, van der Mooren MJ, van Lunsen RH, et al. Efficacy and safety of a testosterone patch for the treatment of hypoactive sexual desire disorder in surgically menopausal women: a randomized, placebo-controlled trial. Menopause. 2006;13(3):387.

16-30 Shifren JL, Davis SR, Moreau M, et al. Testosterone patch for the treatment of hypoactive sexual desire disorder in naturally menopausal women: results from the INTIMATE NM1 Study. Menopause. 2006;13(5):770.

16-31 Blümel JE, Del Pino M, Aprikian D. Effect of androgens combined with hormone therapy on quality of life in post-menopausal women with sexual dysfunction. Gynecol Endocrinol. 2008;24(12):691.

16-32 El-Hage G, Eden JA, Manga RZ. A double-blind, randomized, placebo-controlled trial of the effect of testosterone cream on the sexual motivation of menopausal hysterectomized women with hypoactive sexual desire disorder. Climacteric. 2007;10(4):335.

16-33 Shifren JL, Davis SR. Androgens in postmenopausal women: a review. Menopause. 2017;24(8):970.

16-34 Simon JA, Davis R, et al. Sexual well-being after menopause: An International Menopause Society white paper. Climacteric. 2018;21(5):415-427.

16-35 Achilli C, Pundir J. Efficacy and safety of transdermal testosterone in postmenopausal women with hypoactive sexual desire disorder: a systematic review and meta-analysis. Fertil Steril. Feb. 2017;107(2):475-482.

16-36 Davis SR, Moreau M, Kroll R, Bouchard C et al. Testosterone for low libido in postmenopausal women not taking estrogen. N Engl J Med. 2008;359(19):2005.

16-37 Spoletini I, Vitale C, Pelliccia F. Androgens and cardiovascular disease in postmenopausal women: a systematic review. Climacteric. Dec. 2014; 17(6):625-34.

16-38 Lukanova A, Lundin E, Micheli A, et al. Circulating levels of sex steroid hormones and risk of endometrial cancer in postmenopausal women. Int J Cancer. 2004;108(3):425.

16-39 Braunstein GD, Shufelt CL. Safety of testosterone use in women. Maturitas. May 2009;63(1):63-6.

16-40 Kabat GC, Kamensky V, Heo M, et al. Combined conjugated esterified estrogen plus methyltestosterone supplementation and risk of breast cancer in postmenopausal women. Maturitas. Sep. 2014;79(1):70-6.

16-41 Wierman ME, Arlt W, Basson R et al. Androgen therapy in women: a reappraisal: an Endocrine Society clinical practice guideline. J Clin Endocrinol Metab. 2014;99(10):3489.

16-42 Davis SR, Panjari M, Stanczyk et al. Clinical review: DHEA replacement for postmenopausal women. J Clin Endocrinol Metab. June 2011;96(6):1642-53.

16-43 Scheffers CS, Armstrong S. Dehydroepiandrosterone for women in the peri- or postmenopausal phase. Cochrane Database Syst Rev. 2015;1:CD011066.

16-44 Elraiyah T, Sonbol MB, Wang Z. Clinical review: the benefits and harms of systemic dehydroepiandrosterone (DHEA) in postmenopausal women with normal adrenal function: a systematic review and meta-analysis. J Clin Endocrinol Metab. Oct. 2014;99(10):3536-42.

16-45 Krapf JM, Simon JA. A sex-specific dose-response curve for testosterone: could excessive testosterone limit sexual interaction in women? Menopause. 2017;24(4):462-470.

16-46 Al-Azzawi F, Bitzer J, Therapeutic options for postmenopausal female sexual dysfunction. Climacteric. 2010;13(2):103-120.

16-47 Liang Gao, LuYang, et al. Systematic review and meta-analysis of phosphodiesterase type 5 inhibitors for the treatment of female sexual dysfunction. Int J Gynaecol Obstet. May 2016;133(2):139-45.

16-48 Basson R, Brotto LA. Sexual psychophysiology and effects of sildenafil citrate in oestrogenised women with acquired genital arousal disorder and impaired orgasm: a randomised controlled trial. BJOG. 2003;110:1014-24.

16-49 Billups KL, Berman L, Berman J, et al. A new non-pharmacological vacuum therapy for female sexual dysfunction. J Sex Marital Ther. 2001(27):435-441.

Chapter 17: Estrogen, Your Skin, Joints, Muscles, and More

17-1 Lephart ED. A review of the role of estrogen in dermal aging and facial attractiveness in women. J Cosmet Dermatol. Feb. 2018;13:282-288.

17-2 Brincat M, Moniz CF, Studd JW, et al. The long term effects of the menopause and of administration of sex hormones on skin collagen and skin thickness. Br J Obstetric Gynaecol. 1985;99:256-259.

17-3 Raine-Fenning NJ, et al. Skin aging and menopause: implications for treatment. Am J. Clin Dermatol. 2003;4:371-378.

17-4 Hall G, Phillips TJ. Estrogen and skin: the effects of estrogen, menopause, and hormone replacement therapy on the skin. Journal of the American Academy of Dermatology. Oct. 2005;53:1097-6787.

17-5 Quatresooz P, Piérard-Franchimont C. Skin climacteric aging and hormone replacement therapy. Journal of Cosmetic Dermatology. March 2006;5(1):3-8.

17-6 Emmerson E, Hardman MJ. The role of estrogen deficiency in skin ageing and wound healing. Biogerontology. 2012;13:3-20.

17-7 Watt FE, Carlisle K, Kennedy D, Vincent TL. Menopause and hormone replacement therapy are important etiological factors in hand osteoarthritis: results from a cross-sectional study in secondary care. Maturitas. 2015;81:128.

17-8 Karsdal MA, Bay-Jensen AC, Henriksen K, Christiansen C. The pathogenesis of osteoarthritis involves bone, cartilage and synovial inflammation: may estrogen be a magic bullet? Menopause Int. 2012;18:139-46.

17-9 de Klerk BM, Schiphof D, Groeneveld FP, et al. Limited evidence for a protective effect of unopposed oestrogen therapy for osteoarthritis of the hip: a systematic review. Rheumatology (Oxford). 2009; 48:104-112.

17-10 Watt FE. Hand osteoarthritis, menopause and menopausal hormone therapy. Maturitas. 2016;83:13.

17-11 Xiao YP, Tian FM, Dai MW, et al. Are estrogen-related drugs new alternatives for the management of osteoarthritis? Arthritis Res Ther. 2016;18:151.

17-12 Chlebowski RT, Cirillo DJ, Eaton CB, et al. Estrogen alone and joint symptoms in the Women's Health Initiative randomized trial. Menopause. 2018;25:1313-20.

17-13 Cirillo DJ, Wallace RB, Wu L, Yood RA. Effect of hormone therapy on risk of hip and knee joint replacement in the Women's Health Initiative. Arthritis Rheumatol. 2006;54:3194-204.

17-14 Lou C, Chen H. Association between menopause and lumbar disc degeneration: an MRI study of 1,566 women and 1,382 men. Menopause. October 2017; 24(10):1136-1144.

17-15 Gruber HE, Yamaguchi D, Ingram J, et al. Expression and localisation of the estrogen receptor beta in annulus cells of the human intervertebral disc and the mitogenic effect of 17 betaestradiol. BMC Musculoskelet Disord. 2002;3:4.

17-16 Muscat BY, Brincat MP. Low intervertebral disc height in postmenopausal women with osteoporotic vertebral fractures compared to hormone-treated and untreated postmenopausal women and premenopausal women without fractures. Climacteric. 2007;10:314-319.

17-17 Muscat BY. Menopause and the intervertebral disc. Menopause. Oct. 2017; 24(10):1118-1121.

17-18 Lateef A, Petri M. Hormone replacement and contraceptive therapy in autoimmune diseases. Journal of Autoimmunity. 2012;38:(2-3):J170-6.

17-19 Beydoun HA, el-Amin R, et al. Reproductive history and postmenopausal rheumatoid arthritis among women 60 years or older: Third National Health and Nutrition Examination Survey. Menopause. Sept. 2013;20(9):930-935.

17-20 Chen JY, Stanley P. Ballou SP. The effect of antiestrogen agents on risk of autoimmune disorders in patients with breast cancer. The Journal of Rheumatology. January 2015;42(1):55-59.

17-21 Jung JH, Gwan G. Song GG, et al. Serum uric acid levels and hormone therapy type: a retrospective cohort study of postmenopausal women. Menopause. 2018;25(1):77-81.

17-22 Bruderer, SG, Bodmer M, et al. Association of hormone therapy and incident gout: population-based case-control study. Menopause. Dec. 2015;22(12):1335-1342.

17-23 Tiidus PM et al. Estrogen replacement and skeletal muscle: mechanism and population health. J. Applied physiology. 2013;115:569-578.

17-24 Kovanen V, Aukee P. Design and protocol of estrogenic regulation of muscle apoptosis (ERMA) study with 47 to 55-year-old women's cohort: novel results show menopause-related differences in blood count. Menopause. Sept 2018; 25(9):1020-1032.

17-25 Phillips SK, Rook KM, Siddle NC, et al. Muscle weakness in women occurs at an earlier age than in men, but strength is preserved by hormone replacement therapy. Clin Sci (Lond).1993;84:95-98.

17-26 Qaisar R, Renaud G, et al. Hormone replacement therapy improves contractile function and myonuclear organization of single muscle fibres from postmenopausal monozygotic female twin pairs. The Journal of Physiology. May 2013;591(9):2333-44.

17-27 Lowe DA, Baltgalvis KA, Greising SM. Mechanisms behind estrogen's beneficial effect on muscle strength in females. Exerc Sport Sci Rev. 2010;38:61-67.

17-28 Greising SM, Baltgalvis KA, Lowe DA, Warren GL. Hormone therapy and skeletal muscle strength: a meta-analysis. J Gerontol A Biol Sci Med Sci. 2009;64:1071-1081.

17-29 Pollanen E, Sipila S, et al. Differential influence of peripheral and systemic sex steroids on skeletal muscle quality in pre- and postmenopausal women. Aging Cell. 2011;10:650-660.

17-30 Taaffe DR, Sipila S, et al. The effect of hormone replacement therapy and/or exercise on skeletal muscle attenuation in postmenopausal women: a yearlong intervention. Clin Physiol Funct Imaging. 2005;25:297-304.

17-31 Park Y, Pereira R. Time since menopause and skeletal muscle estrogen receptors, PGC-1α, and AMPK. Menopause. July 2017;24(7):815-823.

17-32 Deschenes MC, et al. Postmenopausal hormone therapy increases retinal blood flow and protects the retinal nerve fiber layer. Invest. Opthalmol Visual Sciences. 2010;51:2587-2600.

17-33 Eye Disease Case Control Study. Risk factors for neovascular age-related macular degeneration. Arch Opthalmol. 1992;110:1701-1708.
17-34 Zetterberg M. Age-related eye disease and gender. Maturitas. 2016;83:19-26.

17-35 Benitez del Castillo JM, et al. Effects of estrogen on lens transmittance in postmenopausal women. Opthalmology. 1997;104: 970-973.

17-36 Dewundara SS, Wiggs JL, Sullivan DA, Pasquale LR. Is estrogen a therapeutic target for glaucoma? Semin Ophthalmol. 2016;31:140-146.

17-37 Hederstierna C, Hultcrantz M, Collins A, et al. The menopause triggers hearing decline in healthy women. Hear Res. 2010;259:31-5.

17-38 Diao H, Zhao L, Qin L, et al. Lower expression of prestin and MYO7A correlates with menopause-associated hearing loss. Climateric. 2019;22(4):361-369.

17-39 Passos-Soares J, et. al. Association between osteoporosis treatment and severe periodontitis in postmenopausal women. Menopause. July 2017;24(7):789-795.

17-40 Han K, Ko Y. et. al. Associations between the number of natural teeth in postmenopausal women and hormone replacement therapy. Maturitas. December 2016;94:125-130.

17-41 Paganini-Hill A. The benefits of estrogen replacement therapy on oral health. The Leisure World cohort. Arch Intern Med.1995;155:2325-2329.

17-42 Grodstein F, Colditz GA, Stampfer MJ. Post-menopausal hormone use and tooth loss: a prospective study. J Am Dent Assoc. 1996;127:370-377.

17-43 Civitelli R, Pilgram TK, Dotson M, et al. Alveolar and postcranial bone density in postmenopausal women receiving hormone/estrogen replacement therapy: a randomized, double-blind, placebo-controlled trial. Arch Intern Med. 2002;162:1409-1415.

Chapter 18: Estrogen and Your GI Tract

18-1 Nelson R, Dollear T, Freels S, Persky V. The Relation of age, race, and gender to the subsite location of colorectal carcinoma. Cancer. 1997; 80(2):193-7.

18-2 Weyant M, Carothers A, Mahmoud N. Reciprocal expression of ERalpha and ERbeta is associated with estrogen-mediated modulation of intestinal tumorigenesis. Cancer Res. 2001;61(6):2547-2551.

18-3 Grodstein F, Martinez M, et al. Postmenopausal hormone use and risk for colorectal cancer and adenoma. Ann Intern Med. May 1998;128(9):705-12.

18-4 Grodstein F, Newcomb P, Stampfer M. Postmenopausal hormone therapy and the risk of colorectal cancer: a review and meta-analysis. Am J Med. 1999;106(5):574.

18-5 Prentice R, Pettinger M, Beresford S, et al. Colorectal cancer in relation to postmenopausal estrogen and estrogen plus progestin in the Women's Health Initiative clinical trial and observational study. Cancer Epidemiol Biomarkers Prev. 2009;18:1531-7.

18-6 Meijer BJ, Wielenga MC, Hoyer, PB, et al. Colorectal tumor prevention by the progestin medroxyprogesterone acetate is critically dependent on postmenopausal status. Oncotarget. July 2018;9(55):30561-30567.

18-7 Tanaka Y, Kato K, et al. Medroxyprogesterone acetate inhibits proliferation of colon cancer cell lines by modulating cell cycle-related protein expression. Menopause. May-June 2008;15(3):442-453.

18-8 Mørch L, Lidegaard Ø, Keiding N, Løkkegaard E, Kjær S. The influence of hormone therapies on colon and rectal cancer. Eur J Epidemiol. May 2016 ;31(5):481-9.

18-9 Simin J, Tamimi R, Lagergren J, et al. Menopausal hormone therapy and cancer risk: an overestimated risk? Eur J Cancer. 2017;84:60-8.

18-10 Symer M, Wong N, Abelson J, Milsom J, Yeo H. Hormone replacement therapy and colorectal cancer incidence and mortality in the Prostate, Lung, Colorectal, and Ovarian Cancer Screening Trial. Clin Colorectal Cancer. June 2018;17(2):e281-e288.

18-11 Clark JM. The epidemiology of nonalcoholic fatty liver disease in adults. J Clin Gastroenterol. 2006;40(suppl 1):S5-S10.

18-12 Florentino GS, Cotrim HP, Vilar CP, et al. Nonalcoholic fatty liver disease in menopausal women. Arq Gastroenterol. 2013;50:180-185.

18-13 Matsuo, K, Gualtieri, MR, et al. Surgical menopause and increased risk of nonalcoholic fatty liver disease in endometrial cancer. Menopause. February 2016;23(2):189-196.

18-14 Holcomb, VB, Hong J, et al. Exogenous estrogen protects mice from the consequences of obesity and alcohol. Menopause. June 2012;19(6):680-690.

18-15 Zhu L, Brown WC, Cai Q, et al. Estrogen treatment after ovariectomy protects against fatty liver and may improve pathway-selective insulin resistance. Diabetes. 2013;62:424-434.

18-16 Brady C. Liver disease in menopause. World J Gastroenterol. 2015; 21:7613-7620.

18-17 Koulouri O, Ostberg J, Conway G. Liver dysfunction in Turner's syndrome: prevalence, natural history and effect of exogenous oestrogen. Clinical Endocrinology. 2008;69:306-310.

18-18 McKenzie, J, Fisher B, Jaap A, et al. Effects of HRT on liver enzyme levels in women with type 2 diabetes: a randomized placebo-controlled trial. Clinical Endocrinology. 2006;65:40-44.

18-19 Rooks JB, Ory HW, Ishak, KG, et al. Epidemiology of hepatocellular adenoma. The role of oral contraceptive use. JAMA. 1979;242(7):644.

18-20 Grodstein F, Colditz G, Stampfer M. Postmenopausal hormone use and cholecystectomy in a large prospective study. Obstet Gynecol. 1994;83(1):5.
18-21 Cirillo D, Wallace R, Rodabough R, et al. Effect of estrogen therapy on

gallbladder disease. JAMA. 2005; 293:330-339.

18-22 Racine A, Bijon A, Fournier A, Mesrine S, et al. Menopausal hormone therapy and risk of cholecystectomy: a prospective study based on the French E3N cohort. CMAJ. 2013;185(7):555.

18-23 Marjoribanks J, Farquhar C, Roberts H, et al. Long-term hormone therapy for perimenopausal and postmenopausal women. Cochrane Database Syst Rev. 2017;1:CD004143.

18-24 Van Erpecum KJ, Van Berge Henegouwen GP, Verschoor L, et al. Different hepatobiliary effects of oral and transdermal estradiol in postmenopausal women. Gastroenterology. 1991;100:482-8.

18-25 Henriksson P, Einarsson K, Eriksson A, et al. Estrogen-induced gallstone formation in males. relation to changes in serum and biliary lipids during hormonal treatment of prostatic carcinoma. J Clin Invest. 1989;84(3):811.

18-26 Messa C, Maselli MA, Cavallini A. Sex steroid hormone receptors and human gallbladder motility in vitro. Digestion.1990;46:214-9.

Chapter 19: Estrogen and Your Life Expectancy

19-1 Min KJ, Lee CL et al. The lifespan of Korean eunuchs. Current Biology. Sept. 2012;22(18): R792-R793.

19-2 Rivera CM, Grosshardt BR, Rhodes DY, et al. Increased cardiovascular mortality after early bilateral oophorectomy. Menopause. 2009;16:15-23.

19-3 Shadyab A, et al. Ages at menarche and menopause and reproductive lifespan as predictors of exceptional longevity. Menopause. Jan. 2017;24:35-44.

19-4 Shuster LT, Rhodes DJ, Gostout BS, Grossardt BR, Rocca WA. Premature menopause or early menopause: long-term health consequences. Maturitas. 2010;65:161-166.

19-5 Bush TL, Barrett-Connor E, Cowan LD, et al. Cardiovascular mortality and noncontraceptive use of estrogen in women: results from the lipid research clinics program follow-up study. Circulation. 1987;75:1102-1109.

19-6 Grady D, Rubin SM, Petitti DB, et al. Hormone therapy to prevent disease and prolong life in postmenopausal women. Ann Intern Med. 1992;117:1016-1037.

19-7 Stampfer MJ, Colditz GA, Willett WC, et al. Postmenopausal estrogen therapy and cardiovascular disease. ten-year follow-up from the Nurses' Health study. N Engl J Med. 1991; 325:756-762.

19-8 Grodstein F, Stampfer MJ, Colditz GA, et al. Postmenopausal hormone therapy and mortality. N Engl J Med. 1997;336:1769-1775.

19-9 Paganini-Hill A, Corrada MM, Kawas CH. Increased longevity in older users of postmenopausal estrogen therapy: the Leisure World Cohort Study. Menopause. Jan-Feb 2006;13(1):12-8.

19-10 Rossouw JE, Anderson GL, Prentice RL. Risks and benefits of estrogen plus progestin in healthy postmenopausal women: principal results from the Women's Health Initiative randomized controlled trial. JAMA. 2002; 288(3):321.

19-11 Anderson GL, Limacher M, Assaf AR. Effects of conjugated equine estrogen in postmenopausal women with hysterectomy: the Women's Health Initiative randomized controlled trial. JAMA. 2004;291(14):1701-12.

19-12 Manson JE, Aragaki AK, Rossouw JE, Anderson GL. Menopausal hormone therapy and long-term all-cause and cause-specific mortality: The Women's Health Initiative Randomized Trials. JAMA. 2017;318(10): 927-938.

19-13 McNeil M. Menopausal hormone therapy: understanding long-term risks and benefits. JAMA. Sept. 2017;318(10):911-913.

19-14 Salpeter SR, Walsh JM, et al. Mortality associated with hormone replacement therapy in younger and older women: a meta-analysis. J Gen Intern Med. 2004;19:791-804.

19-15 Salpeter SR, Walsh JM, Greyber E, Salpeter EE. Brief report: coronary heart disease events associated with hormone therapy in younger and older women. A meta-analysis. J Gen Intern Med. 2006;21:363-366.

19-16 Salpeter SR, Cheng J, Thabane L, Buckley NS, Salpeter EE. Bayesian meta-analysis of hormone therapy and mortality in younger postmenopausal women. Am J Med. 2009;122:1016-1022.

19-17 Schierbeck LL, Rejnmark L, Tofteng CL, et al. Effect of hormone replacement therapy on cardiovascular events in recently postmenopausal women: a randomised trial. BMJ. 2012;345:e6409.

19-18 Boardman HM, Hartley L, Eisinga A, et al. Hormone therapy for preventing cardiovascular disease in post-menopausal women. Cochrane Database Syst Rev. Mar 2015;10;(3):CD002229.

19-19 Tuomikoski P, Lyytinen H, Korhonen P, et al. The risk of fatal stroke in Finnish postmenopausal hormone therapy users before and after the Women's Health Initiative: a cohort study. Maturitas. 2015;81:384-388.

19-20 Xie J, Brayne C, Matthews F. and the Medical Research Council Cognitive Function and Ageing Study Collaborators. Survival times in people with dementia: analysis from population based cohort study with 14 year follow-up. BMJ. Feb. 2008;336(7638):258-62.

19-21 Mikkola R, et al. Reduced risk of breast cancer mortality in women using postmenopausal hormone therapy: a Finnish nationwide comparative study. Menopause. Nov 2016; 23(11):1199-1203.

19-22 Holm M, Olsen A, Kroman N, Tjonneland A. Lifestyle influences on the

355

association between pre-diagnostic hormone replacement therapy and breast cancer prognosis: results from the Danish Diet, Cancer and Health prospective cohort. Maturitas. 2014;79:442-448.

19-23 Yu X, Zhou S, Wang J, et al. Hormone replacement therapy and breast cancer survival: a systematic review and meta-analysis of observational studies. Breast Cancer. Sep 2017;24(5):643-657.

19-24 Sprague BL, Trentham-Dietz A, Cronin KA. A sustained decline in postmenopausal hormone use: results from the National Health and Nutrition Examination Survey,1999-2010. Obstet Gynecol. 2012; 120:595-603.

19-25 Hersh AL, Stefanick ML, Stafford RS. National use of postmenopausal hormone therapy: annual trends and response to recent evidence. JAMA. 2004;291:47-53.

19-26 Steinkellner AR, Denison SE, Eldridge SL, Lenzi LL, et al. A decade of postmenopausal hormone therapy prescribing in the United States: long-term effects of the Women's Health Initiative. Menopause. 2012;19:616-621.

19-27 Crawford S, Crandall C, Derby C. Menopausal hormone therapy trends before versus after 2002: impact of the Women's Health Initiative Study results. Menopause. 2019:26(6):588-597.

19-28 Karim R, Dell RM, Greene DF, Mack WJ. Hip fracture in postmenopausal women after cessation of hormone therapy: results from a prospective study in a large health management organization. Menopause. 2011;18:1172-1177.

19-29 Weissfeld JL, Liu W, Woods C, et al. Trends in oral and vaginally administered estrogen use among US women 50 years of age or older with commercial health insurance. Menopause. 2018;25:611-614.

19-30 Sarrel PM, Njike VY, Vinante V, Katz DL. The mortality toll of estrogen avoidance: an analysis of excess deaths among hysterectomized women aged 50 to 59 years. Am J Public Health. 2013;103:1583-1588.

19-31 Manson JE, Bassuk SS, Merz CN, Kaunitz AM. Menopausal hormone therapy and national time trends in mortality: cautions regarding causal inference. Menopause. Aug 2017;24(8):874-876.

19-32 Nicholas M, Townsend N, et al. Cardiovascular disease in Europe 2014: epidemiological update. Eur Heart J. 2014;35:2950-9.

19-33 Huot L, Couris C, et al. Trends in HRT and anti-osteoporosis medication prescribing in a European population after the WHI study. Osteoporos Int. July 2008;19(7):1047-54.

19-34 Udell JA, Fischer MA, et al. Effect of the Women's Health Initiative on osteoporosis therapy and expenditure in Medicaid. J Bone Miner Res. May 2006;21(5):765-71.

19-35 Penning-van Beest FJ, Goettsch WG, Erkens JA, Herings RM. Determinants of persistence with bisphosphonates: a study in women with postmenopausal osteoporosis. Clinical Therapeutics. 2006;28(2):236-42.

19-36 Modi A, Sajjan S, Insinga R, et al. Frequency of discontinuation of injectable osteoporosis therapies in US patients over 2 years. Osteoporos Int. April 2017;28(4):1355-1363.

19-37 Islam S, Liu Q, Chines A, Hetzer E. Trend in incidence of osteoporosis-related fractures among 40 to 69-year-old women: analysis of a large insurance claims database. 2000-2005. Menopause. 2009;16:77-83.

19-38 Karim R, Dell RM, Greene DF, Mack WJ, Gallagher JC, Hodis HN. Hip fracture in postmenopausal women after cessation of hormone therapy: results from a prospective study in a large health management organization. Menopause. 2011;18:1172-7.

19-39 Empana JP, Dargent-Molina P, Béart G, et al. Effect of hip fracture on mortality in elderly women: The EPIDOS prospective study. J Am Geriatr Soc. 2004;52:685-90.

19-40 Von Friesendorff M, McGuigan FE, Wizert A, et al. Hip fracture, mortality risk, and cause of death over two decades. Osteoporos Int. 2016;27:2945-53.

19-41 Rejnmark L, Mosekilde L. Loss of life years after a hip fracture: effects of age and sex. Acta Orthopaedica. 2009;80:525-30.

19-42 Vestergaard P, Rejnmark L, Mosekilde L. Increased mortality in patients with a hip fracture — effect of pre-morbid conditions in post-fracture complications. Osteoporos Int. 2007;18:1583-93.

19-43 Rosen AB. Incidence and mortality of hip fractures in the United States. JAMA. 2009;302:1573-79.

19-44 Henley SJ, Miller JW. Uterine Cancer Incidence and Mortality — United States, 1999-2016. Morbidity and Mortality Weekly Report (MMWR). December 7, 2018; 67(48):1333-1338.

19-45 Cauley J, Seeley D, et al. Estrogen replacement therapy and mortality among older women. Arch Int Med. 1997;15(19):2181.

19-46 Paganini-Hill A. Estrogen replacement therapy in the elderly. Zentralbl Gynakol. 1996;118(5):255-61.

19-47 Mikkola, TS, Savolainen-Peltonen, M, et. al. New evidence for cardiac benefit of postmenopausal hormone therapy. Climateric. 2017;20(1):5-10.

19-48 Simoncini T, Mannella P, Genazzani AR. Rapid estrogen actions in the cardiovascular system. Ann N Y Acad Sci. 2006;1089:424-30.

19-49 Buber J, Mathew J, Moss AJ, et al. Risk of recurrent cardiac events after onset of menopause in women with congenital long-QT syndrome types 1 and 2. Circulation. 2011;123:2784–91.

19-50 POSITION STATEMENT The 2017 hormone therapy position statement of The

North American Menopause Society. Menopause. 2017;24(7):728-753.

19-51 Baber RJ, Panay N, Fenton A. The IMS Writing Group (2016). 2016 IMS recommendations on women's midlife health and menopause hormone therapy. Climacteric. 2016;19:(2):109-150.

Chapter 20: The Estrogen Question – It's Your Decision

20-1 Sex hormones and your heart. Harvard Heart Letter. May 2019;29(9):1.

20-2 Greek Medicine. Hippocratic Oath. National Library of Medicine. National Institute of Health. https://www.nlm.nih.gov/hmd/greek/greek_oath.html.

Index